Health Professional and Patient Interaction

Health Professional and Patient Interaction

AMY HADDAD, PHD, MFA, RN, FAAN

Professor Emerita
School of Pharmacy and Health Professions
Creighton University
Omaha, NE, United States

REGINA DOHERTY, OTD, OT, OTR, FAOTA, FNAP

Professor and Chair
Department of Occupational Therapy
School of Health and Rehabilitation Sciences
MGH Institute of Health Professions
Boston, MA, United States

With select contributions by:

KESHRIE NAIDOO, PT, DPT, EDD

Assistant Professor and Director of Curriculum
Department of Physical Therapy
School of Health and Rehabilitation Sciences
MGH Institute of Health Professions
Boston, MA, United States

ELSEVIER

Elsevier
3251 Riverport Lane
St. Louis, Missouri 63043

HEALTH PROFESSIONAL AND PATIENT INTERACTION,   ISBN: 978-0-323-83156-7
TENTH EDITION

Content Strategist: Lauren Willis
Content Development Specialist: Shweta Pant
Publishing Services Manager: Deepthi Unni
Project Manager: Sindhuraj Thulasingam
Design Direction: Patrick Ferguson

Printed in India

Last digit is the print number: 9   8   7   6   5   4   3   2   1

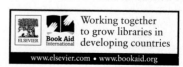

Working together
to grow libraries in
developing countries

www.elsevier.com • www.bookaid.org

With gratitude to the patients, professional colleagues, students, and friends whose insights, stories and scholarship have enhanced the content in this book—and enriched our lives.

Amy and Regina

This slim volume is a gateway to one of the most essential pathways to a satisfying, lifelong journey in any health professional's career. Interactions as a professional are wide ranging; each individual or group one encounters presents opportunities and challenges arising out of their unique life experience. You, too, bring your own history, hopes, constraints, and goals to each one.

This, you say, is true of all significant human relationships, so why spend precious time and energy to add this explicit focus to your studies and other priorities?

Because your success depends on it.

The essence of a professional–patient interaction is unique in several regards. It is not captured by comparing it to a chance meeting of strangers, a friendship, family relationship or a business transaction, yet it includes key characteristics common to all of them The teaching-learning opportunities in this text provide you with basic knowledge, skills, attitudes, and critical thinking that highlight distinguishing features of the health professional–patient relationship, each chapter equipping you with an essential constituent for success in this basically interpersonal experience. But that is not the full story. Health professional–patient interactions also are embedded in society's understanding of the role of professionals in protecting essential values deemed necessary to sustain the wellbeing of individuals and the public good. Over time, the contours of this societally sanctioned role have become expressed in laws, codes and other regulations, shaping reasonable expectations of anyone seeking your services. In summary, each health professional and patient interaction is a private–public venture.

The certainty upon which I am offering such bold claims comes from two sources. First, I am a health professional whose long career as a clinician, administrator, professor, and writer gives me the confidence to speak from my own experience including the sometimes-laborious learning by mistakes that went into shaping my professional interactions. As my experience increased so did my bandwidth of opportunities—as it will yours—notably I added activities to my direct interactions with patients and their support systems. In my case, this included administrative and teaching functions along with policy review and design in the corridors of government. I found my path to sustainable satisfaction in each new setting required attention to and reflection on the relational aspects of my interactions, and it will be so in your career journey. A second source of certainty regarding the importance of the content addressed in this book has its basis in the feedback gleaned over its nine editions. I was the sole author of the first edition (released in c1973), and it is a source of affirmation of its offerings that the 10th edition is going to press with a solid core of educational programs using it. Assuredly, its relevance to today's special situations has not resulted from my sole authorship—many changes and refinements emerged along the way as the health professions themselves continued to evolve. To keep the content current and relevant, several editions ago Dr. Amy Haddad and I became coauthors, the project evolving into a team effort that eventually led to the addition of an excellent third coauthor, Dr. Regina Doherty. In this edition, I am stepping back from authorship. We—and you—are fortunate that Dr. Keshrie Naidoo is contributing substantively to several chapters consistent with her expertise. Thus my attempt to assure you that adding the resources from your study of this text will serve you well derives from realizing that the endurance of major themes throughout nine editions gives heft to their value through the years. At the same time, our changes should be evidence that in making your choice to become a health professional you are entering a continually and dynamically changing aspect of society that will take you on a grand adventure.

Amy Haddad and Regina Doherty asked me to briefly respond to the question, "What if anything is a major change you have witnessed in the health professions since the inception of this book, particularly with an eye to how it has affected the scope and nature of relationships each professional is expected to observe?". Among the many, I believe the most significant generally is the steady—though not always a smooth, unidirectional—progression toward equal societal standing among the wide range of health professionals today. This is in contrast to as recently in the history of the healing professions as the release of the first edition. In the end of the 1960's physicians, and sometimes nurses and dentists, were viewed societally as "health professionals" with members of all the other groups labeled adjuncts, assistants, quasi-professionals, parapro-fessionals, or allied health professionals. It goes beyond the scope of this Foreword to provide more detail, but the reader should take note and be glad that in this edition the core mode of interactions largely is viewed within a framework of interprofessional respect coupled with claims on each individual or group to be accountable for their special area of expertise. At the strictly interpersonal level, recently much more attention is given to the necessity of deeply respecting defining human differences and their effects on every aspect of professional relationships. This generic change reverberates in the theme of respect throughout the text which serves as a defining value today among all parties involved.

I want to add my response to one more question: "What is unique about you?" Each of you is *special* in terms of the gifts and challenges you will bring to the interactions that make up the human core of a professional career. That has been true throughout the history of the health pro-fessions. As a group, you are *unique* compared to almost every professional alive today. You are the generation that prepared to enter or further refined your professional career during the worldwide Covid-19 pandemic, or hopefully, at least during the first years of *post*-pandemic life. You will be given the opportunity to create new or fine-tune old health professions practices and help shape policies fitting for you, your patients and colleagues, and your children's wellbeing. You will also become immersed in devasting long-term effects of the Covid-19 toll on the human spirit and the amazing resiliency of humans to move forward. Hopefully, the undue Covid-19-generated stresses on health professionals that currently are giving renewed attention to the necessity of support for self-care will endure as an essential dimension of your survival and thriving. You can demand it is so.

On a personal note, I am grateful to Amy Haddad and Regina Doherty, the authors of this 10th edition, and to Elsevier, the publisher, for the privilege of offering my reflections in this Foreword. I hope it is an encouragement and I so look forward to meeting you, reader, in the days and years ahead!

Ruth Purtilo, PT, PhD, FAPTA

One joy of preparing this 10th edition of *Health Professional and Patient Interaction* has been the opportunity for us to work together in its development. Our collaborations and collective expertise as interprofessional colleagues with over 75 combined years of experience in health care and education, coupled with the Elsevier team's guidance and support, have enriched our scholarly work.

Each of us also discussed issues examined in the book with students and readers, as well as clinicians, researchers, and faculty members around the country and the world. We thank them for their insights.

Contributing to this new edition is Dr. Keshrie Naidoo. A talented clinician, educator, and scholar, Dr. Naidoo was instrumental in the revision of content for this tenth edition. A physical therapist by professional background, Keshrie' s expertise in care for a diverse society across a wide variety of clinical practice settings has informed our work and will prepare the reader for contemporary practice.

We are also grateful to our dear colleague and friend, Dr. Ruth Purtilo. Ruth's wisdom and vision in authoring the first edition of *Health Professional and Patient Interaction* over 50 years ago have advanced the field, impacting the lives of countless health professionals (and patients who have benefitted from their care). Those who learned from her, were mentored by her, and worked with her are grateful to have seen her mastery and to have felt her appreciation for the impact.

Finally, we extend our heartfelt thanks to our husbands, Steve and Dan, who encourage us in all of our professional projects and enrich our lives, and to Regina's daughter, Olivia, who continues to be a source of inspiration as she charts her path in the world.

As this 10th edition of *Health Professional and Patient Interaction* goes to press, the authors are aware that opportunities in the health professions continue to expand and the level of education for participation in health care is evolving. This book is designed to support readers in their journey to and ongoing development in careers as health professionals. The recent unprecedented challenges in health care due to the COVID-19 pandemic require a different understanding of opportunities and challenges facing health professionals and patients in the coming years. Everyone in health care must gain a basic understanding of the dynamics of human relationships in a variety of care delivery settings. The core of these relationships consists of respectful interactions that shape and influence the success of quality care and thus are the focus of this book.

Readers are guided through the chapter text and related learning activities to help them (1) engage in critical self-reflection; (2) clarify their roles in shaping the health professional and patient relationship; (3) explore effective models of interprofessional communication and collaboration for the delivery of quality, compassionate care; and (4) develop an awareness of the larger health care and societal contexts in which each relationship takes place. Clarification of personal, professional, and societal values sets the stage for exploring the complexity of interactions and the unique perspective that a health professional and patient each brings to their relationship.

Respect is the thread that weaves together discussions regarding relationships in the health care environment. *Health Professional and Patient Interaction* includes evidence-based, respect-generating resources from the foundational disciplines of the humanities, social sciences, communication science, ethics, nursing, medicine, rehabilitation science, and psychology.

The content is designed to apply to everyday clinical experiences across a variety of health professions, considering both discipline-specific and interprofessional perspectives across a range of levels of formal study, from undergraduate to doctoral-level preparation. Competencies and direct accountability differ across professional practice settings, but the human-to-human encounter remains a constant. *Health Professional and Patient Interaction* is your guide to building and improving these encounters. It provides countless tools and highlights how different members of the interprofessional care team can share common challenges, goals, and opportunities for service as they collaborate in the delivery of patient- and family-centered care.

For clarity's sake, we assign meaning to the following key terms: (1) patient—the recipient of and participant in a health care interaction, (2) experiential learning—the portion of formal education that takes place at the type of worksite where a person will likely practice, (3) clinical experience—the accumulation of actual experiences in one's chosen field, and (4) interprofessional collaboration—when multiple health workers (professional, para-professional, and support personnel) from different professional backgrounds work together with patients, families, carers, and communities to deliver compassionate, quality care.

The names of patients, families, health professionals, and other persons in the cases and other examples are fictitious. The cases represent a variety of clinical settings and disciplines to allow the reader to reflect on professional interactions with patients across the life span and throughout the wide spectrum of care delivery settings.

When the last word of a book has been written, its life has just begun. In sharing our extensive research, experiences, and insights about respect in its numerous iterations in health care, we hope that in turn you will be inspired to share yours with others. In this way, we all generate knowledge, making us more skilled in respectful human interactions in health care and beyond.

Amy Haddad and Regina Doherty

Creating a Context of Respect

Introduction

As you enter the pages of this book focused on health professional and patient encounters, the first thing we bring to your attention are some key features of this special relationship wherein health professionals with all their clinical knowledge, experiences, and skills meet patients with their distinct attributes, values, needs, and vulnerabilities. Understanding the central elements of the health professional and patient interaction will ensure the welfare of the patient and balance one's health, well-being, and expectations for longevity in your career.

Chapter 1 introduces the concept of dignity and respect. Respect plays a central function in the professional role as it does in the organization of this book. Respect is essential to a positive working relationship between health professionals and patients and is expressed in everyday actions and attitudes. One indicator or expression of respect is the professional's sincere appreciation for the distinct qualities and lived experiences of each person. Beyond that, respect is expressed through an acknowledgment that the other warrants the professional's considered attention. The ultimate expression of respect toward the other is found in the professional's genuine care for the patient.

Basic values—your own, those of the health professions, and society—constitute a firm foundation for this respect to take root and grow into appropriate conduct and attitudes toward the people and communities you serve.

Chapter 2 describes benchmarks that are standards for measuring respect at the center of the health professional and patient relationship. They include conduct and attitudes that express courtesy and dignity, professional competence and trust, and professional boundaries that shape a healthy professional–patient relationship. The ways in which person-first, identity-first, and inclusive language can honor the positive goals of the health professional and patient relationship are highlighted.

Chapter 3 focuses on developing self-respect in your role as a health professional. Here, we introduce you to the essential skills that serve to sustain resilience and clinician well-being. Self-care practices such as mindfulness, meditation, and communities of practice are presented as tools for building individual and organizational resiliency. Recent research on the link between burnout and compassionate care is highlighted, along with strategies for recognizing and intervening for burnout in one's self and one's interprofessional colleagues to better attend to clinician mental health.

The chapters in Section 1 set the foundation for your role as a health professional. They are optimistic in tone and content, as are we, about your opportunity to honor and help foster respect in the health professions.

Respect in the Professional Role

Prelude

Each and every care encounter is an opportunity to either protect or infringe on patients' dignity.

JOAN OSTASZKIEWICZ[1]

Our earliest understanding of the idea of respect likely began with a parent or other authority figure rewarding us for certain kinds of conduct or correcting us for attitudes or behaviors deemed socially unacceptable. When you were young, you might not have been able to tell the difference between what words or actions were better or preferred by your elders. As you grew older, these teachings were reinforced until you realized that respect is a basic ingredient of getting along well in society. Hopefully, over time, you were guided to understand that respect is part of living a full life and that at the core, respect is relational.

Whether you are preparing to enter a profession for the first time, changing professions, or continuing to seek excellence in a profession through further study, being able to show and receive respect is a critical skill you will continue to develop over the course of your career as a health professional. You might, in fact, think of respect as a linchpin that holds together your professional identity.

What Is Dignity?

Fundamental to all relationships is the recognition that we all are human. Many writers agree that we share a common essence; they term it *dignity*, although it is not always clear what we mean when we use this term. The essence is often referred to as the *intrinsic dignity* of persons, ". . . a worth or value that people have simply because they are human, not by virtue of any social standing, ability to evoke admiration, or any particular set of talents, skills, or powers."[2] Intrinsic dignity is deeply ingrained in the idea of a profession. The assumption being that there is a common thread of humanity that warrants basic regard of a person as such. When dignity is upheld, a person feels included, valued, and appreciated.

An additional conception of dignity, *aspirational dignity*, stands in opposition to intrinsic dignity. Aspirational dignity is a state to which individuals ". . . aspire, rather than a status that they hold simply by virtue of being human. This means that aspirational dignity can be lost, or we can be stripped of it, either through our own actions, the actions of others, or the circumstances in which we find ourselves."[3] Uniting these concepts of dignity is especially helpful in the context of health care. Dignity can be threatened by the actions of others, such as being left on a stretcher in a hallway for an extended time. The physical setting in health care can also threaten dignity by its very structure. A clinic setting that does not allow for private conversations out of earshot of other patients and staff would be an example. It is worth noting that deteriorating health increases vulnerability while decreasing a patient's ability to defend one's dignity.[4] Health professionals must be attentive to the potential of their actions to undermine the standards and principles of their patients and, in particular, the potential for their actions to cause humiliation.[3] Respectful actions to support or maintain a patient's dignity are especially important when patients are unable to speak up about what is important to them. The dignity of our identity is not determined just by our own ability to communicate and maintain our identity.[5] Patients who are incapacitated, that is who lack the mental capacity to make decisions about living according to their standards or values, must rely on not only others, often health professionals, but also family members to uphold their sense of self-worth. This highly vulnerable group of patients includes infants and young children as well as those with cognitive impairment as a result of illness, injury, or disease progression (e.g., advanced dementia). Even if a patient is unable to appreciate how their standards are being upheld, dignity still plays a role in guiding the health professional's approach to such patients. The dignity of the health professional is also at stake and sets limits on how one can act toward other individuals based on certain principles and values such as altruism and compassion. It is only through acting in accordance with such principles that health professionals act with dignity.[3]

What Is Respect?

A simple definition of *respect* is the sum of the actions that appropriately honor and acknowledge a person's dignity.[6] In this context, respect for another conveys, "you matter." Respectful actions indicate to patients that the health professional appreciates the standards and values that shape their patients' identities as important and essential in determining how patients would like to interact with others. For example, consider this brief exchange between a patient, Vivian Bearing, and a technician in radiology from the Pulitzer prize-winning play, WIT by Margaret Edson.[7]

TECHNICIAN 1. *Name.*
VIVIAN. *My name? Vivian Bearing.*
TECHNICIAN 1. *Huh?*
VIVIAN. *Bearing. B–E–A–R–I–N-G. Vivian. V–I–V–I–A-N.*
TECHNICIAN 1. *Doctor?*
VIVIAN. *Yes. I have a Ph.D.*
TECHNICIAN 1. **Your** *doctor.*
VIVIAN. *Oh. Dr. Harvey Kelekian.* (Technician 1 positions her so that she is leaning forward and embracing a metal plate, then steps offstage.) *I am a doctor of philosophy.*

Dr. Vivian Bearing is the main character in WIT. She holds her academic achievements in high regard, so much so that she cannot frame the technician's question of "Doctor?" in any other way than how it refers to her title and her self-identity. The technician does not seem to recognize or care about what is important to Dr. Bearing: she is just another patient who needs a chest X-ray.

No matter how extreme our circumstances, we as humans hope above all that others will not discount our need to be somebody, that they will recognize the standards that are important to us, and that they will be empathetically accompanied through the most difficult and unlikable or threatening aspects of our struggles. And when we rejoice, we hope others will join us in our celebration of happiness or accomplishment.

RESPECT FOR PATIENTS AND FAMILIES

In your study of this book, we will help you look for specific evidence of respect through such everyday actions as the tone of your voice when you address a patient, the adaptation of your pace and body language to meet the needs of a child versus an older adult patient, your trustworthy keeping of patient confidence, your recognition of and attention to cultural differences, your presence during a crisis, and your willingness to work together with a patient's support system, including family, significant others, and care providers. Patients, especially youth and older adults, engage with health professionals in the context of their families and support systems. Respect is best conveyed, and care is compassionately delivered, when this context is attended to and care is a collaborative venture between the family and the interprofessional care team. So important is this concept, an entire chapter is devoted to patient- and family-centered care, the family–health systems approach, and the documented health outcomes related to these approaches in Chapter 7.

Your skilled interventions can foster confidence that each patient is worthy to participate in health-related decisions that protect meaning in their life. Your communications can convey that your intent is to protect them from exploitation or harm and advocate for them in ways that will be to their benefit. Respect as care—and its active form, caring—is the ultimate indicator of respect and goes to the heart of the professional relationship. It invites something of you that includes the appreciation of and attentiveness toward another but goes deeper. Now you commit yourself to providing appropriate measures demonstrating that you genuinely respect a person's worth as a human being. In other words, this indicator of respect involves a willingness to involve yourself as a human being in relationship with another.

Care is conveyed not only by your actions but also by your attitudes that reflect who you really are. When older adults were asked about their patient experiences in acute care settings, the patients and their relatives expressed the most concern about the relational aspects of their care. Patients and their families wanted help with "maintaining identity, 'see who I am' (patients want staff to know what is important to them, and relatives want staff to value what they know about the patient); creating community, 'connect with me' (a connected and two-way relationship with staff gives patients and relatives the reassurance that staff will care for them and meet their needs); sharing decision-making, 'involve me' (patients and relatives want to understand what is happening, and to be given ongoing involvement in decision-making)."[8]

The values of care and its active form, caregiving, are pivotal to realizing the goals of professional practice. Professionals are judged in part by whether they offer competent, quality care appropriate to their area of expertise. In that regard, care expressed as a professional is different in some important respects from caring in a relationship with a spouse, child, friend, or colleague. It is shaped by conscientiously applying clinical knowledge and skill while abiding by ethical duties and rights and demonstrating character traits that describe the proper place of a professional in this relationship. Patients are drawn to the idea of care because the term conveys that a high-stakes human story is taking place, and for them, it always is. Patients have a personal story that holds all their hopes, dreams, and fears. The health professional's caregiving must reflect that the story is heard and that they are prepared to shape a plan of care with the patient's values and goals as an uppermost consideration.[9]

Additionally, in your professional role, your feelings toward a person do not give you permission to limit your responsibility but require you to find a means by which this person's reasonable goals can be met. You must also consider the well-being of the whole person going beyond the sole application of technical skills.

Lack of respect for a patient, whether intentional or not, can have negative consequences beyond bad feelings. When patients perceive that they are being talked down to or being treated unfairly, it can affect whether a patient follows advice from the health professional or obtains needed care. This is especially true among racial and ethnic minority populations and is a known contributor to existing disparities in health care.[10]

There is no one set formula for this core aspect of the caring relationship, though basic characteristics of professional care are addressed later in this chapter and Chapter 2. An exploration of its many expressions is woven into every chapter of this book.

REFLECTIONS

Consider the following case and then reflect on the items that follow:

A patient comes to a doctor's appointment, is greeted, and is brought to an examination room by a medical assistant. Thirty-five minutes later, the patient comes out to ask about the delay in being seen. It is then discovered that her doctor is not in the clinic that day. When the patient asks how this could happen, a staff member responds by saying, "I have no idea. It's not my job to schedule appointments." The patient is so upset by the whole experience that she transfers to another doctor.[11]

- Put yourself in the patient's position and reflect on what conduct or attributes you would deem disrespectful.
- What could the health professionals have done to diminish the patient's experience of being disrespected?

The Relationship Between Dignity and Respect

An international, multidisciplinary group of clinicians explored the application of the concepts of dignity and respect in the intensive care unit (ICU) setting and produced the following key findings.[12] First, in the ICU and other clinical settings, dignity and respect are interrelated; in that, dignity represents the intrinsic worth that every human being possesses merely by being human and holds a certain degree of aspirational dignity that is unique to that person. Respect "represents actions that appropriately honor and acknowledge such understandings of dignity."[12] Fig. 1.1 illustrates the connection between dignity and respect on an interpersonal level as well as at the institutional and societal levels. This practical approach to these complex concepts allows health professionals to identify concrete actions of respectful care and interactions. Additionally, Fig. 1.1 highlights some of the barriers to respectful actions in health care settings that result in the diminishment of dignity. You can see that obstacles to respect can be personal, such as mental health issues like depression or burn-out, but their genesis could also be at the institutional level from heavy workloads or unresolved workplace conflict. The demanding work of implementing measures to encourage respectful interactions must occur on all three levels, personal, institutional, and societal, in which health professionals live and work if it is to be effective. Only then can the moral dimensions of good care be fully actualized.

This introduction to dignity and respect should emphasize some similarities between the function of respect in everyday life and help set the stage for you to further explore how respect factors into what is at stake in being a health professional.

Respect and Values

To embrace and express respect for others, it is essential that you have insight into your own personal values and those of the subgroups and society in which you live. Moreover, there are some values that are especially vital to your role as a health professional. *Values* describe things one

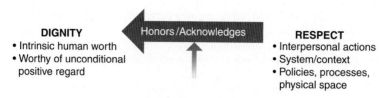

Fig. 1.1 **The relationship between respect and dignity and barriers to the practice of respect.** Used with permission from American Thoracic Society.

holds dear, and everyone can list many things that, on reflection, meet that criterion. We say that something is "of value" when we estimate it to have worth to us. One criterion of a "true" value is that it has become part of a pattern in one's life. Values also provide the content to guide choices. They act as a compass to point where to put your attention and help explain why you care what happens regarding that object, idea, or person.

Taken together, your values constitute your *value system*. Some values in that system are highly specific to you as an individual. Some will be adopted through various formal and informal subgroups to which you belong. Still, others are shared by most humans because of our common human condition. The unique value system for each person reflects a profile of his or her idea of how to survive and flourish. In Chapter 2, the authors focus more fully on how abiding by one's values becomes the fundamental basis of respect for oneself when challenging situations arise. Basic values find expression through the various roles one assumes—in your case, an important one being that of a health professional.

PERSONAL VALUES

Personal values are one's own. Early values are absorbed from familial and social sources. These include parents, grandparents, relatives, childhood friends, caregivers, teachers, religious beliefs and traditions, and other sociocultural influences such as television and social media. Values are imparted, taught, reinforced, and internalized. We incorporate many of them into our lives as a personal value system. We exist in a complex world of bureaucracies and institutions that influence us, too. Our personal value system is dynamic. As we mature, our values may evolve with us to match our insights and experience. Most of us have many personal values, some more clearly defined than others, and go through life trying to realize or balance these personal values simultaneously.

The process of developing self-consciousness about one's values is the focus of values clarification exercises. Values clarification provides the means to discover the values one lives by day to day. An individual who can identify their own values is able to compare the worth of alternatives and make personally satisfying choices. Conversely, if unclear about your values or the connection between them and your choices, poor decision-making and dissatisfaction often result. Sometimes, your personal values will conflict with each other. Consider the value of good health. Other values may challenge the value of good health such as unhealthy practices that provide short-term benefits but long-term harms like smoking, overwork, substance use, lack of exercise, or lack of good sleeping habits.

> **REFLECTIONS**
>
> The following values clarification exercise is helpful in identifying personal values and how these values play out in real life.
> - First, make a list of your 10 most important personal values in order of importance.
> - What sort of picture do these values paint of the kind of health professional you are or hope to become?
> - Compare the list of your own most important values with your own behaviors.
> - To what degree is your behavior consistent with your stated values?
> - What can you do (if anything) to bring your stated values and behaviors into closer alignment?

Understanding more about your personal values is important because they influence the development of your professional values which affect professional actions and how you react to different situations.[13] When patients seek your services, their own personal values are almost always the motivation. They value staying healthy, getting well, or finding relief from pain or comfort during chronic or life-threatening illnesses. They want you to help them restore or maintain their value of health and optimize their functioning. Because health care is concerned primarily with personal values that are addressed through professional and patient relationships, your professional preparation gives you an opportunity to study and think about the challenges your own personal values may pose and identify those that will facilitate your success. If, overall, you conclude that you share similar health-related values with patients, it will help to more easily create a bond with them that reflects your genuine respect for their situation and its challenges. If your situation is so different from theirs that it is difficult to do so, your default during these times is your commitment to the fact that their dignity as a human being must be called on to guide you. A current helpful resource that addresses concrete steps professionals can take in such situations is the Dignity and Respect Campaign started in October 2008 by the University of Pittsburgh Medical Center. The website, under the heading "Dignity & Respect," provides examples and incentives for individuals, organizations, and communities to adopt behaviors that foster a culture in which respect can flourish.[14]

Professional Values and Professionalism

Having chosen to become a health professional requires that you embrace values consistent with what being a professional means and what professional practice entails. Hopefully, many of these values overlap with your personal values or at least do not conflict with them.

WHAT IS A PROFESSION?

Primarily, a *profession* is a societal role, providing service to society, with specific functions. Several criteria are the most often cited, such as describing a profession and how it is different from other societal roles. Supreme Court Justice Louis Brandeis summarized in the early 20th century these elements of a profession:

> *First, a profession is an occupation for which the necessary preliminary training is intellectual in character, involving knowledge and to some extent learning as distinguished from mere skill. Second, it is an occupation pursued largely for others and not merely for oneself. Third, it is an occupation in which the amount of financial return is not the accepted measure of success.[15]*

The number and the type of professions have grown over the course of the last two centuries even if we limit the type of professions to those who work in health care-related fields. Additional requirements have been added to the basic definition of a profession to include autonomy in practice, self-regulation, and specific indications of excellence.

WHAT IS PROFESSIONALISM?

In recent years, professional organizations have devoted growing attention to the idea of *professionalism*. The initiatives geared toward professionalism share the common goal of identifying, protecting, and fostering the appropriate focus of the professional's role in society. Fig. 1.2 provides a conceptual model of the elements of professionalism.[16] Professionalism rests on a solid foundation comprising knowledge and skills that include clinical competence, communication, and ethical and legal understanding. Although Fig. 1.2 specifies "knowledge of medicine," clinical competence applies to all health professions. Each profession has a specialized body of knowledge and more general health-related knowledge that overlap with other disciplines. Communication, with patients, family members, and colleagues, is such an important skill in health care that Chapter 8 is fully dedicated to that topic. Additionally, professionalism increasingly reflects the ability to function effectively as a member of an interprofessional care team. Interprofessional collaboration is the focus of Chapter 8. Ethical and legal understanding also has specific requirements for certain professions and more general ethical obligations for all health professionals that require an understanding of their application in health care.

These foundational elements are necessary but insufficient. Thinking of these foundational elements as columns that support the professionalism pediment or roof of professional aspirations, the following four principles or values that health professionals continually strive to achieve—excellence, humanism, accountability, and altruism—are necessary and sufficient elements of professionalism.

Excellence

The notion of *excellence* is a commitment to striving to do more than the minimum required. A component of excellence is the concept of life-long learning. A new graduate from any health care

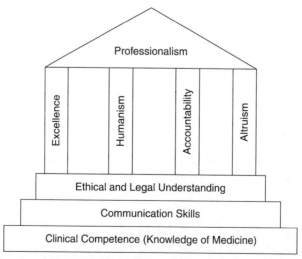

Fig. 1.2 A definition of professionalism. Used with permission from Oxford University Press.

program spends the first few years developing competency in basic skills, procedures, etc. When basic competence is achieved or when the not-so-new graduate feels comfortable with the fundamentals, they might think, "I would really like to learn more about . . ." and that is the beginning of going deeper into a particular specialty, earning a certificate, attending continuing education sessions, etc. on the road to excellence. Self-improvement is not the only area in which achieving excellence is possible. Efforts to improve interprofessional collaboration, reduce errors, or engage in scholarship to measure and improve the quality of care are all examples of striving for excellence on a professional or institutional level.

Humanism

It seems obvious that people who choose health care as their profession should be interested in working with and helping people. As one famous medical educator wrote, more than 90 years ago, "One of the essential qualities of the clinician is interest in humanity, for the secret of the care *of* the patient is in caring *for* the patient."[17] Contemporary health care associations, educators, and clinicians carry on the work of advancing and documenting the outcomes of humanism in health care. For example, the Arnold P. Gold Foundation and the Schwartz Center for Compassionate Care emphasize humanism and compassion through educational programs allowing health care professionals the opportunities to continually reflect on, and understand that to deliver the best care to their patients, compassion and empathy must be the hallmark of their clinical practice. As noted earlier in this chapter, respectful actions that support human dignity are at the very heart of humanism, the recognition of the worth and value of another human being.

Accountability

Health professionals are *accountable* or responsible to many parties, including the patients and families they serve, colleagues within their own profession, and those on the interprofessional care team, to their profession beyond those with whom they work, and to the public. Self-regulation as an individual health professional includes keeping current with clinical practice, licensure, documentation of services rendered, and ethical obligations. At the level of a health profession, accountability involves developing, updating, and upholding a code of ethics, setting standards of practice and self-policing including acceptance of external scrutiny by third parties such as payers or licensing boards, and remediation and discipline of members who fail to meet professional standards.[18] Health professionals also have a duty to serve the public which increasingly includes advocating for access to quality health care not only for individual patients but also for those populations who are marginalized and historically underserved. The principle of solidarity speaks to this type of responsibility; in that, it requires the privileged to be accountable to the vulnerable among us.[19]

Altruism

In health care, *altruism* means putting the needs of the patient first. Since patients rarely live a solitary life, the needs of the patient and their family or immediate support system should take precedence over the interests of the health professional. To advocate for the needs of another person before one's own does not mean that health professionals must sacrifice their well-being or abandon self-care. A balance must be struck between these two moral goods. The importance of self-care is explored in Chapter 3.

Much more could be said about these four principles of professionalism, but the basic definitions supplied here should serve as a sufficient introduction to guide professionalism in health care. Since adding other principles in support of professionalism can emphasize discipline-specific values, we now turn our attention to the concept of core professional values.

PROFESSIONAL VALUES

Many health professional organizations articulate basic core values that undergird their specific identity. These values help explain the reasonable expectations that society can count on regarding all members of that profession. For example, the National Association of Social Workers lists the following core values, claiming them to be the foundation of social work's unique purpose and perspective: service, social justice, dignity and worth of the person, the importance of human relationships, integrity, and competence.[20] Another example is the list of core values developed by the American Physical Therapy Association Academy of Education. It includes accountability, altruism, compassion and caring, excellence, integrity, professional duty, and social responsibility.[21] The International Council of Nurses notes the following core values for all nurses regardless of the setting or country where they practice: compassion, empathy, trustworthiness, integrity, respect, justice, and responsiveness.[22] It is worth your effort to identify the values that your own professional organization has generated. You will readily see areas of overlap among the health professions and begin to observe a general profile of professional values. For instance, several include ideals of selfless conduct, trustworthiness, and commitment. Many of these professional values and skills, including the values for interprofessional practice, are discussed in greater detail in different chapters of this book. All these professional values are multifaceted and complex.

There are also barriers to acting on professional values both external and internal to the profession as a whole and individual professionals. External concerns include financial arrangements, technological advances, structural barriers such as length of visits, and the time it takes to complete the necessary documentation. There are also underlying concerns that larger forces outside of the professions themselves such as changes in the health care delivery and reimbursement systems that place undue pressure on professionals. Internal challenges for individuals and professions include conflicts of interest that go unrecognized or are minimized, greed, arrogance, bias, unwillingness to collaborate with other professions in the health care system, and impaired providers.

A key question for a health professional, then, is, "Do I really value what is required of me in this type of human relationship to work toward fully expressing 'I care' for the wide variety of patients I will encounter?"[23] If a health professional does not hold this value as essential in their own professional identity or a key to career satisfaction over time, professional service is not a good fit for this person. As this book unfolds, specific skills needed for effective care in diverse kinds of situations and many examples of care are explored in more detail.

The task for you, the reader, is to incorporate appropriate values of professionalism into your value system. You may wonder why so much time is devoted to values like this that seem obvious in many regards. The authors have found the preparation is well worth the effort because all health care providers will have conflicting claims placed on them and be involved in extremely complex situations such as the recent COVID-19 pandemic. During such times, the ability to ground yourself in your own and the profession's values, undergirded by your commitment to professional responsibility, creates a valuable foundation for informed, intentional movement forward.[24]

Societal Values

The third set of values that make up your value system derives from the larger society. One well-recognized characteristic of the human condition is that we, as human beings, organize ourselves into complex interactions as groups of individuals called *societies*. You belong to many communities made up of smaller numbers of people within the larger society already. Each subgroup has values that you are aware of and may accept, reject, or question how they support your attempt to lead a good life. One of these communities and its values is especially important that of the institution or organization where you are employed in your work as a health professional. Organizational structures and values as well as issues of respect and privacy at work at the organizational level are the focus of Chapter 5. The principle of respect, when it operates at an organizational or societal level, requires a broader perspective and different skills on the part of the individual and professionals.

The scope of societal values that influence value choices has expanded in the past few decades. Millions have immediate access to societal values expressed through resources on the Internet, such as social media, television news, search engines, websites, and podcasts, as well as older technology such as radio. These broadening circles of access and influence have led some to conclude that we are all indeed members of a global society and to survive must come to grips with the common values that will help all lead a good life. All societies experience social division and reunification as values are publicly debated and evolve. As you will see in Chapter 9, the public has taken advantage of the wide variety of communication modes available and other means of data gathering to gain health care and clinical information not previously accessible to them.

Despite the increased exposure to new and ever-expanding sources of values, there continues to be a belief among many that some basic societal values are so fundamental that they can be deemed universal. Their argument is that human beings are fundamentally social beings and therefore rarely find satisfaction outside the social context of living in a society, so they agree to abide by basic values that apply to all.

REFLECTIONS

Consider whether you believe the following are universally held societal values and what supports your conclusion:
- Protection of human life
- Rights and liberties
- Having power and opportunities
- Financial security
- Adequate food and shelter
- Self-respect
- Health and vigor
- Intelligence and imagination
- Autonomy/self-governance

What additional values would you add or substitute?

Some major sources of mainstream Western values are laws, philosophical inquiry, and shared experiences. For example, lawmakers in such societies rely on the principle that human life itself is a basic value and therefore ought to be protected and nourished by rules of law or institutional policies and guidelines.

Philosophers are an ongoing source of input as well. John Rawls, one of the most influential American philosophers near the end of the 20th century, argued that humans value several primary goods. *Social primary goods* include rights, liberties, powers, opportunities, income, wealth, and self-respect. (Self-respect is necessary for a person to feel assured that one's life plan is worth carrying out or capable of being fulfilled.) The realization of these goods is at least partially determined by the structure of society itself. *Natural primary goods*, also partly determined by societal structures but not directly under their control, include health, vigor, intelligence, and imagination.[25] Together, he says, these social and natural primary goods provide a sort of "index of welfare" for individuals in any society. However, there are other interpretations of universal value sets, not just those advanced by persons in the dominant culture of a society. Contextual factors, such as education, religion, identity, and others, discussed in greater depth in Chapter 4, influence understanding of what is to be valued on the personal and professional levels. The greatest difficulties in values' clarification arise at the societal level when one tries to identify values that everyone can agree upon.

Whether there are universally held societal values, they do have the power to affect well-being positively or negatively on large groups of adherents. Whatever one's lot in life, most individuals possess the need to be accepted within society and be able to embrace and live by its most basic values.

Integration of Values

In this chapter, you have encountered examples of three spheres of values: personal, professional, and societal. Their differences have been highlighted, but in everyday life, a person usually adopts a set of personal values that overlap in part and are harmonious with role-related values and larger social values. Motivation for this integration usually arises to reap personal and societal benefits that derive from doing so. It is possible to say of persons who live according to their value system, "That person has a good life." However, when a person's value system includes respect for values that help to uphold and further society as well, we say, "That person *leads* a good life."

Of course, not everyone adopts a set of personal values compatible with societal values or even with those in their own social or cultural subgroups. In the extreme form, this person has never integrated any societal or other cultural values into a value system or rejected them over time. Such a person likely believes that there are no benefits to be derived from living in harmony with society's values. Some examples are the recluse, the outlaw, and the saint or martyr. The recluse and outlaw reject societal values and replace them with their own; the saint or martyr rejects societal values and replaces them with a "higher" set of values.

Most people experience value conflicts from time to time, and a default tendency may be to not "rock the boat," no matter how unsatisfactory the situation, until it is judged to be a crisis. And so, it is jarring when something compels a person to reflect on their own values and decide that they do not suffice. For the health professional, a disconnect can occur when professional values that have been incorporated into legal and other institutional practices come into conflict with personal values or what the professional believes are appropriate societal values. A current example of a conflict in health care practices and policies was evident during the COVID-19 pandemic when there was a marked rise in the number of critically ill patients and a lack of appropriate professional protection equipment. Health professionals had to make decisions between their own personal risk and the welfare of patients. Any time a professional cannot conform in good conscience to practice and policy norms, it can become not only a source of discomfort for all but also an occasion for thoughtful reflection, discussion, and action. Also, it is essential to manage value conflicts early as this generally leads to better outcomes rather than waiting and not "rocking the boat."

Summary

Genuine respect involves both attitudes and actions that acknowledge your regard for another person's dignity, no matter what their attributes and circumstances are. Indicators of respect can be found in appreciating the distinctiveness of each individual, directing considered attention to their needs and values, and choosing action consistent with professional standards of care. Our values constitute the content of what we hold dear and important. Values influence whether we will want and be able to express genuine respect for patients, their families, and other professionals. Some values arise from personal preferences, whereas others become internalized over time through the influences of our affiliations and societal forces. Professional values are transmitted through professional identity formation that is the substance of clinical and educational experiences. A professional identity based on respect will guide you back to the understanding that, in your relationships with patients, their assurance that they are being respected will depend on your ability to convey that you understand that the stakes are high for them. They will also be reassured that you will devote your energy to addressing their needs appropriate to your professional role.

You convey care through respectful, patient- and family-centered actions. You can make substantial progress on your road to respectful interaction by reflecting on your own values and developing a genuine interest in others.

References

1. Ostaszkiewicz J. Defending patients' dignity: an under recognised and under resourced nursing role. *JARNA*. 2019;22(2):4–6. p. 5. https://doi.org/10.33235/jarna.22.2.4-6.
2. Sulmasy DP. Dignity and bioethics: history, theory, and selected applications. In *Human Dignity and Bioethics: Essays Commissioned by the President's Council on Bioethics*. Washington, DC: President's Council on Bioethics; 2008:473.
3. Killmister S. Dignity: not such a useless concept. *J Med Ethics*. 2010;36:160–164. https://doi.org/10.1136/jme.2009.031393. p. 161.
4. Barclay L. In sickness and in dignity: a philosophical account of the meaning of dignity in health care. *Int J Nurs Stud*. 2016;61:136–141. p. 139.
5. Nordenfeldt L. The concept of dignity. In: Nordenfeldt L, ed. *Dignity in Care for Older People*. Chichester: Wiley-Blackwell; 2009:26–53.
6. Sokol-Hessner L, Folcarelli PH, Annas CL, et al. A road map for advancing the practice of respect in health care: the results of an interdisciplinary modified Delphi study. *Jt Comm J Qual Patient Saf*. 2018;44:463–476. p. 463.
7. Edson M. *WIT*. New York: Dramatists Play Services, Inc; 1999:15–16.
8. Bridges J, Flatley M, Meyer J. Older people's and relatives' experiences in acute care settings: systematic review and synthesis of qualitative studies. *Int J Nurs Stud*. 2010;47(1):89–107. p. 105.
9. Purtilo RB. What interprofessional teamwork taught me about an ethics of care. *Phys Ther Rev*. 2012;17:197–201.
10. Blanchard J, Lurie N. R-E-S-P-E-C-T: patient reports of disrespect in the health care setting and its impact on care. *J Family Pract*. 2004;53(9):721–729. p. 721.
11. Sokol-Hessner L., Folcarelli P.H., Annas C.L., et al. A road map for advancing the practice of respect in health care: the results of an interdisciplinary modified Delphi Consensus Study. *Jt Comm J Qual Patient Saf*. 2018;44:463–476. p. 464.
12. Brown SM, Azoulay E, Benoit D, et al. The practice of respect in the ICU. *Am J Respiratory Crit Care Med*. 2018;197(11):1389–1395.
13. Luciana M, Rampolidi G, Ardenghi S, et al. Personal values among undergraduate nursing students: a cross-sectional study. *Nurs Ethics*. 2020;27(6):1461–1471. p. 1461.
14. Dignity and Respect Campaign. https://www.dignityandrespect.org. Accessed October 13, 2022.
15. Brandeis LD. *Business: A Prof*. Boston, MA: Small, Maynard & Company; 1914:2.
16. Arnold L, Stern DT. What is medical professionalism? In: Arnold L, Stern DT, eds. *Measuring Medical Professionalism*. New York: Oxford University Press; 2016:15–37. p. 19.
17. Peabody JW. The care of the patient. *JAMA*. 1927;88:877–882. p. 877.
18. Cassell CK, Hood V, Bauer W. A physician charter: the 10th anniversary. *Ann Intern Med*. 2012;157(4):290–292.
19. Garlington SB, Collins ME, Bossaller MRD. An ethical foundation for social good: virtue theory and solidarity. *Res Soc Work Pract*. 2020;30(2):196–204. p. 199.
20. National Association of Social Workers. *Preamble to the Code of Ethics*. Washington, DC: National Association of Social Workers; 2017. https://socialworker.org/About/Ethics/Code-of-ethics. Accessed January 7, 2021.
21. American Physical Therapy Association. *Core Values for the Physical Therapist and Physical Therapist Assistant*. Alexandria, VA: American Physical Therapy Association; 2021. https://apta.org/apta-and-you/leadership-and-governance/policies/core-values-for-the-physical-therapist-and-physical-therapist-assistant. Accessed October 13, 2022.
22. International Council of Nurses. *Code of Ethics for Nurses*. Geneva: ICN; 2021. tenet 1.8. https://www.icn.ch/.
23. Doherty RF, Purtilo RB. The ethical goal of professional practice: a caring response. In: *Ethical Dimensions in the Health Professions*. 6th ed. St. Louis, MO: Elsevier; 2016:27–50 [Chapter 2].

24. Doherty RF, Peterson EW. Responsible participation in a profession: fostering professionalism and leading for moral action. In: Braveman B, ed. *Leading & Managing Occupational Therapy Services: An Evidence-Based Approach*. 3rd ed. Philadelphia, PA: FA Davis; 2021.
25. Rawls J. *A Theory of Justice*. 2nd ed. Cambridge, MA: Belknap Press of Harvard University; 1971.

Professional Relationships Build on Respect

OBJECTIVES

The reader will be able to

- Describe how trust and trustworthiness serve as a benchmark to gauge respect between patient and health professional;
- Examine professional competence as the foundation of a trust-based connection between health professional and patient;
- Recognize professional behaviors that meet the benchmark of respect in care delivery;
- Explain how acknowledging and responding to the phenomenon of transference or countertransference in the health professional and patient relationship serves as a benchmark of respect;
- Describe three types of situations in which setting and maintaining professional and emotional boundaries are crucial to effective care delivery;
- Define overidentification and describe its negative effects; and
- Articulate ways in which person-first, identity-first, and inclusive language can honor the positive goals of the health professional and patient relationship.

Prelude

I asked Mike to comment on his experience with providers' use of language. His answer added even more nuance to my understanding of how words matter. He expressed that he was grateful for the nurses' and doctors' nonstigmatizing word choices. "No one ever said, 'You're an alcoholic,'" he explained. "It was always, 'You are in the hospital,' 'You are in withdrawal.'" But when I pointed out that he had used the word alcoholic to describe himself, Mike affirmed that word choice. "I know that I am an alcoholic," he said. "It's different if I say it versus if a doctor says it."

J. SALWAN[1]

In this chapter, you have an opportunity to take the insights about respect you have gained from Chapter 1 and put them more specifically into the context of your relationship with patients. In the reflection above, you get a feel for the health professional's desire to make a fuller human connection with her client—in her words, to find out more about the patient's experience related to the use of language. She believes correctly that words matter. They contribute to recovery and control over illness, and perhaps most importantly, effectively express respect for a patient's unique situation.

The health professional and patient relationship is determined by what you have subscribed to by becoming a professional and what the patient is experiencing that has brought this person to you instead of seeking out a friend, loved one, or business associate for help. Therefore, although respect is the foundation of any relationship, a good professional relationship has special respect considerations built into it because of your respective roles.

The phrase *patient-centered* or *person-centered* is an apt example of terms and concepts used in the health professions literature to keep an appropriate focus on the provider–patient relationship. Patient-centered care recognizes the experience of each patient as unique and conceives the patient as a person first.[2] It is respectful of and responsive to individual patient preferences, needs, and values and ensures that patient values guide all clinical decisions.[3,4] The goal of being patient-centered involves honoring the indicators of respect in its three forms—appreciation of a patient's distinctness among persons, attention to that person's health-related need, and commitment to conscientiously providing your professional knowledge and skills to address that need. In meeting this goal, health professionals and patients alike benefit from observable and measurable *benchmarks*. Benchmarks serve as standards and points of reference to assess whether an activity is in fact accomplishing its intended purpose. A respect benchmark measures observable actions that demonstrate that respect is operating at the core of a health professional and patient relationship. Important respect benchmarks include evidence that the relationship is based on trust and expressions of professional, inclusive, and courteous behavior toward patients and their support networks.[5,6]

Build Trust by Being Trustworthy

Legally and ethically the health professional and patient relationship is based on trust. In the law, it is categorized as a *fiduciary relationship* in contrast to one that depends solely on the terms of a contract between two persons. The term *fiduciary* comes from the root *fides*, meaning "faith in someone or something." In this instance, it rests on an assumption that one of the two parties, the patient, cannot be expected to have all the relevant facts that would allow them to contract as equals.

Trust is the patient's sense of security that he or she is being respected by you, including confidence in your intent to provide your best professional services and take the patient's interest and concerns seriously. The patient and others deem you *trustworthy*. Traditionally, providers were judged not only on mere physical presence but also that there was a personal connection with the patient and family who were soothed by the professional's benevolence and compassion.

Modern interpretations of the role of trust in human relationships are molding the understanding of how it is recognized in health professional and patient interactions. In the view of developmental psychologists, trust plays a central role in every person's developmental task of figuring out when and why to depend on others. Underlying this is the belief that no one knows fully what is best for another individual and that to turn over that responsibility completely to someone else, even a professional, is not in a person's best interests. Therefore health professionals are considered trustworthy when a patient is helped to feel secure not only in the professionals' technical skills and decisions but can rely on them to support fuller participation in decisions about personal health and well-being.

Trust in the health professional–patient relationship goes beyond reliance. It involves an expectation that the health professional has goodwill toward the patient and will take their interests seriously.[7] When health professionals meet this expectation through the implementation of patient-centered care, the patient feels confident that the professional's clinical decision is being guided by an underlying respect for that person's basic human dignity.

TRUST BUILT THROUGH LISTENING

Respect conveyed through listening is a primary manifestation of trust. Patients come from all different cultures, backgrounds, faiths, races, genders, and sexual orientations. Upholding trust means you accept patients for who they are, treat them according to their needs, and meet them with competence.[8] Health professionals and patients who build trusting relations work to understand each other's expectations and experiences. Tools for effective listening are described in more detail in Chapter 9. As you develop your skills, you will appreciate that when health professionals listen to their patients, they become better diagnosticians and more attuned providers.[9] Other chapters in this book emphasize that trust and distrust do not arise solely in the one-on-one professional and patient interaction.

PROFESSIONAL COMPETENCE AND TRUST

Trust building cannot be achieved fully without a patient's and others' confidence in your ability to apply skills specific to the unique modalities of your chosen profession.

Your *professional competence* includes

1. knowing what you know and are skilled to do within your specific area defined by your formal training and referred to in the literature and regulations as your "scope of practice";
2. a commitment to lifelong learning and continuing competence to ensure you stay current on the research and management of conditions within your scope of practice;
3. awareness of your professional and personal shortcomings that could negatively affect optimum patient outcomes; and
4. continual reflection and discussion with other professionals for self-improvement.

A patient's request for services in your scope of practice is usually generated by the presence of injury or illness resulting in a lack of ability to function, or some other disquieting physical, cognitive, or mental symptom. People also seek your counsel about how to stay healthy and prevent health-related difficulties. The patient counts on you and other members of the interprofessional care team to clinically assess the patient's problem, what it means for his or her everyday life, and what he or she needs to do to initiate and follow a clinical process leading to restoration or maintenance of the highest quality of life possible in the situation.

A trust-based professional relationship guided by the professionals' areas of competence builds over time, but that alone is not enough. Some challenges to trust result from the way the health care system itself is set up or the social institutions or environments in which services are offered. It has been well documented that mistrust leads to racial disparities and inequity in care delivery.[10,11] When mistrust is present, the burden falls on members of the group with greater power to assume responsibility for building trust. This may be achieved by creating a safe space to ask questions, documenting injustices, working to change ineffective or unfair policies or practices, and in other ways participating in building a continuum of care respectful of patients' needs and preferences.

Health professionals and institutions are so familiar with the professional setting that sometimes they become insensitive to unintended messages that get conveyed, causing patients and other laypeople to be wary of how patients are viewed. For example, commonly used signs and terms such as the "bone clinic," the "allergy office," or "cardiac surgery," all can conjure patients' images of body parts or procedures rather than living, breathing human beings, leading one cartoonist to take this patient concern to the extreme (Fig. 2.1).

Some have called this phenomenon *thinging*. In it, the patient fears being more valued for the "interesting thing" that he or she brings to the health professions setting than, above all, being a person with a human need. This is a serious challenge for health professionals because a necessary part of professional training is to look for the abstractive meaning of a condition: the chest sound, laboratory findings, X-ray films, the sight of the skin or tone of the muscle, and so forth. Common sense suggests that patients should not trust you if you seem more interested in their diagnosis or symptom than in what these mean to their well-being as persons. To the extent that you recognize

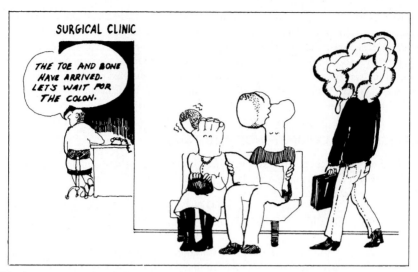

Fig. 2.1 At one extreme, the patient may feel that the health professional is interested only in the body part or symptom. From the Swedish translation of Health Professional and Patient Interaction: Vård, Vårdare, Vårdad.

the mistake of "thinging" and being sensitive to language that can be erroneously interpreted, you will have taken a giant step toward engendering a genuine bond of trust.

Clinically unattainable patient or family expectations also can be a barrier to trust. For example, you may be in a situation where you and the interprofessional care team are uncertain of the best course of treatment for a patient. In these instances, the patient and loved ones need to know that the situation surpasses clinical knowledge at this point so as not to rest their trust on false hopes.[12] Some patients have complex conditions involving several bodily systems or symptoms that cause varying degrees of uncertainty among care providers. The uncertainty may be about the patient's actual diagnosis, the best plan of treatment, the likelihood of unanticipated complications, the expected timeline of results, or the eventual outcome (prognosis) even if all goes well.[13] The process of maintaining a trust-based relationship in these situations starts with offering any snippet of information that you can stand behind with certainty. Reassurance also may take the form of your willingness to respond compassionately to difficult questions about areas that are causing anxiety for patients or their families because abandonment is a common fear. Beyond that, though, are some challenges that are more difficult for many health professionals. For instance, many are very reticent to say "we don't know ourselves what to expect in your situation—it's not going as we hoped" because they worry that this admission will destroy the patient's hope. On the contrary, an honest admission usually does not have a lasting deleterious effect if this bad news is shared with compassion and deep respect for its significance to the patient and family.[14] One reassurance that can always be offered is, "You can count on us to continue to put our best effort forward on your behalf, and we will stand by you in the process."

REFLECTIONS

Think of a time in your life when someone tried to reassure you.
• What did the other person say or do that worked?
• Can you recount an example of when someone tried to reassure you but it did not work?
• Why did their attempts fail?

Concentrate on Caring

A benchmark of respect in the health professions is to go beyond competently applying the modalities of your profession to exhibiting an approach that embodies care. This broader expression includes conduct based not only on your technical knowledge and skill sets but also on how your attitudes, experience, and reflection apply to an authentic human relationship with a particular individual.[15] What then are some markers that you and the patient can use to measure the success of meeting the respect benchmark of care? We offer several practical ones here, and others are woven throughout the pages of this book.

STAY FOCUSED—ON THE PERSON

Health professionals must infuse each patient professional relationship with convincing evidence that the patient is seen as a person first. The undergirding of respect also operates on your behalf when you are faced with external challenges that threaten to deter you from your focused attention on what you have learned about the patient and how your professional care can best be expressed in your relationship. Recall from Chapter 1 that an indicator of respect is to be mindful that the distinct person who has become your patient deserves your attention. At the same time, almost everyone struggles with effective time management in today's fast-paced care delivery settings. Your commitment to not cut corners in patient care helps keep you focused on fostering a relationship that goes beyond the mere minimum of caring behaviors. There is nothing more upsetting to a patient than feeling that you are seeing him or her simply as another case on the long list of cases, to be filed as "completed" at the end of the day (Fig. 2.2).

But this commitment is sometimes difficult to keep. When you must take shortcuts, a patient is more likely to maintain their assurance that you care if you explain the reason for an unfortunate or exceptional circumstance. Your commitment to foster respectful care can be effective if at the outset you remind the patient of the amount of time you have to be with them and work together to discuss what you hope the two of you will accomplish in that time. Every health professional knows that on some days a particular patient needs extra time to work through a problem, which can wreak havoc on a schedule. Then, there are patients who for good (or poor) reasons are late, linger, or divert your time and energy from other patients. Setting your daily schedule against a backdrop of differing patient needs will help to keep you on as clear a path as possible through the

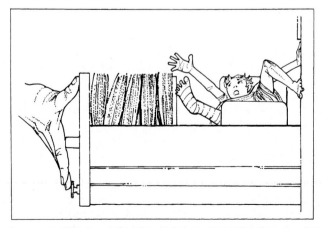

Fig. 2.2 Nothing is more upsetting to a patient than to feel you are treating them as a "case" to be filed or entered in the computer before you go on to the next patient or commitment on your schedule.

day. Although some patients you have kept waiting will become impatient, your focused attention on doing all that you are able to do for them when their turn comes will support their feeling that your behavior remains consistent with your respectful caring for them. Some waiting areas today list the professionals who are seeing patients, whether they are on schedule, and, if not, how long it appears it will be before the next patient can be seen. This can be effective to a point, especially if the professional apologizes for a delay and the waiting patient has an opportunity to learn something about the cause for delay when their turn comes.

Managing time with the goal of giving full attention to the patient can be aided by additional clues about how to conduct yourself with the patient during the time you are actually together:

- Remove the person from areas where distractions are likely to impinge on your time together.
- Sit down or in other ways convey your intent to give full attention to the person.
- If you are hurried, take a mindful pause before entering the patient encounter. Approach the person slowly and graciously.
- Look the person in the eye while conversing. A lack of direct eye contact communicates a lack of interest.
- Place a clock in an area where you can be aware of the time without being obvious about it.
- Let others know you are engaged and should not be disturbed. For example, turn your cell phone to do not disturb mode and silence pagers.

This section on staying focused on the person who is a patient would not be complete without including a guideline for how you speak of and to patients. The disability rights movement has led attention to the power of words in their emphasis on *person or people-first language.*

> *The language a society uses to refer to persons with disabilities shapes its beliefs and ideas about them. People First Language emphasizes the person, not the disability. By placing the person first, the disability is no longer the primary, defining characteristic of an individual, but one of several aspects of the whole person. It eliminates generalizations and stereotypes, by focusing on the person rather than the disability.*[16]

An example is to use the phrase "a person who has Parkinson's disease" instead of "a Parkinson's patient" or a "person with schizophrenia" instead of a "schizophrenic." This may seem a subtle shift, but the latter does not equate the person with a diagnosis but communicates that this person has the diagnosis among their many other traits and characteristics. Although person-first language is ideal, some communities and groups have different preferences. Just as some prefer person-first language, others see disability as part of their identity and culture. *Identity-first language* is preferred by some communities. For example, in select autistic communities, it is seen as a source of empowerment representing a cultural shift toward neurodiversity.[17] So how do you know which to choose? As in the case of asking patients their preferred name or gender pronoun/s, asking the preference of a patient/group is best practice. In fact, attending to the patient's declared language preferences is one of the best ways to convey the core of respect. Communicating through nonstigmatizing language and using words that focus on strengths show your commitment as a health professional to understand the human experience.[18] Fig. 2.3 provides suggestions of sample alternate terminology to consider in your patient interactions.

RESPECT FOR LITTLE THINGS

An important way to support a patient's feeling of self-worth and confidence in the caring relationship is to acknowledge little personal details that too often go unnoticed. The poet William Blake noted, "He who would do good to others must do it in minute particulars." If you think about your own life, there are times when "minute particulars" have counted as essential expressions of deep respect shown by another. Thoughtful little details take many shapes, but a few common ones are discussed here that apply to the health professional and patient relationship.

Table
Alternate Terminology to Consider. With Patient's Preference Always Taking Precedence

Instead of	Consider
Diagnosis-first language (schizophrenic)	Person-first language[a] (person with schizophrenia)
Noncompliant, resistant, refusing	Declined, chose not to, is not in agreement with
Illegal, foreigner	Undocumented
Frequent flyer	Person who uses services
Abuser, addict, junkie	Has a substance use disorder
Sweetie	Mr./Mrs./Ms. X
Committed suicide	Died by suicide
Failed/unsuccessful suicide attempt	Survived a suicide attempt
Suicide survivor	Suicide attempt survivor or suicide loss survivor (differentiate)
Suffers from/is a victim of	Experiences, he lives with, has a history of
Being clean/getting clean	Sober, in recovery. has a negative test result
Narcotic	Oplaid
Opioid substitution therapy	Treatment or pharmacotherapy
Transsexual	Transgender

[a] With some exceptions, detailed in the text.

Fig. 2.3 Sample alternate terminology that puts the patient first. From Carroll SM. Respecting and empowering vulnerable populations: contemporary terminology. *J Nurse Pract*. 2019;15(3):228–231.

Personal Hygiene and Comfort Measures

When a patient has a straightforward hygienic need that can easily be relieved, your attention to it before any other activity or exchange will be deeply appreciated. It is surprising how embarrassed a person may be to admit that he needs to use the bathroom or needs a tissue to wipe a runny nose but cannot do it independently. A simple unsolicited act on your part makes the difference between an embarrassed or fidgety person and one ready to focus on the clinical issue at hand. Comfort-enhancing details not only matter greatly to patients, but they also demonstrate respect for their dignity. Asking "Are you comfortable?" or "Is there anything else I can do for you while I am with you to make you more comfortable?" expresses respect that will be interpreted as a genuine caring act.

REFLECTIONS

- Have you been stuck in a situation where you could not get comfortable? Describe how it made you feel.
- What did you have to do to remedy the situation?

Personal Interests and Landmark Events

Almost everyone has some area of interest, whether it be a hobby, job, family, or other focus. Showing interest in the person does not require probing unduly into his or her personal life. Some patients will want to chat about life outside of the moment, and others will not. At the same time, asking a hospitalized patient about the noon menu, complementing an ambulatory care patient on something he or she is wearing, reminding a teenager that her favorite rap artist has a special show on television that night, and spelling Mr. Schydlowski's name correctly on his appointment slip count as personalized care. Landmark events in the person's life often involve birthdays and anniversaries, and usually, it is accepted as a sign of respect by this person if you mark it. For instance, if you think that he would enjoy the attention, on Mr. Arnold's birthday write "HAPPY BIRTHDAY, DICK ARNOLD" in bold letters on his lunch tray or let other staff know so that they can acknowledge it, too. You will think of other expressions of this type of respect to put into everyday action (Fig. 2.4).

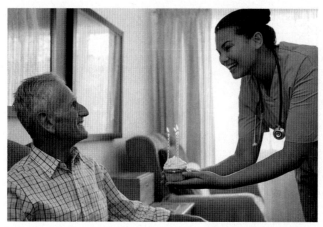

Fig. 2.4 A birthday is often an important opportunity to recognize a patient. © http://Wavebreakmedia/iStock/ Thinkstock.com.

In addition to personal events, most patients are very aware of holidays or even the passing of the seasons as holding special meaning they may or may not be able to acknowledge in ways they would like or remember doing. Asking them to share such memories can be interpreted as an expression of genuine care.

A special challenge arises for patients and residents who have been confined to a home, hospital, or other long-term care facilities. You know how quickly one can lose touch with the rest of the world once schedules and everyday surroundings change. By sharing an incident observed on the way to work, reviewing a play seen the evening before, or taking the patient to a window to see a child and dog playing together, you can extend the patient's environment beyond the immediate setting, bringing him or her into contact with the outside world. The passing of the seasons can have significance for patients too. One of the authors once brought apple blossoms into a four-bed room in an assisted living facility only to have two of the residents burst into tears, saying they missed the sweet smells of spring more than anything else since being forced to make this their permanent home. This simple act opened the door to a discussion about springtime memories and was a reminder of how much such seemingly small things can be conducive to meeting the benchmark of care.

RESPECT FOR THE PATIENT'S AGENDA

Earlier in this chapter, we introduced the notion of a patient-centered relationship and that in it the patient's say-so is essential for their being. We pick up this theme again to underscore that a patient's perception of the life challenges they are experiencing understandably can be quite different from that of the health professional's interpretation of the situation. This insight relies on the fact that patients are concerned primarily with what their clinical condition signifies in terms of their daily lives, loves, and activities. Hardly ever is the technical aspect of what is wrong the governing concern; rather it is "How does this affect the quality of my life?"

Because the professional's intent to partner with the patient will always involve blind spots, *humility* is one basic character trait all professionals must cultivate. Humility acknowledges one's limits; thus respect for the patient partially is realized through humility in the form of acknowledgment of the patient's autonomy and authority in the relationship. *Autonomy* is the principle of self-determination. It means that the patient is an active participant in health care decisions and, as such, has the say-so or self-governance regarding health care decisions. Health professionals demonstrate trust by affirming the patients' expertise about their health, circumstances, and abilities.[9] When a care plan reflects a patient's values and preferences, the patient can trust that the interprofessional care team respects their wishes and contributions. This reciprocal trust honors the patient–provider relationship and is the foundation for shared decision-making.

In the United States and many other countries, the mechanism of informed consent is a useful legal and ethical tool. *Informed consent* is a means to facilitate effective communication and trust, placing the onus of responsibility on the professional to level the playing field through a process of informing and being sure that the patient understands and consents (or not) to a proposed course of action. This contract between you and the patient is just the beginning. Everything after that either reinforces or sets up barriers to the person's ability to participate confidently in details that give his or her life its content, texture, and meaning, many of them realized through participation in daily activities that the professional may think are not that important. Humility teaches us to behold the gift of listening that is entrusted to us by our patients. When we do so, we not only provide information but fully support deliberation and decision-making for patients and families.

Distinguish Courtesy From Casualness

You might think that everyday niceties such as "Hello, how are you today?" are such an obvious component of a respectful relationship that it need not be discussed. However, as important as a warm initial greeting is, the type of social exchange that is relevant as a benchmark of respect in a professional relationship is more akin to the idea of *courtesy*, which has a subtle level of formality to it. You can begin to see the difference in this simple dictionary definition of courtesy as ". . . elegance . . . of manners; graceful politeness or considerateness."[19] It includes but goes beyond minding your manners in the superficial sense that you were taught to do as a child. Professional courtesy requires doing so with words, attitudes, and gestures that convey your genuine acknowledgment of the other's dignity. Patients take their initial cues about whether they matter as people from the courtesy they receive when they first come through the door (or, in the case of home health care, when you pass through theirs). Although we must also strive to embed courteous conduct into the deeper understandings of care in the health professional and patient relationship, the patient's first, and often lasting, impression is connected to courtesies they receive (or do not receive) from you and others in the environment.

REFLECTIONS

Take a minute to reflect on the last time you visited a physician, dentist, therapist, or other health professional. Picture the environment as you first entered.
- What led you to feel confident that you were welcomed and that the staff had given some thought to what would make you as comfortable as possible?
- How could the environment and conduct of the staff have been improved to make it a more comfortable and inclusive place?
- Now try to picture yourself being visited in your home by a home health care provider during your recovery from a serious accident. List some professional courtesies you would expect.

Respect, Contract, and Covenant

Although a patient must successfully carry his or her share of responsibility for developing a flourishing relationship with you, the health professional must take leadership in the process of building a relationship that meets the benchmark of care based on respect. Toward realizing that result, ethicist

William May proposes that thinking of ourselves as being bound by a *covenant* includes the contract elements of professional mechanisms such as informed consent and the items detailed in professional codes of ethics but goes further. Covenants place the parties in a situation of mutual benefit at the human level. Just as humility highlights areas of the professional not being all-knowing, covenants allow the professional to acknowledge benefits derived from health care practice and from the opportunity to be with a particular patient who arrives not only with signs or symptoms but also with talents, gifts, and histories. Affirming these talents and celebrating a patient's expertise about their health, circumstances, and abilities build trust. Therefore an element of *professional gratitude* enters the relationship, empowering patients to do their best and encouraging professionals to go beyond the bare minimum of expectations that are agreed upon in a strict contract approach.[20]

INTEGRITY IN WORDS AND CONDUCT

Covenants set the foundation, but conduct reveals integrity in action. *Integrity* comes from the French root *integritas*, meaning "whole or undivided." The cultivation of integrity is your commitment to first and foremost know yourself thoroughly. A large part of this task is realized through living according to your value system as discussed in Chapter 1. Only then can you confidently demonstrate to others that your values and commitments are seamlessly aligned with your conduct, so others experience a high level of consistency between what you say and what you do. We have been emphasizing examples of how trust does not build automatically in the health professional and patient relationship: it is the patients' judgment call as to whether they view you as trustworthy in declaring that you have their best interests at heart. Your integrity means that you project an authentic wholeness in your attitudes, words, purpose, and actions, providing evidence that they may confidently place their trust in you.[21,22]

The patient's reliance on the professional's integrity also extends to his or her experience with the interprofessional care team in the form of collective integrity across systems of care. When there is an absence of collaboration, interventions offered by team members can be confusing to the patient, leaving room for distrust to take root. We offer three general guidelines as preparation for your further study in Chapter 8 of interprofessional care teams to help patients see you as trustworthy.

1. Be respectful of all team members' contributions and decide among yourselves who will be the primary spokesperson in different situations that arise.
2. Be an alert and active participant in team decisions. Provide your expertise and listen to the perspectives and expertise of others.
3. If a patient or family caregiver has a question that goes beyond your area of expertise, immediately convey this information to the appropriate team member, and let the patient know you are going to tap the expertise of others in response to their question.

In summary, trust and trustworthiness are central components of the success of any health professional and patient relationship. Having introduced you to several details of what is involved in meeting this important benchmark of respect, we turn now to another type of benchmark—namely, your acknowledgment of, and attention to, boundaries in professional relationships.

What Is a Professional Boundary?

Professional boundary is a term developed in the professional literature and practice guidelines to provide guidance regarding appropriate, prudent physical and emotional constraints to intimacy. Although most benchmarks of respect involve positive action, this one calls for understanding where and when to exercise constraint. The general rule is that the physical and emotional boundaries between you and patients must always be guided by the goal of facilitating a patient's well-being and maintaining profound and caring respect in the interaction (Fig. 2.5). But knowing the general

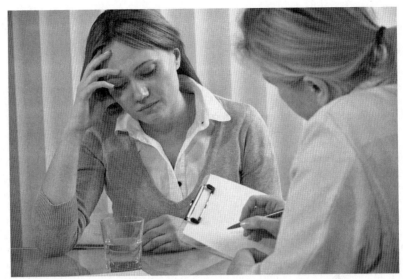

Fig. 2.5 Maintaining professional boundaries helps put the goal of facilitating a patient's well-being at the forefront of the professional and patient relationship. © Alex Raths/iStock/Thinkstock.com.

rule will not necessarily always help you with the complex human stories you face in the line of work you have chosen. For one thing, relationships are dynamic, and there are changes in them with every encounter. Boundary issues may arise from physical or psychological/emotional sources. An extreme example is when health professionals lose their licenses or in other ways are sanctioned for engaging in sexual misconduct with patients. We discuss this type of breach in a section that broadly describes physical boundaries. Guidelines regarding emotional boundaries are designed to prevent psychological dynamics that are harmful to the patient or to you during the relationship. We discuss these, too. It is easy to see that breaches may involve aspects of both. Some boundary guidelines have arisen from external considerations (e.g., the time you spend in the encounter), whereas others are internal (i.e., characteristics you and the patient bring to it).

Guidelines for physical and psychological or emotional boundaries are derived from several sources. Some come from professional codes of ethics. These draw on a long history of differentiating the role of the professional from that of a citizen. Others come from institutional codes of conduct, laws, and regulations that have grown out of the experience of health professionals and patients and serve to regulate conduct and protect the public trust. Sometimes, guidelines change based on insights from psychology regarding tensions that may arise from human needs for privacy, intimacy, power, and acceptance.

One way the wisdom of maintaining boundaries has been dramatized in the past is through advancing the erroneous idea that being professional requires one to be aloof, objective, and efficient at the price of personal warmth and affectionate conduct. But to suggest that respect entails aloofness is a distortion of the highest goals to which professionals aspire.[23]

PSYCHODYNAMICS IN PROFESSIONAL RELATIONSHIPS

We have shown that maintaining professional boundaries is not achieved by employing a cold or impersonal approach because such an approach may increase patients' conviction that you are being disrespectful of them and their situation. At the same time, the line between behaviors and expectations in your personal versus your professional relationships can be stretched thin in some situations. At times, emotional responses and actions may lead to challenges in person-centered care. We turn our attention to a few of these challenges now.

Tease Out Transference Issues

The psychotherapeutic notion of *transference* can help you understand certain kinds of behaviors some people exhibit toward you in your professional relationship with them. How you respond and use this insight serves as a respect benchmark. Transference has its root in the theories advanced by Sigmund Freud and further developed by other psychologists who employ this term to convey the process of shifting one's feeling about a person in the past to another person.[24] A young man, angry that his father brutally ruled with an iron hand, might conclude, "Here it comes again!" and respond aggressively to a male health professional as soon as something about the professional triggers a negative memory of his father. Or consider the example of Ray, a male nursing student who prepared extensively and carefully for his interaction with his first obstetrics-gynecology patient. Part of the clinical evaluation was to conduct a basic history and do a general physical examination. On entering the patient's room, he said, "Good morning. I'm Ray Abrams, a student nurse who is going to be caring for and examining you today." The patient took one look at this bearded, 6-foot-plus student and said, "Oh, no you're not! You look too much like my son, honey!" His supervisor, who had just stepped into the room, caught this woman's reaction and judged that to disregard the patient's discomfort would be a sign of disrespect, although she may have mis-understood what the student meant was not a gynecological examination. Instead, the student's clinical instructor privately used the occasion as a teaching moment with the student, explaining that this type of transference sometimes happens. The instructor then informed the patient that in this case the examination simply included taking vital signs such as temperature, blood pressure, and pulse. Still, the patient was relieved when she was reassigned a different student nurse.

Transference can be negative or positive. Examples of negative transference are the aggres-siveness of the young man who "saw" his father in the professional and the discomfort stimulated by the similarity of the male nursing student to the woman's son. For reasons, patients sometimes cannot identify or express, their comfort level is low and their guard is up. At the other end of the spectrum, positive transference, the good feelings a patient transfers to the health professional, usually can promote a well-working relationship.

It is not always easy to tell whether the transference will create a problem. A young occu-pational therapist caught a new male patient staring at her. Finally, he shook his head and said, "Man oh man, I could have sworn my first wife walked in when you came into the treatment area. Whew!" The man seemed a bit shaken, and of course, this raised some questions for the therapist who responded by saying, "Well, is that a good or bad thing?" He said, "Both!" So, she was still in the woods on this one. She felt she had no choice at this moment but to continue with the patient, watching for further signs that this man's association seemed to be inappropriately affecting his responses and their relationship. (There were none, and the matter never came up again.)

The patient is not the only party in the relationship who experiences transference. *Countertransference*, a professional's tendency to respond to a patient with associations of others in his or her life, takes place every bit as often. A health professional may transfer feelings to the patient based on name, physical appearance, voice, age, or gestures that conjure up powerful associa-tions of other people. It is up to you to be self-aware about such associations and adapt your con-duct to correct for any negative or other troubling feelings and responses you think might be issuing from your mental association of the patient with someone in your past or present relationships.

At the same time, total neutrality is not required. If you have served on a jury, you know that the judge's concern is that the jurors' past experiences and associations do not in any discernible way adversely come into play to unduly sway the juror's judgment when the facts of the case and the identification of the defendant and plaintiff are made known. The basic concern is similar in the health professional and patient relationship. You can learn to listen for signs that such associations may be occurring. Fundamentally, what is necessary for maintaining respectful professional relationships with patients when this dynamic is taking place is to acknowledge transference or countertransference and try to respond to it in a way that honors it for the benchmark of respect that attending to it is. Your actions can range from simple awareness to providing for the patient to be referred to a colleague who is equally suited for the clinical challenges.

Overidentification With the Patient's Predicament

Maintaining appropriate emotional boundaries and psychological distance can become a challenge when you have had an experience so like the patient's that you believe your experiences to be identical. Such a reaction of overidentification is a little different from transference as discussed above. Transference highlights an association you have of that person with someone else you know or have known. Overidentification puts you personally into very close alignment with the other and is a variety of enmeshment. Enmeshment includes the emotional responses and psychological attachments of the health professional or patient which can interfere with respect for the patient and damage the therapeutic relationship.

At first, it seems a mistaken idea that having had similar experiences may actually hinder the effectiveness of a respect-based health professional and patient relationship. But everyone has had the experience of beginning to relate a traumatic (or exciting) event only to have the other person interrupt with "Oh! I know exactly what you mean!" and then go on to describe his or her own story. One feels cheated at such times, thinking, "No, that's not what I meant, but you are more interested in telling me about yourself than in listening to me!" The way such overidentification works within the health professions can be illustrated in the following Case Study.

CASE STUDY

Mrs. Rita Garcia, an elementary school teacher, became interested in teaching language skills to hearing-impaired children after her third child, Lucia, who was born deaf, successfully learned to communicate by attending special classes for those with hearing impairment. Mrs. Garcia enrolled in a health professions course directed toward training teachers of hearing-impaired persons.

In her first position, she was surprised and alarmed that some of the mothers requested that she not be assigned to their children. Finally, she approached one of the mothers whose child she had been working with and with whom she felt comfortable. "What's wrong?" she asked. "Do they think I'm incompetent because I was older when I went back to school or am new in my field? Is it my personality or the fact that I have a Spanish accent? I want so much to help these children, and I can't understand what I'm doing wrong." The embarrassed mother replied, "Well, since you asked, I'll give you a direct answer. I don't feel this way, but some of the mothers think that you don't understand their children's unique challenges because every time they start to tell you something about their child, you immediately interrupt with an experience you have had with your daughter."

Unfortunately, Rita Garcia's intent was a good one, but her effectiveness as a teacher was hindered by her own experiences and, likely, her need to share what she had been through. She would benefit from recognizing that the tendency to overidentify is bound to be present because of her own situation. It also will be helpful to remind herself periodically that attempts to relate to the patient (or in this case the parent of the patient) by pointing out superficial similarities between her own experience and theirs may be interpreted as her desire to talk about her own problem. Overidentification, once it becomes a part of the caregiver's thinking, cannot be easily erased. But giving the other an opportunity to fully describe his or her unique experience and express the feelings attached to it before superimposing any similarities can help convey respect for the other's unique situation and decrease the deleterious effect on the relationship. Coworkers also can be valuable when a health professional's close relationship with the patient prevents him or her from seeing the patient's situation clearly. They may see what is happening and thus provide insight into the challenge occasioned by one's own similar, intense experience.

The task for all professionals who encounter a patient's situation that lends itself to overidentification is to be on the lookout for and honor the unique details and differences as well, thereby meeting the benchmark of respect.

RECOGNIZING A "MEANINGFUL DISTANCE"

In everyday life, we seldom are consciously aware of the distance between oneself and the other; rather, we automatically position ourselves among others to maintain our comfort zone. However, in human interactions, psychological and physical distances have societal and often personal meanings determined by the degree of intimacy it represents for both parties. At one pole, there may be a complete sense of separateness such as accidentally being physically pressed against each other in a crowd, and, at the other, there is a realm of togetherness that is highly personal, informal, and familiar (i.e., intimate). At any point along this continuum, certain messages and expectations are put into play, whereas others remain in the background. The nuances with which the appropriate boundaries of respect must be maintained are the impetus for many of the reflections on this topic. We present the most fundamental ones for your learning and reflection.

PHYSICAL BOUNDARIES

As a rule, mainstream Western societies do not condone much touching, especially among strangers. You may find a clerk in a store who physically touches the palm of your hand in returning change. You may shake a stranger's hand in meeting. Among some contexts, strangers may impulsively hug the man or woman next to them during an important sports event. However, the occasions when touching among strangers is socially sanctioned can probably be counted on one hand. At the same time, many tasks in the health professions environment require caregivers to be in close physical contact with strangers who are their patients and to do so respectfully. In addition, displays of affection expressed by a pat on the shoulder, a gentle hug, or other signs of support are behaviors you may be comfortable engaging in as a part of your interaction if you feel confident that the patient is welcoming it.

All cultures and subcultures have socially constructed rules about when and between whom touching (or even visual access) is condoned. Such rules often extend to the acceptable conduct between health professionals and patients. For example, in some cultures, a male caregiver may not touch or even look at a woman's bare body. At the same time, when taken seriously, appropriate touch can be an effective means of establishing rapport or showing reassurance and may be required for diagnostic or treatment regimens. In short, acceptable contours of physical contact between health professional and patient require considered attention.

Unconsented Touching

Informed consent, mentioned earlier in this chapter, is one of the most basic societal acknowledgments that professional contact may permissibly depart dramatically from general accepted social norms of physical contact. By giving informed consent the patient is saying, in effect, I give you—and others involved in my care—consent to hold, stroke, rub, poke, or even puncture or cut me, depending on the scope of practice in your professional role. Obviously, the permission to make physical contact already puts the health professional and patient relationship into a special category in which usual socially acceptable distances are breached on a regular basis.

Your right to make physical contact does not give you permission to impose on a patient's sensitivities or dislikes regarding physical contact. Cultural, social, and personal factors come together to create a patient's comfort zone regarding physical contact, and the health professional must be guided by a sensitivity to these individual differences.

Inappropriate Touching

Some types of physical contact are deemed unacceptable in the health professional and patient relationship under any conditions, even with the consent of the patient or client. Under law, you cannot make contact with a patient with an intent to harm them physically or psychologically. If you do, you will be charged with abuse.

The type of inappropriate touching that has received the most attention is physical contact delivered with an intent to excite or arouse the patient sexually. Although sexual intimacies are the most prohibited of inappropriate touching between a health professional and patient, the prohibitions are not limited to them. For example, the American Physical Therapy Association states explicitly, "Physical therapists shall not engage in any sexual relationship with any of their patients/clients, supervisees, or students."[25] In this case, the boundary is tied to the value of maintaining professional integrity. You might wonder why it is forbidden if a competent, adult patient consents to or even seems to invite sexual contact. The strongest argument against this type of contact is that it betrays the reasonable expectations built into the essence of the health professional and patient relationship. Patients have a right to receive the best care possible without having to satisfy the professional's needs. The reasoning is that sexual activity is never free from other types of claims on the other person, so both patient and health professional may begin to alter the conditions of the relationship considering the power of its sexual dimensions rather than the conditions under which a patient sought professional care in the first place. In short, it is never considered fair that the patient would have to meet your need for sexual pleasure, sexual intimacy, sexual fulfillment, dominance in a relationship, or any other gain, no matter what either you or the patient believes would be gained.

SEXUAL HARASSMENT

The importance of the idea that sexual boundaries must be maintained in public settings is aired in the notion of *sexual harassment*. The US Equal Employment Opportunity Commission defines harassment as unwelcome sexual advances, requests for sexual favors, and other verbal or physical conduct and includes activity that creates a hostile or unwelcome work environment for the person who feels "harassed." Harassment can consist of a single act or multiple persistent and pervasive acts. A more specific description follows:

Sexual harassment is a form of sex discrimination that violates Title VII of the Civil Rights Act of 1964. Unwelcome sexual advances, requests for sexual favors, and other verbal or physical conduct of a sexual nature constitute sexual harassment when this conduct explicitly or implicitly affects an individual's employment; unreasonably interferes with an individual's work performance; or creates an intimidating, hostile, or offensive work environment. Sexual harassment can occur in a variety of circumstances, including but not limited to the following: The victim and harasser may be a woman or a man. The victim does not have to be of the opposite sex. The victim does not have to be the person harassed but could be anyone affected by the offensive conduct. The harasser's conduct must be unwelcome. It is helpful for the victim to inform the harasser directly that the conduct is unwelcome and must stop.[26]

Although harassment was developed within the context of employer–employee and related situations, most state licensing acts governing health professionals have similar provisions prohibiting such behavior toward patients or others, and many institutions include prohibitions in their policies. You will have ample opportunity to learn more about the particulars of the legal and regulatory issues involved in this area of professional practice, and it is in your best interest to do so.

Summary

This chapter presents basic instructions on how to translate professional respect into specific everyday relational actions and offers benchmarks of respect to assess the success of this goal. Through the remainder of the book, the reader will delve more fully into these general forms of evidence that the health professional and patient relationship can help realize the well-being of each patient and be a welcome ingredient in fostering a flourishing society.

The benchmark of a trust-based relationship is met when both parties are free to move forward with confidence that the best possible course is being offered to the patient and that the professional's actions come from a place of integrity. A second benchmark is manifested by courteous behaviors based on true respect for the human dignity of each individual and offered in everyday words and actions experienced by the patient and his or her support systems. The professional's acknowledgment of and considered response to the psychological dynamics of transference and countertransference is a third benchmark that allows the specific contours of a health professional and patient relationship to remain true to its intended purposes. Finally, the benchmark of professional caring behaviors is the ultimate measure of what the health professional and patient relationship should look like. The previously mentioned three benchmarks are instrumental in meeting this goal because each reflects an aspect of respectful care in action. Many expressions of professional care are possible, and even those that appear mundane at first glance are in fact essential considerations. Such expressions of care include everyday personal details that help give each patient hope for maintaining a meaningful quality of life. Taken together, these benchmarks of respect provide an overall measure of how health professionals and patients can effectively work together to achieve common goals. The test of the ideas presented in this chapter is the extent to which any of them supports genuine respect toward patients, their families, and the ideals of the health professions. Professional relatedness builds on basic human relational characteristics such as trust, sensitivity to the effects of psychological dynamics at play, behaviors assuring the patient that he or she is a person deserving of keen attention, and care offered in ways that embody genuine human respect.

References

1. Salwan J. Person first and patient first: tailoring language to individual patient needs. *Subst Abuse.* 2019;40(2):146–147.
2. Ilardo ML, Speciale A. The community pharmacist: perceived barriers and patient-centered care communication. *Int J Environ Res Public Health.* 2020;17(2):536. https://doi.org/10.3390/ijerph17020536.
3. The American Geriatrics Society Expert Panel on Person-Centered Care. Person-centered care: a definition and essential elements. *J Am Geriatr Soc.* 2016;64:15–18.
4. Scholl I, Zill JM, Harter M, Dirmaier J. An integrative model of patient-centeredness—a systematic review and concept analysis. *PLoS ONE.* 2014;9:e107828.

5. Rassouli M, Zamanzadeh V, Valizadeh L, Asghari E. Limping along in implementing patient-centered care: qualitative study. *Nurs Pract Today*. 2020;7(3):217–225.
6. Drossman DA, Ruddy J. Improving patient–provider relationships to improve health care. *Clin Gastroenterol Hepatol*. 2020;18(7):1417–1426.
7. Sullivan LS. Trust, risk, and race in American Medicine. *Hastings Cent Rep*. 2020;50(1):18–26.
8. Carlström R, Ek S, Gabrielsson S. 'Treat me with respect': transgender persons' experiences of encounters with healthcare staff. *Scand J Caring Sci*. 2021;35(2):600–607.
9. Grob R, Darien G, Meyers D. Why physicians should trust in patients. *JAMA*. 2019;321(14):1347–1348.
10. Gupta N, Thiele CM, Daum JI, et al. Building patient–physician trust: a medical student perspective. *Acad Med*. 2020;95(7):980–983.
11. Nguyen AL, Schwei RJ, Zhao YQ, Rathouz PJ, Jacobs EA. What matters when it comes to trust in one's physician: race/ethnicity, sociodemographic factors, and/or access to and experiences with health care? *Health Equity*. 2020;4(1):280–289. https://doi.org/10.1089/HEQ.2019.0101.
12. Jacobs BB, Taylor C. Medical futility in the natural attitude. *Adv Nurs Sci*. 2005;28(4):288–305.
13. Robinson E, Hamel-Norduzzi M, Purtilo RB, et al. Complexities in decision making for persons with disabilities near end of life. *Top Stroke Rehabil*. 2006;13(4):54–67.
14. McGuigan D. Communicating bad news to patients: a reflective approach. *Nurs Stand*. 2009;23(31):51–56.
15. Doherty R. *Ethical Dimensions in the Health Professions*. 7th ed. St. Louis, MO: Elsevier; 2021.
16. *The Arc*. The Power of Words: People First Language, 2021. http://www.thearc.org/who-we-are/media-center/people-first-language.
17. Vivanti G. Ask the Editor: what is the most appropriate way to talk about individuals with a diagnosis of autism? *J Autism Dev Disord*. 2020;50(2):691–693.
18. Carroll SM. Respecting and empowering vulnerable populations: contemporary terminology. *J Nurse Pract*. 2019;15(3):228–231.
19. *The Shorter Oxford English Dictionary*. 5th ed. Vol. 1 (A–O). Oxford: Oxford University Press; 2002.
20. May WF. Code and covenant or philanthropy and contract? *Hastings Cent Rep*. 1975;5:29–35.
21. Hardingham LB. Integrity and moral residue: nurses as participants in a moral community. *Nurs Philos*. 2004;5(2):127–134.
22. Freud S. *The Ego and the Mechanisms of Defense*. New York: International Universities Press; 1966.
23. Swisher LL, Page CG. *Professionalism in Physical Therapy Practice*. Philadelphia, PA: Saunders; 2005.
24. Rich RA, Hecht MK. Staffing considerations. In: Haddad A, ed. *High Tech Home Care: A Practical Guide*. Rockville, MD: Aspen; 1987.
25. American Physical Therapy Association. *Principle #4.C American Physical Therapy Association Code of Ethics*. Fairfax, VA: American Physical Therapy Association; 2020. Available at: https://www.apta.org/siteassets/pdfs/policies/codeofethicshods06-20-28-25.pdf.
26. U.S. Equal Employment Opportunity Commission. *Fact Sheet: Sexual Harassment Discrimination*. EEOC-NVTA-0000-2. Title VII, 29 CFR Part 1601, 29 CFR Part 1604. Issue date 1.15.97 https://www.eeoc.gov/laws/guidance/fact-sheet-sexual-harassment-discrimination.

Respect for Self in the Professional Role

The reader will be able to

- List some positive goals related to self-respect that can be realized by attending to one's own needs and healthful habits;
- Describe some reasons why striking a balance between socializing and solitude is important for a lifetime of professional vitality;
- Define professional resilience and explain why it is a critical trait to support a career in the health professions;
- Identify essential professional practice skills that serve to sustain self-respect and resilience;
- Name two types of bonds that can develop among work colleagues to help create a network of support and mutual respect;
- Understand the psychological and physical health benefits of gratitude;
- Describe guidelines to assess how supportive an employer and future colleagues are likely to be;
- Distinguish intimate from personal relationships and therapeutic from social relationships;
- Identify the benefits of mindfulness as it relates to self-care and the health professional and patient interaction;
- Identify the three hallmarks of burnout in the health professions;
- Exercise tools for supporting oneself and one's interprofessional colleagues in times of personal or professional struggle; and
- Evaluate why addressing one's anxieties and accepting responsibility for one's actions are essential to maintaining self-respect and realizing professional satisfaction.

Prelude

Dignity can be considered as two values: other-regarding by respecting the dignity of others, and self-regarding by respecting one's own dignity or self-respect.

ANN GALLAGHER[1]

In this chapter, we stand back from some specific aspects of your professional role and identity formation to examine the fundamental question of how you can care for yourself and make physical and psychological space for optimal professional functioning.

Sustaining Self-Respect Through Nurturing Yourself

Nurturing comes from root words meaning "feeding," "taking loving care of," and "bringing into full bloom." In Chapter 1, you were introduced to the idea that a professional life guided by respect depends in part on the ability to identify and shape your own life according to your personal values and those that help to build a stronger community. The basic question we ask for your reflection in this chapter is, "What kinds of activities and attitudes can you cultivate to stay authentically you—healthy, happy, satisfied with your job, and able to integrate your professional and personal values and goals?"

There is the issue of who is responsible for your well-being. Today, the consensus is that individuals ultimately are responsible for their own health. Do you agree and, if not totally, what are some exceptions? It certainly is the case that people feel better, look better, and can function more fully when nurturing their own sense of well-being, seeking balance in their lives, and mapping a life course that has the opportunity for changing priorities.

None of these goals comes easily for most! The positive results of keeping life-affirming habits, practices, and goals in the forefront of your life plan as new situations arise seem obvious. However, if you are among the millions who make New Year's resolutions each year, you know that acknowledging the benefits of staying healthy physically, mentally, and spiritually and being successful in doing so are not the same. Consider with us some insights and suggestions to help you succeed in staying happy and healthy through enjoying self-respect in your professional role.

Self-Respect and Self-Care

You were introduced to care in previous chapters as an essential benchmark of respect in professional practice. You will recognize some themes about professional care in the following paragraph:

> *Everyone talks about care as a positive feature of human relationships. It is. But care has a much more serious function in sustaining them than often we acknowledge. It is the link we make with another human being in distress, taking their suffering and well-being into account. At its core, care is not limited to the warm sentimentality so often expressed on the inside of greeting cards. True caring requires us to choose among our priorities and may become a challenge or even a burden. Caring always requires involved concern about the specific barriers to the other person's well-being and the action required to relieve them.*

What do you notice about this statement? It is about care of *others*. This is not surprising, because professionals' reason for being is to determine and provide a caring response to a patient's plight. At the same time, this emphasis on caring for others points to a deeper issue. The emphasis on caring for others is so deeply rooted in professional identity that the care of oneself can easily get left out of the equation. In fact, many health professionals are so attuned to being caregivers or care *providers* that they perceive themselves as immune to needing care themselves.

The health professions have been slow to incorporate policies that respect the importance of self-care even though a professional obviously is in a better position to serve others well when acting from a position of personal strength gained through self-respecting habits and activities. In the words of Eleanor Brownn, a contemporary self-care workshop leader, "Rest and self-care are so important. When you take time to replenish your spirit, it allows you to serve others from the overflow. You cannot serve from an empty vessel."[2]

You can get a fuller picture of what is at stake by looking at the paragraph about care on the previous page but this time thinking of it in terms of self-care:

> *Everyone talks about care as a positive feature of human relationships. It is. But self-care has a much more serious function in sustaining me than often I acknowledge. It is the link each of us makes with our own inner selves in distress, taking suffering and well-being into account. Often it is not limited to the warm sentimentality so often expressed on the inside of greeting cards. True caring requires me to choose among my priorities and may become a challenge or even a burden. Caring for myself always requires involved concern about the specific barriers to my well-being and the action required to relieve them.*

Note that none of this attention to the self deflects from the realization that being in a professional relationship with patients means putting their specific health-related needs at the center of your professional decisions. At the same time, self-care gives you a measuring rod of qualities that allows you to fully engage in a person-centered approach with patients without being in a constant state of alert self-protection. The gift of this effort is a feeling of well-being.

Noting self-care activities is a great start because in declaring them you are taking a conscious step toward the self-respect that results from seeing yourself worthy of care. However, we also reminded you earlier in this chapter that many good ideas remain in the realm of "resolutions" that fall away. Starting with right now, take a few minutes to follow up on what you have just listed as some things that will help you experience well-being as a normal state. Reflections like this can help health professionals identify what is important to oneself and find ways to follow them through into everyday choices, exercising the discipline to remain true to self-care over time.

Professional Resilience

Resilience is an essential attribute to survive and thrive in the health professions. It has been defined in the literature as the ability to bounce back, positively adjust, and adapt in the face of adversity, trauma, tragedy, threats, or significant sources of stress.[3-5] Resilience is both a quality and a process. It is the positive resources an individual possesses that can be activated during stressful life events and is key to the prevention of negative mental health outcomes. At a practical level, resilience arises from professional self-care and serves to sustain professional identity.

REFLECTIONS

- What are your "go to" strategies for coping with stressful situations?
- How might these strategies support or inhibit your resilience as a health professional?
- What are two positive habits of mind or habits of body that you might integrate into your own professional self-care plan to foster resilience?

BUILDING RESILIENCE AS INDIVIDUALS AND INTERPROFESSIONAL CARE TEAMS

In the reflection above you identified some strategies to help support you in your journey as a health professional. Building resilience for professional practice in today's ever-changing health care delivery settings is both an individual, team, and organizational commitment. As an individual, developing a personal self-care plan that supports professional well-being is a key step. Your plan should have specific goals, and strategies for achieving those goals, serving as a practical tool along your career trajectory. A personal self-care plan is an important step, but even more important is an organizational approach to clinician well-being. This means that there are structures in place to support you and your intra and interprofessional colleagues in the professional practice environment. What do these supports look like? They start with basic structures, such as values statements and leadership, and expand into formal services and activities such as peer support groups, ethics rounds, and employee assistance programs. See Table 3.1 for examples of evidence-based resilience strategies at the individual and organizational levels.

Striking a Balance Between Socializing and Solitude

One step in following through on choices that demonstrate self-care is to recognize the importance of setting a balance between being with others and having time to yourself for spacious self-reflection. To fail to strike such a balance undermines the self-respect that you assiduously have honored in making choices that show you care about yourself.

TABLE 3.1 ■ **Resilience Building Strategies and Supports at the Individual and Organizational Levels**

Individual	Organizational
Self-Care Plan	Employee Assistance Programs with 24-hour Access and Mental Health Counseling Services
Mindfulness/Mind–Body Practices (body scan, purposeful pause, progressive muscular relaxation, intentional breathing)	Interprofessional Communication and Team Building Programs
Structured Mentorship	Peer Support Groups
Attention to Sleep/Sleep Hygiene	Workplace Wellness Programs (including those that target workload and schedule)
Routine Self-Screening of Well-Being	Regular Leadership Communication and Presence at the Point of Care
Meditation Practices	Narrative Sharing and Meaning Making

Socializing yields both important professional and personal benefits. Of the former, the language often used in the description of what happens in the process of becoming and being professional is that the person becomes *socialized* into this identity. Professional *communities of practice* are an opportunity for such socialization. A community of practice is made up of a group of people who share common interests and who interact regularly in a process that builds and shapes knowledge. They provide health professionals with an opportunity to network; developing reflective practices, collaborative meaning-making, and an enhanced a sense of belonging.[6] It follows that a key component of communities of practice is the development of professional competence and critical thinking. Thinking about one's own thinking is critical to professional reasoning development and models best practice across a variety of care delivery settings.

It goes almost without saying that personal benefits gained from informal socializing, such as leisure and relaxation activities, are for most readers an essential component of their self-care. Why, then, be concerned with the importance of striking a balance between constant interactions of socializing and reflective aloneness as a criterion of self-care? One compelling reason is that the professions are a *reflective practice*, not just a direct application of material you have absorbed. Benner[7] and others have shown that the process of going from being a *clinical novice* to becoming a *clinical expert* is a self-reflective dimension of learning. In self-reflection, you fly solo and need time and open space to do so without continuously charging ahead to the next activity or responding to who or what calls for your immediate attention.

A second reason is that personalities differ in their need for internal "quiet time" to grasp and integrate material and feelings.[8] Even the most extroverted person needs some solitude. Some of you will need it to survive, while others can practice it for their own self-enrichment as well as not always imposing on others one's extroverted need to be connected.

What is solitude and why is it important? *Solitude* is a time to *be with yourself only*, not responding to others, and to engage in reflections and restorative activities. Some people are active in their solitude, finding walking, jogging, biking, reading, or other solitary activities a time for honoring oneself. Others prefer the stillness of meditation, yoga, or just sitting quietly as a positive, active state of being. The experience of solitude is not identical to happiness and may even be "bittersweet" (accompanied by sorrow or anger) because it reveals parts of ourselves to ourselves that we otherwise may never recognize even though they are influencing our health. It is a form of self-respect realized by embracing the necessity of not always responding to other people whenever they need or want it and not reacting to every circumstance that comes one's way. As one health professional commented when she began to turn off her cell phone for an hour each day, "I realized over time that I had been acting like a service organization by always interrupting what I needed to do to respond to someone else!" Unlike loneliness, which is a form of suffering, solitude is a life-affirming and self-respect–supporting activity.

REFLECTIONS

- List here the things you most like to do by yourself.
- If you do not currently make or have enough time for some of these activities, make two columns, one listing the reasons why you do not do them and the other making some suggestions about how you might make more opportunities to enjoy them.

Some ideas to help you make time for yourself include the following:

1. Set a time and place, and rigorously try to adhere to it.
2. If needed, identify to others what you are doing during these solitary activities and how they contribute to your well-being.
3. Breathe, think, and breathe again.
4. Take notes on your reflections or keep a log of your solitary activities.

Remind yourself often that a basic minimum requirement for many other health-supporting activities is to take time and make space to be with yourself. In addition, you can help others have their own time alone by learning to recognize this need in others and encouraging it.

With this backdrop of self-care and some aspects of your environment to help realize it, we turn to other issues that incur self-respect and offer suggestions for ways to support and enrich it.

ATTITUDES AND CHARACTER

Your attitudes toward caring for others, responses to persons who may be different from yourself, and the qualities you believe make life worth living all are part of how your feelings of self-respect are either supported or diminished by challenges in the health profession environment. In most instances, your intuitive responses are a great resource. Attitudes that seem to keep you at a distance from being able to engage wholeheartedly in your professional tasks warrant deep reflection.

Some basic attitudes and character traits needed for successful professional practice were outlined as core professional values in Chapter 1. Almost all of them are other-directed as resources for care of others. They apply to self-care as well. In addition, a career in the professions requires lifelong learning, and so it follows that one important attitude to cultivate at the outset is a love of learning and discerning what matters most for your own sustenance and growth at any period of your career. Keeping abreast of key opportunities to enhance your expertise is rewarded with the self-respect that comes with professional competence.[9]

Self-Respect and Acceptance of Support

We turn now to several additional considerations; among the most important is the necessity of being willing to graciously accept support when you need it and set priorities that keep the most important people in your close circle of caring. Family and friends are at the top of the list. Professional colleagues are close behind.

BALANCE PERSONAL AND PROFESSIONAL LIFE

Because professional life can be so involving, family and friends outside of your work environment are at risk for being left out of your life in important ways unless you make conscious efforts to include them. Still, there is much evidence that the support of family and friends is key to thriving in almost all walks of life. Often, they are taken for granted and may get the leftover part of your days, the majority of the best hours having been spent in workplace activities.

> **REFLECTIONS**
>
> This reflection is aimed to help you consider your personal support network. Draw two concentric circles (a circle within a circle) on a piece of paper or your electronic device. In the center circle, write the name of the most important person (or persons) in your life. Add those who are in a second tier in the outer circle. Finally, add those around the periphery, but still in the mix outside the second circle.
> - What do you find encouraging about naming the individuals in your circle of care?
> - What habits do you already have that will serve you well in your attempts to nurture the inner circles of your support system?
> - Are there individuals in the outer, second circle who might nurture you in your role as a health professional?

Your challenge is to establish priorities and conduct that will reflect the rhythms needed for your family members and friends to be able to support you when you need it. A young lawyer shared this comment as he recounted the choices he began to exercise when he felt himself being consumed by his work:

> *There were a few things that helped to restore my sense of equilibrium. The first was to make a conscious effort to spend time with my wife. In the beginning, I resisted when my wife would plead, cajole, and sometimes push me out the door of our apartment so that we could spend a few hours watching a movie or going to dinner. Eventually, I realized how important this time was. It strengthened our relationship by keeping the lines of communication open between us. Not only that, it also made me a better worker by giving my anxious mind a much-needed rest.*
>
> *A second source of balance came from getting together with other people who were facing similar pressures at work. Two or three times a month I would meet with a few friends from law school who were working in other firms around town. Our get-togethers were combination lunches and b.s. sessions. These meetings did wonders for my perspective. I found myself becoming less anxious and self-absorbed as I discovered that my friends were dealing with the same worries and concerns I was facing. We helped ourselves by helping each other[10]*

In short, this young professional used the resources of family, friends, and his own form of solitude for spiritual reflection to create the balance he felt slipping away from him. In the process, he created a support network that not only benefited his work but also helped him maintain a balance that showed respect for himself and those closest to him. He also mentions his professional colleagues as a resource. This is so important that we now examine it in more detail.

HONOR BONDS WITH COLLEAGUES

One source of support is that persons working in a health care setting have several common bonds, all of which help establish rapport and mutual support. Of special importance and sometimes easy to overlook in the hubbub of everyday tasks are the professional colleagues in one's immediate workplace.

Bond of Shared Concerns

At your worksite, self-care and self-respect can be realized through having a place to air common concerns about a particular patient's clinical problems, about the department, about what is happening in one's field, and about health services in general. This can be achieved while respecting confidentiality regarding specific patients or others and refraining from gossip. As health professionals, we voluntarily place ourselves in the mainstream of human suffering. No one commits us to this role. We choose to be there because we care enough about human well-being to want to effect certain changes using our professional skills. But this life you chose makes intense demands on you, and an essential resource is to know there is a trusted group with whom to share your common worries, uncertainties, moral dilemmas, and questions.

Gratitude

Gratitude has been characterized in the literature as an emotion, a character trait, a psychological characteristic, a disposition, a material gesture, and a politeness response.[11] In the crush of everyday work, colleagues often take less time telling one another directly that they appreciate and care about them than they do sharing their concerns. Creating a generous atmosphere of thankful expression helps transform a workplace from a worksite only to a true community. It accentuates the positive, boosts self-esteem, and fosters empathy so that the interprofessional team can stay resilient and cope with workplace stress. Since gratitude is a prosocial motivator, it has a positive impact on patients, families, informal caregivers, and health professionals. Health professionals who express gratitude not only enhance their own well-being but also augment their capacity

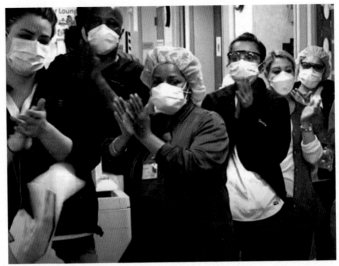

Fig. 3.1 Sharing good news and recognizing the efforts of colleagues at work helps build strong working relationships and an environment of congeniality in which team resilience can flourish. https://www.aha.org/

for patient-centered care.[12] Gratitude has also been found to reduce perceived stress, increase job satisfaction, increase teamwork and collaboration, decrease work absences, and protect against burnout.[13-17]

REFLECTIONS

- What are some ways in previous jobs you have held or currently hold that you and your colleagues have shown appreciation for each other's contributions?
- What ideas do you have for helping to create a happy and supportive workplace for yourself and your colleagues?

Many gestures of gratitude are quite simple to implement. Remembering when colleagues complete a milestone in their professional studies such as passing a board examination or attaining certification in their discipline is one example. Performing other "random acts of kindness" creates a general environment of congeniality in which the language of mutual respect for the efforts and gifts of one another's skills and presence can flourish (Fig. 3.1).

SEEK SUPPORTIVE INSTITUTIONAL ENVIRONMENTS

The bonds of shared concern, caring, and gratitude work together to encourage the realization of mutually shared goals and values. However, it is not enough for individuals alone to desire to create a respectful environment—respect also must be reflected in the structure and values of those who have policy authority. One group of health care administrators suggest the following for the design of organizational structures that meet the requirement: "Optimally there is full alignment among (1) the moral identity of individuals, which informs and shapes their behavior as they work in an organization; (2) the implicit values of the organization as embodied in the organizational culture and stated and unstated practices; and (3) the organization's explicit social purpose and stated mission."[18]

It is a good idea, then, when considering a position to seek at least one person who appears to be a potential source of support when problems arise that could challenge your self-respect in your position. You should be bold in asking questions that will allow you to gain some understanding of how support is expressed within the department and larger institution. To make an assessment, the following guidelines may be useful:

1. Inquire of your future employer whether there are meetings or other sessions in which problems associated with the everyday workplace stresses of health care delivery are discussed. If so, how regularly do they take place?

2. Ask potential colleagues what they think the sources of the most intense stressors in that environment are and how the group typically handles them.

3. Ask about resources in place for workplace wellness. Include in this inquiry an example of an outcome of a particular wellness program or quality improvement related to employee wellness.

4. Make a mental note of those who appear to be potential sources of support or if no one appears to be. If everyone denies that problems exist or become defensive about such questions when they are tactfully posed, this probably signals a setting in which stresses are dealt with alone, without the support of one's colleagues or the institution.[9]

Fortunately, only in rare situations are no support mechanisms available. In fact, being a support to others is often the key to finding support from them when it is needed. The adage "To have a friend is to be one" almost always holds true in the workplace.

CULTIVATE JOY AND PRACTICE MINDFULNESS

No one can—or should—keep self-respect if they unnecessarily put up with or contribute to an atmosphere of doom and gloom. Persons in the health professions are fortunate to be in a line of work in which they know they are usually making a positive difference in patients' lives. That in itself is a reason to enjoy their work.

But there's more. Shortchanging the joy that can come from remembering to put some levity and fun into the environment is doing yourself a disfavor. It does not take much—a cartoon, a good joke, a lighthearted story that a colleague or patient is trying to tell, or some other type of pleasure can do the job. One author, himself a health professional, observes:

> *Joy is only possible for persons who are attentive to the present. One cannot be happy if one is continually ruminating about what might have been or fretting over whether wishes will come to pass. Americans have a tough time with real joy. Americans are oriented toward outcomes, expectations, and the future; toward ever more competition in proving that they deliver the best results, and anxiously pondering how things might have turned out if only they had chosen differently. This makes it hard to be happy. In health care, these tendencies are exaggerated. Worries about what will happen next to the patient and worries about their own future careers blot out the possibility of joy for many health care professionals. Joy is a present tense phenomenon. It is possible only if one attends to the moment.[19]*

Attending to the moment is a key component of *mindful practice*. Mindfulness is setting an intention to "pay attention systematically and nonjudgmentally to the present moment for whatever arises."[20] It cultivates self-awareness and compassion through an attitude of curiosity, openness, and acceptance.[21] Mindful practices such as mind-body awareness, purposeful pauses, breathing exercises, body scans, and informal and formal meditation have been correlated with resilience in the health professions.[21–25] They lead to increased emotional regulations and self-awareness, which in turn honors self-respect. The words of a health professional who was new to the practice of mindfulness capture the benefits aptly "the thing that I got out of this was

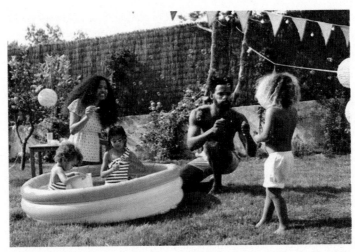

Fig. 3.2 Health professionals should remember to make time for family and friends. © monkeybusinessimages/iStock/Thinkstock.com.

reflecting on some of those more emotional things, psychological sort of things, that you don't necessarily specifically talk about or think about or debrief about in your day-to-day work."[26] Sometimes, mindful activities such as yoga outside of work hours enhance the ability for coworkers to enjoy one another in a more relaxed environment as well as enhance the time spent with family and friends (Fig. 3.2).

Refining Your Capacity to Provide Care Professionally

The development of basic professional competencies discussed earlier in this chapter is not only a requirement for self-respect but also a splendid opportunity for your continued growth and flourishing. Chapters 1 and 2 provide basic building blocks of professional identity and benchmarks of respect and boundary setting that help give further shape to the professional role. We offer some additional refinements here to those basic foundations. Consider with us some distinctions between intimate and personal modes of caregiving and important differences between strictly social and therapeutic relationships. The former focuses on the depth of a relationship and the latter on the avenues of expression.

INTIMATE VERSUS PERSONAL RELATIONSHIPS

Acts of caregiving, both intimate and personal, depend on the depth of involvement in which the persons engage in each other's lives. *Intimate care* is what you offer to someone you love or for whom you care deeply. Most often that inner circle of intimate relationships is limited to a few such as family members or beloved friends. One test is that the offer of intimate forms of assistance in its most extreme form means that you would be willing to risk personal danger to yourself for this person. In contrast, *personal care* is what you are willing to offer colleagues, friends, acquaintances, or strangers whose human needs you see you can respond to without getting more deeply entwined in their lives. It takes many forms in everyday interactions from giving directions, assisting a person physically, or donating money to a good cause. Random acts of kindness express care of this sort. Both types of relationships demand an investment in the well-being of others, and the boundaries are not always hard and fast between the two. For example, in a group of acquaintances you may over time become closer to one and find yourselves increasingly more engaged in each other's lives.

Professional caring belongs to the category of personal rather than intimate relationships. Maintaining the respectful conduct that characterizes personal helping in health professional and patient interaction is the primary focus of this book.

REFLECTIONS

Reflect on the past couple of days of your encounters with family, friends, and others with whom you have come into contact.
- Which of the encounters would you say were intimate?
- Which ones met the general criteria of personal caring conduct toward the other(s)? Why?

SOCIAL VERSUS THERAPEUTIC RELATIONSHIPS

A related way to view your relationships as a care provider emphasizes the types of activities rather than degree of involvement with the other person. Any care you provide in which your resources are not prescribed by specific, well-defined professional skills that maintain boundaries specific to the professional–patient relationship are examples of *social relationships*. Social caregiving takes many forms because the numbers of resources you can use are as numerous as your imagination and your willingness to extend yourself for someone else's benefit. One helps a child cross the street, lessens an old man's loneliness by paying him a visit, or lends $5 to a neighbor in need. On the face of it, this example of caring could stem from wanting to benefit someone else while feeling the benefit of self-respect as well, and in most cases this is true. But offers of the social help variety are not always welcomed by the recipient and, in fact, may not be interpreted as showing genuine care at all. A study by several scientists interested in altruism concluded this is especially true if the recipient perceives the offer as being motivated primarily by the person supposedly offering care but needing only to fulfill his or her own needs.[27] Persons with disabilities are often victims of this displaced motive. Consider this experience recounted by a health professions student.

CASE STUDY

On weekends, the student cared for a 15-year-old boy with paraplegia who mobilized with the help of a wheelchair. One Saturday, the student and boy were shopping in a large department store and paused at a vending machine for a Coke. First, the student bought a soft drink for his young friend and then turned to buy one for himself. The boy had just taken the first sip and was resting the can on the arm of his wheelchair when a woman laden with bundles rushed up and dropped a dollar in his lap. She patted the astonished boy on the head and exclaimed, "Poor, poor boy. I hope that helps you get better." She then gathered up her packages and scurried away.

REFLECTIONS

- What seems not to be caring behavior in this woman's actions?
- Supposing her motives were indeed to show personal care toward this young man, what should she have done that would have made a difference?

In short, the carer in the social relationship may use any available means to offer assistance rather than depending on specialized skills, but how the offer of care is perceived by the recipient will be determined in part by what the motive seems to be and how sensitive the caregiver is to the effects of the offer. There is another kind of care available and when put into the relational context is recognized as a therapeutic relationship.

A *therapeutic relationship* develops when the professional caregiver performs professionally competent acts designed to benefit the person who needs his or her services. Therapeutic caring is personal but not intimate. At times, this is a difficult difference to grasp because often there are aspects of the therapeutic relationship that involve the patient's sharing of deeply intimate details of his or her life and that impinge on the usual physical boundaries of propriety. The prosthetist may rub the stump of a patient's bare thigh in order to be sure the muscles are relaxed sufficiently for a prosthesis mold to fit accurately; a dietitian may interview a patient about deeply personal eating habits to evaluate nutritional status and plan the dietary regimen; nurses, assistants of all kinds, therapists, and others regularly touch, probe, hold, and stroke patients. Some ways in which close physical contact requires attention were addressed in Chapter 2 regarding how to understand and honor professional boundaries. The common denominator is that your unique professional role determines what is permitted for truly therapeutic care to be provided.

Anxiety, Burnout, and Accountability

This chapter has focused on several tools and some key insights that can help you maintain your self-respect. Still, as authors, we know from experience that some stresses are inevitable because nothing that presents worthwhile challenges comes without its burdens. When you care enough about yourself to take the time to pay attention to stressors and act accordingly, you are actualizing your role as an accountable health professional.

RESPONDING TO ANXIETY

Anxiety is a psychological response to a stress that is calling for attention. It is the result of unresolved stresses, some of which can lend themselves to resolution but, if not attended to, may gnaw at one's confidence, happiness, and, most important, self-respect. Anxiety arising from deep uncertainty or unresolvable situations is more difficult to bring to a full resting place but does not have to remain destructive to one's well-being.

Anxiety may arise from situations in your workplace ranging from feeling unprepared for some of the challenges facing you with particular types of patient situations to feeling frustrated with institutional conditions that are not allowing you a sense of satisfaction. At another level, the troublesome feeling may be pointing to something deeper in yourself. For example, one of the most difficult things to admit is that you find you are not cut out for the type of work you are preparing—or have prepared—to do. If you take the time for solitude and reflection, you may hear that inner voice saying, "You do not want to be—or stay—in this type of work." Not everyone is cut out for what the health professions demand. Maintaining self-respect must not hinge on trying to do the impossible for whatever reason or deceiving oneself into believing that because you began a career, or were encouraged to do so, you made the right choice. Not everyone can just change careers midstream, but dropping out prematurely would be a tragedy if the source of unease is temporary and there is a way through an unsettling period characterized by anxiety.

Anxieties arising from personal issues can engender disabling effects too. An impending divorce, a serious illness, an unexpected or unwanted pregnancy, the news that a loved one is seriously ill, sudden changes in financial viability—these and many other personal, family, and other relational problems can threaten a person's feeling of well-being and affect workplace performance.

It is also important to note that the overlap of one's professional life and personal life can serve to compound anxiety. For example, during the COVID-19 pandemic, health professionals and other front-line workers suffered distinct sources of anxiety compared to the general public. In the early stages of the pandemic, these included not having sufficient personal protective equipment, high levels of uncertainty, and the fear of taking the virus home to their families. Since health professionals are often self-reliant and do not ask for help, it was even more important that health care organizations listened and provided emotional and psychological support for staff.[28]

If anxiety persists, it should be addressed. The following are three suggestions on how to respond constructively out of your commitment to well-deserved self-care:

1. *Identify the source:* One of the most important steps in dissipating the destructive tension associated with anxiety is to identify its source if you can do so on your own. Is it directly work related? Is there some other obvious reason that anxiety has descended on you, or is the source too diffuse to identify? Are there times when you are free from it and, if so, when? What activities seem to help allay it?

2. *Share feelings with a trustworthy friend or family member:* The sting of anxiety is that it can alienate you from others who know that something is wrong but do not know what or why. Keeping the source to yourself can baffle them when they observe your change in conduct or become aware of your self-deceit that obviously is covering a deeper problem. They may even think it is something they have done. In sharing your anxiety with a trusted person, you have overcome the isolation of the experience and in most cases have gained an ally who can help you address it. An unintended but encouraging side effect of this process is that you may find out how common your feelings are. By knowing that others, too, are feeling stressed, you feel less "out of joint" with the rest of the world.

3. *Seek professional help:* Talking with a trusted friend or family member is often not adequate, and it is becoming increasingly necessary for health professionals to seek professional help. In such cases, an instructor or counselor can help you discover why you feel anxious. Many workplaces today provide such services, knowing that anxiety affects the mental health, resilience, and productivity of their employees. The treatment for stress may require an extended course of intervention over weeks or months. Your well-being is at stake, and this is an area of caring for yourself that, when acted on, will help bolster your self-respect for what you took the time to do.

BURNOUT

Burnout is a syndrome resulting from chronic workplace stress. It has been described by the World Health Organization as an "occupational phenomenon" and, as of May 2019, burnout is included in the International Classification of Diseases. The rising rate of burnout in the health professions has led many to refer to it as a public health crisis. The hallmarks of burnout are emotional exhaustion (being emotionally depleted or overextended), lack of personal accomplishment (feeling one cannot make a difference), and depersonalization and detachment (characterized by difficulty empathizing and making personal connections).[29] In addition to burnout, witnessing trauma, disease, injury, suffering, death, disability, and social injustices can lead to psychological stress for health professionals caring for individuals and families with complex needs.[9] Health professionals who experience burnout are more likely to take shortcuts, make diagnostic errors, communicate poorly with their patients and colleagues, suffer from emotional exhaustion and experience mental health conditions.[30]

The COVID-19 pandemic and global public health emergency have led to increasing rates of anxiety, depressions, burnout, and other mental health concerns in health professionals. According to the National Institute for Health Care Management Foundation, 76% of health care workers reported exhaustion and burnout in September 2020.[31]

This alarming trend has led many to a call to action for a national and systems-based approach to clinician well-being.[32] Extensive resources to promote clinician well-being have been curated by the National Academy of Medicine Action Collaborative on Clinician Well-Being and Resilience. This network of more than 200 organizations is committed to reversing trends in clinician burnout and has three main goals: (1) raise the visibility of clinician anxiety, burnout, depression, stress, and suicide; (2) improve baseline understanding of challenges to clinician well-being; and (3) advance evidence-based, multidisciplinary solutions to improve patient care by caring for the caregiver. You can learn more about the collaborative at https://nam.edu/initiatives/clinician-resilience-and-well-being/.

RECOGNIZING AND INTERVENING FOR BURNOUT

Recognizing burnout in oneself and one's colleagues is an important part of self-care. Burnout manifests differently in different people, some with experiencing physical symptoms such as pain, chronic fatigue, substance use disorders, or headaches; others experiencing psychological or emotional symptoms such as depression, anxiety, anger, or irritability; and still others experience changes in appearance, interactions or expressions of thought. Regardless, most symptoms translate to job performance so you may note yourself or a colleague being more detached, apathetic, or cynical in one's patient care interactions. The authors feel it is vitally important to familiarize readers with these signs given the impact on both health professionals and patients. One does not need to diagnose burnout in a colleague but should feel comfortable supporting them by asking if they are okay. In fact, a characteristic of effective interprofessional teams is to have mutual trust and feel safe enough to ask a question or admit a struggle without fear of embarrassment or punishment.[33]

Sometimes, planting a seed can raise awareness on the topic and allow the opportunity for a trusted colleague to share their difficulties in a supported way. Validate your colleague and let them know that they are not alone in their experience. It's not always easy when someone says they're not okay, but it could change a life. The "R U OK?" campaign is a national suicide prevention initiative that many organizations use to help destigmatize conversations regarding mental health struggles. You can learn more about the campaign at https://www.ruok.org.au.

ACCOUNTABILITY

In Chapter 1 you were introduced to the basic ideas of knowing and remaining true to your values and those that are expected of you as a professional. The reward for doing so is that you will be sustained over a lifetime of challenges to your personal and professional integrity. In a word, you can remain whole in the presence of destabilizing situations and forces that threaten your very core of being.

Accountability means taking responsibility for one's actions and is the key to maintaining your integrity. A professional is viewed as an *agent*—that is, one who has the specialized knowledge, skills, and other authority to be held legally and ethically responsible for his or her professional judgment and actions taken on behalf of patients. This includes the pleasure of taking credit for a job well done but also readily admitting mistakes or errors in judgment. Fortunately, almost all institutions and your professional codes of ethics have guidelines for how clinical or other errors in the professional role must be reported and steps taken. In addition, your professional educational experiences teach you in more detail how to honor this requirement.

An important aspect of health care is the legal and ethical responsibility of professionals to report unethical, unsafe, or impaired conduct observed among one's peers. This type of accountability signals the trust that society places in the health professions to police themselves when wrongdoing is observed and is taken up in more detail in Chapter 5, in which institutional policies within care delivery systems are emphasized. Strict procedures to protect all involved during the process of discovering, reporting, and following through on such allegations have been developed in the very structures of health care to emphasize the weight society places on the professionals' expanded role as protectors of the cherished value of health.

Summary

This chapter highlights how to realize self-respect for your choice of profession and implement self-care throughout your career. All along the trajectory from student to experienced professional, self-respect and the caring it generates are cherished resources to be used. A balance between socializing and taking time for reflection and solitude is essential. So too is the cultivation of gratitude, mindful practice, and resilience.

Showing respect toward and accepting support from family, friends, and the people you work with daily are invaluable resources. Their support of you is essential to break your fall should you ever feel like you are losing your footing. The appropriate nature of your relationships with patients is basically personal and therapeutic, not intimate and social, providing additional guidance for respect to be honored all around. Addressing understandable bouts of anxiety and embracing areas of professional accountability will help keep you focused on the necessity of including care of yourself while expressing professional care toward interprofessional colleagues, patients, and society. Remember to enjoy the benefits of this type of work, including the opportunity to participate in a basic type of goodness as its own reward!

References

1. Gallagher A. Dignity and respect for dignity—two key health professional values: implications for nursing practice. *Nurs Ethics*. 2004;11(6):587–599.
2. Brownn E. Eleanor Brownn Quotes. https://www.goodreads.com/author/quotes/10614034.Eleanor_Brownn. Accessed May 29, 2021.
3. Brown T, Yu M-L, Hewitt AE, Isbel ST, Bevitt T, Etherington J. Exploring the relationship between resilience and practice education placement success in occupational therapy students. *Aust Occup Ther J*. 2020;67(1):49–61. https://doi.org/10.1111/1440-1630.12622.
4. American Psychological Association. APA dictionary of psychology. https://dictionary.apa.org/resilience; 2020.
5. de Witt PA, Monareng L, Abraham AA, Koor S, Saber R. Resilience in occupational therapy students. *S Afr J Occup Ther*. 2019;49(2):33–41. https://doi.org/10.17159/23103833/2019/vol49n2a6.
6. Marcolino T, Kinsella E, Araujo A, et al. A community of practice of primary health care occupational therapists: advancing practice-based knowledge. *Aust Occup Ther J*. 2020;68. https://doi.org/10.1111/1440-1630.12692.
7. Benner P. *From Novice to Expert: Excellence and Power in Clinical Nursing Practice*. Commemorative edition. Upper Saddle River, NJ: Prentice-Hall; 2005.
8. Cain S. *Quiet. The Power of Introverts in a World That Can't Stop Talking*. New York: Random House; 2013.
9. Doherty RF. *Ethical Dimensions in the Health Professions*. 7th ed. St. Louis, MO: Saunders; 2021.
10. Allegretti JG. *Loving Your Job, Finding Your Passion: Work and the Spiritual Life*. New York/Mahwah, NJ: Paulist Press, Inc.; 2000. Reprinted by permission of Paulist Press, Inc. http://www.paulistpress.com.
11. Day G, Robert G, Rafferty AM. Gratitude in health care: a meta-narrative review. *Qual Health Res*. 2020;30(14):2303–2315. https://doi.org/10.1177/1049732320951145.
12. Rao N, Kemper KJ. Online training in specific meditation practices improves gratitude, well-being, self-compassion, and confidence in providing compassionate care among health professionals. *J Evid Based Complement Altern Med*. 2017;22(2):237–241. https://doi.org/10.1177/2156587216642102.
13. Aparicio M, Centeno C, Robinson C, Arantzamendi M. Gratitude between patients and their families and health professionals: a scoping review. *J Nurs Manag*. 2019;27(2):286–300. https://doi.org/10.1111/jonm.12670.

14. Burke RJ, Ng ESW, Fiksenbaum L. Virtues, work satisfactions and psychological wellbeing among nurses. *Int J Workplace Health Manag*. 2009;2(3):202–219. https://doi.org/10.1108/17538350910993403.

15. Jans-Beken L, Lataster J, Peels D, Lechner L, Jacobs N. Gratitude, psychopathology and subjective well-being: results from a 7.5-month prospective general population study. *J Happiness Stud*. 2018;19(6):1673–1689. https://doi.org/10.1007/s10902-017-9893-7.

16. Stegen A, Wankier J. Generating gratitude in the workplace to improve faculty job satisfaction. *J Nurs Edu*. 2018;57(6):375–378. https://doi.org/10.3928/01484834-20180522-10.

17. Sawyer KB, Thoroughgood CN, Stillwell EE, Duffy MK, Scott KL, Adair EA. Being present and thankful: a multi-study investigation of mindfulness, gratitude, and employee helping behavior. *J Appl Psychol*. 2022;107(2):240–262. https://doi.org/10.1037/apl0000903.

18. Rambur R, Vallett C, Cohen JA, et al. The moral cascade: distress, eustress, and the virtuous organization. *J Org Moral Psych*. 2010;1(1):41–54. with permission from Nova Science Publishers, Inc.

19. Sulmasy DP. *The Healer's Calling: A Spirituality for Physicians and Other Health Care Professionals*. Mahwah, NJ: Paulist Press; 1997.

20. Kabat-Zinn J. *Full Catastrophe Living: Using the Wisdom of Your Body and Mind to Face Stress, Pain, and Illness*. New York: Dell Publishing; 1990.

21. Chmielewski J, Łoś K, Łuczyński W. Mindfulness in healthcare professionals and medical education. *Int J Occup Med Environ Health*. 2021;34(1):1–14.

22. Rees CS, Craigie MA, Slatyer S, et al. Pilot study of the effectiveness of a Mindful Self-Care and Resiliency program for rural doctors in Australia. *Aust J Rural Health*. 2020;28(1):22–31. https://doi.org/10.1111/ajr.12570.

23. Sawyer KB, Thoroughgood CN, Stillwell EE, Duffy MK, Scott KL, Adair EA. Being present and thankful: a multi-study investigation of mindfulness, gratitude, and employee helping behavior. *J Appl Psychol*. 2021. https://doi.org/10.1037/apl0000903. Advance online publication.

24. Pidgeon AM, Ford L, Klaassen F. Evaluating the effectiveness of enhancing resilience in human service professionals using a retreat-based Mindfulness with Metta Training Program: a randomised control trial. *Psychol Health Med*. 2014;1:355–364.

25. Barattucci M, Padovan AM, Vitale E, Rapisarda V, Ramaci T, De Giorgio A. Mindfulness-based IARA Model ® proves effective to reduce stress and anxiety in health care professionals. a six-month follow-up study. *Int J Environ Res Public Health*. 2019;16(22). https://doi.org/10.3390/ijerph16224421.

26. Rees CS, Craigie MA, Slatyer S, et al. Pilot study of the effectiveness of a Mindful Self-Care and Resiliency program for rural doctors in Australia. *Aust. J. Rural Health*. 2020;28(1):22–31. p. 27. https://doi.org/10.1111/ajr.12570.

27. Dugatkin LA. *The Altruism Equation: Seven Scientists Search for the Meaning of Altruism*. Princeton, NJ: Princeton University Press; 2007.

28. Shanafelt T, Ripp J, Trockel M. Understanding and addressing sources of anxiety among health care professionals during the COVID-19 pandemic. *J Am Med Assoc*. 2020;323(21):2133–2134. https://doi.org/10.1001/jama.2020.5893.

29. Trzeciak S, Mazzarelli A. *Compassionomics: The Revolutionary Scientific Evidences That Caring Makes a Difference*. Pensacola, FL: Studer Group, LLC; 2019.

30. Epstien R. *Attending: Medicine, Mindfulness, and Humanity*. New York: Simon and Schuster; 2017.

31. National Health America, Inc. The mental health of health care workers in COVID-19, 2020. https://mhanational.org/mental-health-healthcare-workers-covid-19 Accessed May 29, 2021.

32. Dzau VJ, Kirch D, Nasca T. Preventing a parallel pandemic – a national strategy to protect clinicians' well-being. *N Engl J Med*. 2020;383(6):513–515. https://doi.org/10.1056/NEJMp2011027.

33. Smith CD, Balatbat C, Corbridge S, et al. *Implementing optimal team-based care to reduce clinician burnout*. *NAM Perspectives. Discussion Paper*. Washington, DC: National Academy of Medicine; 2018. https://doi.org/10.31478/201809c.

Respectful Interactions in Institutional Settings of Health Care

Introduction

Respect involves awareness of and appreciation for individual and group differences in the interactions that are part of healthcare delivery. Chapter 4 focuses on respecting others who may have a different value system from one's own. Culture and cultural biases are explored. The health professional is provided with resources to examine personal biases and their effect on attitudes and conduct. Primary and secondary cultural characteristics such as race, ethnicity, gender identity, sexual identity and orientation, socioeconomic status, age and intergenerational diversity, education, occupation, environment, religion, and spirituality are described. The health professional is presented with strategies for respecting these differences in the health care environment and resources that support the delivery of culturally responsive care.

Chapter 5 examines the variety of settings in which health care is delivered including acute care, long-term and rehabilitative care, ambulatory clinics, and other outpatient services. The specific setting in which health care is delivered has an impact on respectful interactions between patients, coworkers, and others. The physical and administrative structures of the work setting also affect how responsibilities are assigned to individuals and interprofessional teams and how lines of communication work in a health care institution. The chapter also explores the influence of policies, accreditation standards, laws, and regulations on health care institutions and those who provide care and receive it.

Respect in a Diverse Society

The reader will be able to

- Provide a working definition of culture and its relevance to the health professional and patient relationship;
- Recognize primary and secondary characteristics of culture;
- Examine various types of diversity in health care settings and society at large;
- Distinguish cultural bias, personal bias, and implicit bias;
- Define prejudice and how it relates to discrimination and health disparities;
- Describe how discrimination of all types affects patients and health professionals and identify some ways you can counter their disrespectful dimensions;
- Contrast racism and microaggressions, appraising their connections to health, illness, and social participation;
- Describe the differences between sex and gender and strategies for inclusive communication with individuals with different expressions of gender identity;
- Discuss the dimensions of culturally responsive care; and
- Define cultural humility and describe the process of viewing the health professional and patient relationship in this manner.

Prelude

We are striving to forge a union with purpose,
to compose a country committed to all cultures, colors, characters and
conditions of man.
And so we lift our gazes not to what stands between us,
but what stands before us.
We close the divide because we know, to put our future first,
we must first put our differences aside.
We lay down our arms
so we can reach out our arms
to one another.
We seek harm to none and harmony for all.

AMANDA GORMAN[1]

Section 1 of this book focused on creating a context of respect in one's professional role. Respect also involves awareness of and appreciation for individual and group differences in the interactions that are part of health care delivery. In Chapter 1, you completed a value's clarification exercise, where you listed 10 of your values in order of importance. However, even with a deep understanding of your personal values and clarity about building relationships and setting boundaries, respectful patient interaction still does not result. It requires a lifelong commitment to look below the surface at the differences that affect interactions with patients and devise strategies to overcome barriers and facilitate respectful dialog.

Culture Defined

In your career as a health professional, you will care for a wide variety of patients and interact with different population groups. Many group and individual differences are often attributed to *culture*. But what is culture? For our purposes, an apt working definition of culture is:

> *behaviors and values that are learned, shared, and exhibited by a group of people. Culture is also evidenced in material and nonmaterial productions of a people. Culture as a set of characteristics is neither fixed nor static*[2]

Culture can be viewed in terms of primary characteristics such as race, ethnicity, gender identity, sexual orientation, or age and secondary characteristics such as place of residence, education, or socioeconomic status (SES). All are part of the web of social interactions in daily life, and many influence health.

Yet to be considered in your examination of the health professional and patient relationship is the fact that each person interprets another's actions, verbal and non-verbal communication, and other characteristics according to their cultural conditioning and experience, social context, and other factors that shape how they view the world. From the perspective of culture, our interactions occur within a society that, at least within the United States, has long been described as a "melting pot" in which all the various cultures blend. The melting pot metaphor has its origins in the days of vast numbers of immigrants entering the United States at the turn of the 19th century to help explain the relationship between the dominant culture and the new arrivals in America. However, this metaphor hints at a view of US society that forces assimilation, which strips immigrants and refugees of long-standing cultural traditions and practices and requires the adoption of the cultural practices of the dominant culture. The melting pot analogy is misleading and inaccurate because cultures, which are rich and dynamic and steeped in tradition, cannot be melted down like metal.[3] However, some still hold to the melting pot description of the United States, and you often hear this view when people say something like, "They (the immigrant population in question) could at least learn to speak English."

With increased global migration, the assimilation concept has been challenged with a move to think about how to incorporate diverse citizens into a shared value system.[3] Rather than expect newcomers to a society to lose all connection to their cultural traditions or ethnic identity, the argument is made for America to be seen as a salad bowl rather than a melting pot savored both for the character of the individual ingredients (ethnically derived differences) and for the combination of flavors (social integration).

Furthermore, members of cultural groups can individually or collectively adapt traditions or borrow traits from other cultures, which is quite common when members of diverse cultures are in prolonged contact.[4] The phenomenon of merging cultures is called *acculturation*. In this chapter, we examine the diversity you will encounter in clinical practice and the barriers (e.g., implicit bias, prejudices, and discrimination) that get in the way of appreciating differences and hence inhibit respectful interaction.

Bias, Prejudice, and Discrimination

A *cultural bias* is a tendency to interpret a word or action according to the culturally derived meaning assigned to it. Cultural bias derives from cultural variation, discussed later in this chapter. For example, maintaining eye contact during social interaction differs according to culture. While maintaining eye contact is viewed positively by Western cultures, East Asian cultures view too much eye contact as a sign of disrespect.[5] In health care, attitudes toward pain, methods of conveyance of bad news, management of chronic illness and disability, beliefs about the seriousness and causes of illness, and death-related issues vary among different cultures. These different kinds of beliefs about disease and illness impact health care–seeking behavior and acceptance of the advice, status, and intervention of health professionals. Understanding a patient's concept of health and illness is critical to developing interaction strategies that are clinically sound and acceptable to the patient.

A *personal bias* is a tendency to interpret a word or action in terms of a personal significance assigned to it. Personal bias can derive from culturally defined interpretations and originate from other sources grounded in personal experience. The individual internalizes the cultural attitudes until they believe them to be entirely personal. The bias can lead to more favorable or less favorable judgments than are warranted. This process is similar to internalizing societal values described in Chapter 1.

Understanding how personal biases influence us and their effect on our attitudes and conduct is important to the health professional. Whenever bias is present, it affects communication between the persons involved and, therefore, must be recognized as one determining factor in respectful interaction. In some cases, personal bias may produce a positive bias, or "halo effect," on specific individuals; that is, a single characteristic or trait leads to positive global judgments about a person. For example, a patient who is pleasant and cooperative during office visits also could be thought by the health professional to be adherent with therapy because of the halo effect, even though the opposite could be true. Although showing favoritism based on personal bias alone is inappropriate in the patient and health professional relationship, shared interests can, of course, have legitimate positive effects on the relationship between two persons working together and thus improve the health professional and patient relationship.

Just as personal biases can lead to positive effects, they can also lead to negative ones, including discrimination. *Discrimination* is negative, different treatment of a person or group. It is usually derived from bias or prejudice. Gordon Allport, in his definitive work, *The Nature of Prejudice* (which, although written over 60 years ago, is still widely considered an authoritative study), describes *prejudice* as "an aversive or hostile attitude toward a person who belongs to a group, simply because he belongs to that group, and is therefore assumed to have objectionable qualities ascribed to that group."[6] In this way, we see how prejudicial attitudes of health professionals tend to manifest discriminatory behavior that can have concrete implications for patients and the care they receive.

In short, every exchange between a patient and health professional will undoubtedly be influenced by cultural differences and other sources of personal bias. Sometimes, these feelings will create an attitude of prejudice and a desire to discriminate. And, despite attempts to eliminate discrimination in the health care environment, it occurs craftily and evasively. You must watch for it in yourself and others because both parties involved are inevitably injured by the interaction. At the same time, treating people differently because of race, religion, ethnicity, gender identity, or other attributes does not necessarily imply prejudice and discrimination. Respect for differences includes understanding when those differences should count to benefit patients, how they inform the responses of people, and the process of providing patient-and-family-centered, culturally responsive care.

The cultivation of respectful attitudes and conduct begins with self-examination and consideration of what cultural and other differences mean to you. In Chapter 1, you explored your values and worked on aligning your stated values and behavior, requiring you to reconsider long-held assumptions about individuals and groups that raise questions about your values and beliefs.

We will continue this challenging but rewarding work in this chapter with a focus on respecting others who have a different value system from one's own. We explore differences, both obvious and subtle, that exist among people, such as differences in language and why, for example, even when we speak the same language, we may hear what a patient says but not understand its true meaning. Once you become aware of your often *unconscious biases*, you can more easily avoid being influenced by them in your interactions with others.

Unconscious (or implicit) biases are associations that we make without awareness or intention that influences our interpretation of what we hear and see to conform with previously established beliefs.[7] In health care, if we wish to fulfill the goal of delivering just and equitable care, we must avoid any type of negative association because of a group a patient may belong to. Particularly concerning are the biases against those who are already vulnerable such as racial and ethnic minority populations, sexual and gender minorities, older adults, or those with low health literacy.[8] By becoming aware of your hidden biases, you will be less likely to form inappropriate judgments about patients, colleagues, and others and more likely to remain sensitive and open to differences that influence and inform your interactions with them.

Respecting Differences

A cursory look around almost any community in the United States or most other countries would indicate that we live in multicultural societies. Each of us belongs to multiple groups (or microcultures) and therefore has multiple identities.[3]

REFLECTIONS

Consider the various microcultural groups that you belong to. They may be based on your:
- racial identification
- national origin
- gender identity
- birth order
- health professional identity—both specific to your profession and that of the interprofessional team

Use the diversity wheel to help you identify other identities (see Fig. 4.1). Next, try and rank your identities in terms of what is most important to you just as you did with your values clarification exercise in Chapter 1.
- Would someone be able to tell the important aspects of your identity just by looking at you?
- What aspects of your identity might be more or less visible to those interacting with you? How might those contribute to their interactions?

The need for awareness of cultural differences today has increased owing to the various underrepresented minority rights' movements over the past several decades,[3] the recent increase in displaced persons from war-torn countries,[9] and the growing percentage of ethnic minorities in the United States.[10] According to population estimates in 2019, the national population was approximately 328,239,523. Of this total, 18.5% self-identified as Hispanic or Latino; 13.5% as African American or Black; 5.9% as Asian; and about 1.5% as American Indian, Alaskan native, Hawaiian native, or Pacific Islander.[10] This growing diversity also has strong implications for the provision of health care.

Although the patient population is growing more diverse, the composition of health professionals remains overwhelmingly White with Northern Hemisphere cultural and ethnic roots.

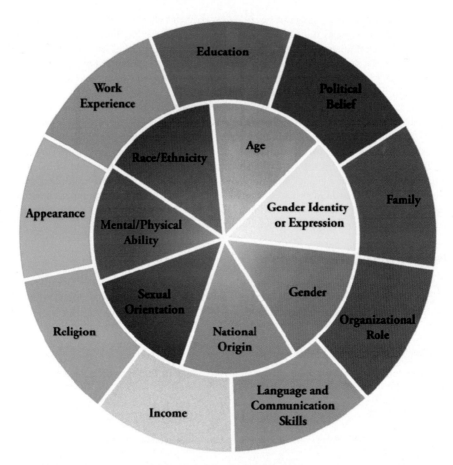

Fig. 4.1 Wheel of diversity. From Hawkins BW, Morris M, Nguyen T, Siegel J, Vardell E. Advancing the conversation: next steps for lesbian, gay, bisexual, trans, and queer (LGBTQ) health sciences librarianship. *J Med Lib Assoc: JMLA.* 2017;105(4):316–327. doi:10.5195/jmla.2017.206.

While 40% of the US population identify as a racial/ethnic minority, only 10% of health care professionals are people of color.[11] The significant underrepresentation of racial and ethnic minorities in the health professions contributes to the disparity in the health status of minority groups.[12] The challenge in the health professions is to bridge from a predominantly White perspective to meet the needs of a racially and culturally diverse population. However, while the health professions work to diversify the profession, it is not only up to professionals from minoritized backgrounds to provide culturally responsive care but all health professionals.

In almost every health care setting, you will interact with patients of backgrounds different from your own. Certain differences are apparent, and others are hidden. The iceberg model (Fig. 4.2) illustrates how much remains below the surface at various levels that others cannot see or discern. For example, we may notice that a new patient is wearing a scarf that completely covers her hair and quickly conclude that she is Muslim. The head covering is "above the waterline" in that we can see that symbol. When we look at her, we might be able to tell if she is a young or older woman but not accurately arrive at her age. When we speak to her, we might be able to tell if English is her first language. However, we cannot know without further inquiry what values or

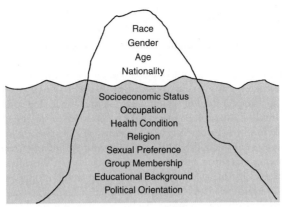

Fig. 4.2 Iceberg model of multicultural influences on communication. From Krepp GL. *Effective Communication in Multicultural Health Care Settings*. New York: Sage Publications; 1994. © 1994. Reprinted by permission of Sage Publications.

beliefs lie below what we see and hear or how they could affect health care decisions. We may not be as accurate as we think in determining exactly who the person sitting in front of us is. With limited information about potential differences, a professional can take steps in the right direction to adjust communication patterns and approaches accordingly. However, it is more difficult to assess hidden differences that can have as profound an effect on a patient's health beliefs or behavior. Differences that are hidden may create more stress than those that can be more readily identified. These considerations are what have led sociologists and others to develop the notion of culture to better grasp our variations and their importance.

Cultural practices and beliefs can have a significant effect on the following health-related issues: diet, family rituals, healing beliefs, understanding of illness symptoms and causation, communication process and style, death rituals, spirituality, values, art, and history. The National Center for Cultural Competence notes the following reasons why cultural competence is so critical in contemporary health care: to respond to the demographic changes in the United States, improve the quality of health outcomes, and comply with the growing number of regulatory and professional mandates including accreditation standards.[13] We turn our attention to specific primary and secondary cultural characteristics beginning with race.

RACE

Race is one characteristic of culture almost always mentioned in discussions about cultural differences. Even though racial categories are based on arbitrary physical attributes such as skin color and hair color/texture, race is the characteristic or descriptor most fraught with controversy. The 1999 Institute of Medicine Report edited by Haynes and Smedley[14] stated that in all instances, race is a social and cultural construct based on perceived differences in biology, physical appearance, and behavior. An editorial in *Nature Genetics* flatly stated, "Scientists have long been saying that at a genetic level there is more variation between two individuals in the same population than between populations and that there is no biological basis for race."[15]

However, while it may be tempting to dismiss the concept of race, it is associated with privilege. *Privilege* is defined as "the perception of choices and opportunities in a given context as well as an individual's expression of rights and opportunities afforded to her/him/them in our society"[16] highlighting that while some have the opportunity to dismiss the concept of race, others do not. Ignoring the construct of race does a disservice to our patients whose experiences with health and the health care system may be greatly affected by their race. Take, for example, the disproportionate effect Black and Brown communities experienced during the COVID-19 pandemic. Majority Black counties saw three times the infection rate and almost six times the death rate compared to counties with majority White residents.[17] Also, consider the violence and microaggressions toward people of Asian and Pacific Islander descent during the pandemic.[18]

If there is no biological basis for race, you might ask, why is race closely connected with health and well-being? One contributor is racism. Dr. Camara Phyllis Jones, Past President of the American Public Health Association defines racism as "a system of structuring opportunity and assigning value based on the social interpretation of how one looks (which is what we call 'race'), that unfairly disadvantages some individuals and communities, unfairly advantages other individuals and communities, and saps the strength of the whole society through the waste of human resources."[19] Racism works at many levels of society driving health inequities by influencing the social determinants of health (explored later in this chapter) including housing, employment, and education. Racism in all its forms can impact health. Structural racism (built into organizations and systems), interpersonal racism, and internalized racism all have implications for health (both physical and mental) and well-being.

While overt racism is closely connected with health, so too are *microaggressions*. Microaggressions, a term first coined in 1970, refer to "verbal, nonverbal, and/or environmental slights, snubs, or insults that are either intentional or (most often) unintentional; they convey hostile, derogatory, or otherwise negative messages to target persons based upon their membership in a structurally oppressed social group."[20] One example of a microaggression includes when Asian-Americans are asked "Where are you from?" and the aggressor refuses to accept the answer of say "Boston" thereby emphasizing the difference between a White person and a person of color who is also from the United States. While subtler than overt racism, microaggressions contribute to poorer health by leading to elevated levels of depression and trauma among persons from minoritized backgrounds.

In a national study conducted by the Institutes of Medicine on disparities in health care, evidence indicated that stereotyping, biases, and uncertainty on the part of health care providers could all contribute to unequal treatment.[21] Additionally, there are ample historical reasons for minoritized populations to mistrust the health care system. For example, in the not-too-distant past, Black and African American patients were refused treatment at "Whites-only" hospitals. Other members of the Black and African American population were undertreated and deceived in the now infamous Tuskegee syphilis study. Mistrust in the health care system on the part of Black and African Americans and others who identify with the treatment of Black Americans continues to this day because of these historical events and continuing discriminatory events in health care.[22]

Understanding race and how structural racism is manifested in health care is the first step toward advocating for social justice. However, health professionals must advance beyond "not being racist" toward being an "antiracist."[23] *Antiracism* is "the practice of identifying, challenging, and changing the values, structures, and behaviors that perpetuate systemic racism."[7] While dismantling structural racism seems like an overwhelming task for the health professional, a good starting place is acknowledging the presence and impact of structural racism.[24] The health professional can then consider where to intervene: at the individual, interpersonal, or institutional level (e.g., the clinical environment). At an individual level, we can work on identifying and mitigating our implicit biases and being conscious about using inclusive language. Implicit biases are by nature unconscious, so we need to gain awareness about our attitudes, judgments, and stereotypes. One helpful resource is Project Implicit by Harvard Medical School. "Project Implicit is a non-profit organization and international collaboration between researchers who are interested in implicit social cognition – thoughts, and feelings outside of conscious awareness and control. The goal of the organization is to educate the public about hidden biases."[25]

REFLECTIONS

Consider the following: You have a new awareness of a bias that was previously unconscious. What should you do next?

Once aware of an implicit bias, the health professional benefits from asking themselves difficult questions about their biases:

- Where did I learn this belief?
- What fear is hiding behind this belief?
- How does this belief serve me?
- Who is harmed by this belief?

Next, listen for all-or-nothing thinking when using words like "all" and "always" to avoid placing people into false or harmful categories.

Then embrace alternative thinking:

- What other perspectives can I take?
- What else could I choose to believe?
- How might I explore this patient's experience rather than rushing to judgment?

Gaining the trust of patients whose racial identity is different from one's own can sometimes be a challenge but is not an insurmountable one if health professionals show that they are trustworthy through dignity, respect, and providing optimal care while working to eliminate racial disparities and health inequities. Enhanced health care provider diversity can also impact health disparities among minoritized groups as racial concordance between patient and health care provider is associated with increased patient participation in the care process, greater adherence to treatment, and higher patient satisfaction.[12] However, this does not mean that patients must always be treated by members of the same race to receive quality care. First, this would not be possible because few health professionals are racial and ethnic minorities. Second, it is essential for all health professionals to learn how to work effectively with patients different from one's own racial and ethnic backgrounds through sensitivity, knowledge, and cross-cultural communication skills, especially when informed by the virtue of humility.

While the health care industry continues its work toward being antiracist, we must also acknowledge that the health professional may encounter biased and racist patients.[26] There is a tendency to treat biased patients as a nonproblem because "the patient is always right," and it is our job to care for them. However, health professionals also have the right to be treated with dignity and respect in their workplaces. It is often the most vulnerable health professionals (such as students and those from minoritized backgrounds) who encounter the biased patient with little recourse, often resulting in feeling unsupported and invisible after an unpleasant patient encounter. Health professionals who spend more time with patients (e.g., nurses, personal care attendants, therapists) may also be at higher risk of facing bias and discrimination from patients.[27] In the last decade, there has been a 110% spike in violent incidences reported by health care workers.[28] In one study, 76% of registered nurses reported experiencing physical or verbal abuse by patients.[29] A useful framework for responding to biased patients is offered as follows:

1. Assess for three characteristics in the encounter: clinician safety and well-being, patient's medical condition, and reason for the patient's request or biased behavior.
2. Act depending on what the assessment revealed: if the health professional feels unsafe, they exit the encounter and transfer care; if the patient is unstable, the health professional must treat and stabilize the patient first; or the health professional determines whether the patient's behavior is ethically justifiable and makes the decision how to proceed.
3. After the incident, the health professional informs their supervisors and administration and debriefs the incident.[27,30]

Additional resources for health professionals can be found in Table 4.1.

TABLE 4.1 ■ Web Resources that Support Delivery of Culturally Responsive Care

Organization/Resource	Web Address
ALTA Language Services	http://www.altalang.com
American Society on Aging	http://www.asaging.org
Black Mamas Matter Alliance	https://blackmamasmatter.org/
Center for Applied Linguistics	http://www.cal.org
The Cross Cultural Health Care Program	https://xculture.org
Cultural Humility: People, Principles and Practices	https://www.youtube.com/ watch?v=_Mbu8bvKb_U&t=184s
Dignity and Respect Campaign	https://dignityandrespect.org
Findhelp.org Resources for food assistance, housing, transit, and legal needs	www.findhelp.org
Institute for Health Care Improvement	http://www.ihi.org
Institute for Diversity and Health Equity	https://ifdhe.aha.org
National Center for Cultural Competence	https://nccc.georgetown.edu/
Project Implicit	https://www.projectimplicit.net
TedEd Talk Dr. R. Williams. How racism makes us sick	https://ed.ted.com/lessons/oRaEODBk
The Cross Cultural Health Program	http://www.xculture.org
The Macy Foundation Racist Patients: Taking Action on Harmful Bias and Discrimination in Clinical Learning Environments	https://macyfoundation.org/ news-and-commentary/taking- action-on-harmful-bias-and-discrimination- in-clinical-learning-environments
The National LGBTQIA + Health Education Center	https://www.lgbtqiahealtheducation.org
Racial Trauma Guide. Department of Psychology, University of Georgia	https://www.psychology.uga.edu/ racial-trauma-guide
Stanford Geriatric Education Center	http://sgec.stanford.edu
U.S. Administration on Community Living	http://www.aoa.gov
U.S. Department of Health and Human Services— Indian Health Service LGBTQ and Two-Spirit Health	https://www.ihs.gov/lgbt/

ETHNICITY

Ethnicity refers to a person's sense of belonging to a group of people sharing a common origin, history, and set of social beliefs. Ethnicity also may refer to an individual's place of geographical or national origin. While in the not-too-distant past, it may have been unusual for a health professional to treat patients from different countries, the world often seems much smaller today with the displacement of large groups of people due to war and famine. Health professionals may now encounter refugees in their own communities and be faced with unfamiliar beliefs, traditions, and values. Note this excerpt from Anne Fadiman's comprehensive work on the Hmong refugees who immigrated to Merced County, California from Laos, in *The Spirit Catches You and You Fall Down:*

> none of the doctors at MCMC [Merced County Medical Center] had ever heard of the word "Hmong," and they had no idea what to make of their new patients. They wore strange clothes— often children's clothes, which were approximately the right size—acquired at the Goodwill. When

they undressed for examination, the women were sometimes wearing Jockey shorts and the men were sometimes wearing bikini underpants with little pink butterflies. They wore amulets around their necks and cotton strings around their wrists (the sicker the patient, the more numerous the strings).[31]

Although the United States has a history of immigration from various parts of the world, global migration is at an all-time high. The United Nations Refugee Agency reports that, by the end of 2019, 79.5 million people have been forcibly displaced with the top source countries, including Syria, Venezuela, Afghanistan, and South Sudan.[10] A result of the influx of immigrants and refugees is often more challenging to sort out and identify specific cultural differences that modify behavior in various ethnic groups.

Sometimes as a health professional, you may have a difficult time remembering that members of an ethnic group are not homogeneous. Ethnicity is only one characteristic of the culture or cultures that our patients bring to their present experience. At times, each of us becomes aware of cultural beliefs held by an individual that, on the surface, seems to be incongruent. For example, a Chinese American may be highly assimilated into the majority culture and seeks mainstream health care for a gastrointestinal disorder, yet also seeks care from a traditional Chinese healer who might prescribe herbs, teas, or other therapies appropriate for their culture. Because we can identify with individual variations in our own cultural beliefs and the blending of seemingly opposite beliefs that can occur within us as individuals, we must appreciate the profound variability in cultural groups.

One of the broadest cultural gaps you will encounter in your role as a health professional is created by the "ethnocentrism" of health professionals. (Although separate professions often are not thought of as cultures in themselves, they are.) *Ethnocentrism* is the belief that one's cultural ways are superior. Health professionals often believe that their way is best and so may be guilty of medical ethnocentrism. While you are a student, you are learning and adopting the culture and identity of your chosen health profession. The culture of a health professional encompasses the interrelationships of professional values, beliefs, customs, habits, and symbols. You are learning the cultural meaning your profession gives to concepts such as pain, disability, independence, disease, and illness. You will find that even within the culture of the health professions, there are different meanings and understandings of identical phenomena. Thus, as an individual, you may share the same ethnic origin, race, and gender identity as the patient you are working with and yet not hold the same beliefs and perspectives about some essential values related to what their health care or treatment should involve. The alignment of patient-centered values and evidence is called *values-based practice*. In this practice model, the unique preferences and expectations of patients are integrated into clinical decisions based on evidence-based care.[32]

GENDER IDENTITY

In your role as a health professional, you will encounter various gender identities. Many people confuse sex and gender and use the terms interchangeably assuming that sex defines gender. Sex is the classification of a person as male, female, or intersex. Sex assignment occurs at birth based on chromosomal, gonadal, and anatomical characteristics. However, sex assigned at birth may not correspond with gender. Gender describes our internal understanding and experience of our own gender identity. Each person's gender identity is personal and cannot be known simply by looking at a person (see iceberg example). Gender identity is a living, growing experience that can be either fixed or fluid.[33] Gender nonconformity describes those whose gender identity or expression differs from that which was assigned at birth. A person may be cisgender if they accept the category of boy/man or girl/woman assigned at birth or may be transgender if they belong to a gender category different from assigned at birth. Transgender individuals include transgender females (who identify as female but assigned male at birth), transgender males (who identify as male but assigned female at birth), and those who identify as male or female and may describe their identity as nonbinary.[34] Providing respectful care to all patients requires recognizing the complexity of gender identity and education about how people self-identify according to gender-related distinctions.

Similar to the experience of racism, transgender individuals face discrimination and stigma at three levels within a society: structural, interpersonal, and individual.[33,35] Consider the recent societal debate about transgender people's use of public restrooms in schools and attempts to legally restrict such usage because of alleged safety risks to others as an indicator of how strongly some people react to those who are transgender. Transgender individuals have complex health needs, and language used in medical settings can further marginalize trans individuals.

One way that health professionals can show respect to their patients on a personal and interpersonal level is by acknowledging a patient's gender identity and using the correct pronouns. She/her/hers, he/him/his, or they/them/theirs are the most common pronouns encountered, although this list is not exhaustive. Many medical records include information on sex but do not record gender identity, resulting in the health professional misgendering patients based on outward appearance. *Misgendering* occurs when we address patients using language that does not match their gender identity and can negatively impact their experience in the health care system. At an institutional level, the health professional can advocate for more inclusive intake forms which ask patients about their preferred pronouns. However, one way to determine the appropriate pronouns is to ask the patient. Health professionals can also get into the habit of introducing themselves and their pronouns, thereby setting the stage to allow the patient to share their pronouns. If you find yourself in a situation where you unintentionally misgender a patient, it is best to avoid making excuses. Instead, apologize and offer reassurance to do better in the future.

Gender inequities in health status, access, and treatment exist worldwide and are strongly related to other social determinants of health such as education and economic status. In the United States, women have a history of unequal access to sources of economic and political power that has an impact on access to health care resources.[36] This is especially true for women of color or older women who experience the combined impact of race, gender, and age discrimination. The health professional may encounter the term *intersectionality* that examines the relationship between race, gender, and class, with one not seen as more salient than the other.[37,38]

One way to explore how gender can inform the health care experience is by exploring patients' preferences regarding the gender of their physician. In a systematic review of studies among women seeking gynecological or obstetrical care, a large number of women preferred a female physician.[39] Because many women feel uncomfortable and perhaps embarrassed during a gynecological examination, they may choose female physicians because they are familiar with the female body and have firsthand experience with the examination. It follows that if women are more comfortable with the examination, they will be more likely to follow through with checkups and follow the physician's recommendations. Patients in this study reported that outside of gender, other factors such as experience, knowledge, communication skills (particularly patient-centered communication skills),[39] and clinical competence are also important to patients seeking a gynecologist–obstetrician.[40] Another study shows that outside of the specialty of obstetrics and gynecology, communication skills were the most important factor for female patients with regard to their interaction with a physician.[40] The take-away lesson here is that all health professionals need to adopt patient-centered behaviors and communication styles to compensate for any differences from their patients.

A patient's preference for a health professional of the same gender may also be culturally or religiously grounded.[41] Many cultural groups are concerned about modesty and may require that only a female health professional examine a female patient's breasts and genitalia or be present when they are undressed. The importance of modesty can have its origins in culture, religion, or personal preferences and is especially important to consider in the health care environment in which patients are often subjected to being unnecessarily exposed. Regardless of the reason for modesty, inattention to respecting a patient's modesty can lead to poor follow-through with preventive procedures or follow-through with agreed-upon treatment or therapy.

SEXUAL IDENTITY AND ORIENTATION

Sexual self-identity or orientation is another characteristic of culture that may elicit bias and discrimination. As Dr. Nivet, the Chief Diversity Officer for the Association of American Colleges, highlights, "significant legal and societal advances have resulted in encouraging improvements in the health and well-being of lesbian, gay and bisexual (LGB) members of the population. Still, disparities persist both in the delivery of quality health care and in the health outcomes experienced by people in these populations. Transgender individuals and people born with differences of sex development (DSD) face even greater difficulties in obtaining compassionate, evidence-based, and patient-centered care."[34]

Patients who are LGBT, gender nonconforming, or born with DSD experience inadequate or inappropriate care which can range from implicit bias to overt discrimination. In addition to the negative attitudes expressed by health professionals toward patients with a sexual orientation different from their own, gay, lesbian, transgender, and bisexual patients find themselves in a health care system built on heterosexual assumptions. Common examples include women seeking gynecological or obstetrical care who may not even be asked about their sexual history and lesbian and gay patients' partners not being formally acknowledged in family education or care planning. Patients who identify as LGBTQIA+ ("Q" for genderqueer, questioning, or gender nonconforming and "I" for intersex) are not homogenous and have very different health needs. Challenges interacting with the health system may translate into decreased quality of care received and ultimately health disparities.[34]

Providing sensitive, culturally appropriate care requires understanding that each of the populations represented by a letter in the acronym LGBTQIA+ is complex and distinct. This complexity is heightened when we consider the addition (and *intersectionality*) of other primary and secondary cultural characteristics such as age, race, ethnicity, SES, religion, and geographic location. We must take the patient's sexual orientation fully into account and ensure that information is used to optimize the quality of care. Often, equitable care begins with appropriate terminology, as discussed earlier in this chapter.

AGE AND INTERGENERATIONAL DIVERSITY

Stigma associated with being old is related to the prejudices of an ageist society. The word *ageism* was coined to designate the discriminatory treatment of older people. Older adults living in mainstream Western societies are confronted continuously with ageist conduct in their day-to-day interactions with others. Unfortunately, ageist conduct occurs in the health care environment as well. Older patients often receive less attention or are denied services based on age alone. Physical and psychological problems may not be addressed because health professionals assume that they are normal for an older person. Additionally, older patients are highly complex regarding the numbers and types of health problems they possess, so more time is necessary when diagnosing and treating them. Older patients are prime targets for overmedication and frequently experience the effects of poorly coordinated care. Regardless of their state of health or physical ability, a patient who is an older adult is frequently met with a condescending attitude. Ways in which you can overcome the tendencies to engage in ageist behavior are discussed in more detail in Chapter 13.

Intergenerational diversity is another aspect of patient care that is different from discriminatory behavior on the part of the health professional based on age. Working across the generations is a very common occurrence between young health professionals and older patients that can cause misunderstanding for both. Adjustments in communication tactics and exploration of differences in values or meanings express respect in contrast to responding to older patients with negative stereotypes, such as assuming hearing loss or diminished mental capacity, resulting in the health professional's use of inappropriately loud or oversimplified language. Another important point to consider is that LGBT older adults (born before 1946) are less likely to disclose their sexual orientation and gender identity as they came of age when homosexuality and nonnormative gender identities were stigmatized.[42] As we have discussed elsewhere in this chapter, the health professional must avoid categorizing patients and making assumptions, this time purely based on the patient's age.

SOCIOECONOMIC STATUS

As we have been exploring in this chapter, there are a wide range of personal, social, economic, and environmental factors that contribute to health (i.e., the *social determinants of health*). The World Health Organization defines the social determinants of health as the "non-medical factors that influence health outcomes. They are the conditions in which people are born, grow, work, live, and age, and the wider set of forces and systems shaping the conditions of daily life."[43] SES is closely linked with health as patients with quality education and stable employment, who live in safe neighborhoods, tend to be healthier.[44] While race, ethnicity, and SES can combine to contribute to health and disease patterns,[45] the health professional should avoid assuming that a patient who belongs to a racial/ethnic minority group automatically has a low SES status.

As mentioned previously in this chapter, a vast majority of US and Canadian health professionals are White, with average incomes in the upper-middle to high economic range when considered globally. The income level and accompanying higher social status of health professionals can create barriers in their relationships with many patients. The difference in SES may hinder patients from asking you important questions, hinder you from empathizing with patients, and limit your knowledge of the practical everyday obstacles that prevent or facilitate the ability of patients to pursue, and adhere to, medication or treatment regimens. The following example highlights the challenges some patients face accessing care.

CASE STUDY

A young mother and her two small children, a toddler and a 3-month-old, leave their apartment at 7:00 a.m. for a 9:00 a.m. clinic visit. In the rush to leave the apartment to get to their appointment, the mother forgot her cell phone. With the baby in a stroller and the toddler at his mother's side, they head for the bus stop that is four blocks from their home. The first bus is late because of icy conditions. She must transfer three times to get to the clinic and walk two blocks to the clinic building. She arrives at the clinic 45 minutes late for her 9:00 a.m. appointment. The medical assistant at the intake desk looks at the clock as the mother signs in and says, "Couldn't you have called if you were going to be late?"

We will address different interpretations of time in Chapter 10, but in this case, there is no disagreement between the clinic staff and the patient about what "on time" is. The medical assistant is either insensitive to or does not understand the complications that arise from having to be dependent on public transportation or the hassle of finding a payphone today. The fact that this patient made it to the clinic is a testament to her desire to receive care. Yet this fact becomes lost in complaints about the patient's tardiness and lack of consideration for the clinic staff. Health professionals may take for granted owning a car or a cell phone, items that could be entirely beyond the financial means of some patients.

Differences in social class and economic status also affect the type and frequency of interaction between patient and health professional outside the health care setting. Informal networks in neighborhoods and communities provide opportunities to establish cooperation, exchange information, and determine appropriate behavior. Health professionals who have mainly been socialized in largely White, urban middle-class values may see patients as "noncompliant" and fail to appreciate the complexity of the patient environment and context. For example, a patient may be told to increase their exercise and go on daily walks, which sounds easy for someone who lives in a safe neighborhood. But in a crime-ridden area, a walk around the block could in fact danger one's health.

Health professionals can make unintentional errors in judgment because they underestimate the effects of race, ethnicity, age, or SES on patient's engagement with the health care system. Even gaining enough trust to adequately treat a patient is not enough to understand what goes into staying afloat on a minimum-wage salary or holding down two or three part-time jobs to make ends meet.

EDUCATION

The level of education is another social determinant of health. Adults with a college degree live on average 5 years more than those with less than a high school education.[44] Education can also serve as a barrier between health professionals and patients. Patients may be too intimidated to ask questions or admit when they do not understand something. Also, they may fear that they will be seen as ignorant or superstitious, and neglect to mention that they are also seeking alternative methods of care or providers. Even when patients are well educated, they may not speak the dominant language well enough to express themselves adequately. You may understand what this feels like if you have struggled to make yourself understood across a language barrier. It is important to remember that the "language" of health care is often foreign to patients as well. In Chapter 10, we discuss in more detail how language, vocabulary, and health literacy can facilitate or limit what patients perceive as respect from you.

OCCUPATION AND ENVIRONMENT

One of the first questions we often ask a new acquaintance in a social setting is, "What do you do?" This deep identification with occupations is mainstream in American culture. Some would go so far as to say that their occupation defines who they are more than their ethnicity or other primary characteristics. Consider where you ranked your occupation when you completed the reflection on identity. Occupations shape how people see the world, what they value, and how they spend their time. The importance of a person's occupation is sometimes seen more clearly when illness, injury, disease, disability, or retirement forces a change in occupation. How patients occupy themselves, whether they spend their time in the formal workforce or not, can give important cultural clues that impact health beliefs and decisions.

We do not often think of place of residence as a cultural variable in our interactions with patients, yet there is increasing evidence that place of residence has an impact on how patients think about health. For example, certain health beliefs and practices sometimes differ between urban and rural patients. People who live in rural areas must often travel a considerable distance to see a health professional because of their environment. Thus, rural patients are often more independent regarding the use of health care services than their urban counterparts. Another significant difference between rural and urban dwellers is the way health needs are viewed. Rural dwellers, from a variety of locations, tend to determine health needs primarily in relation to work activities.[46] It is therefore important to consider where someone lives and the other cultural values they bring to their place of residence.

Rural areas tend to have poorer access to health care services.[47] Rural residents tend to value self-reliance more than urban residents. Rural residents, particularly farmers and ranchers, often are required to maintain a higher level of physical fitness as they take care of their land, tend animals, manage the maintenance of and use heavy machinery, etc. Their ability to accomplish these tasks is tied to their self-identity and self-worth.[46]

Regardless of neighborhood and community contexts where the patient resides, you will show respect when mindful of the impact that place of residence can have on your interactions with patients and their health-related routines. This is especially true when the patient does not have a permanent place of residence or is unhoused. The challenges of working with patients without housing include not only significant issues such as ensuring the safety and basic well-being of the patient but also practical considerations such as the need for access to a bathroom, warmth and dry clothing, or a source of clean drinking water. Persons who lack stable and consistent housing either by choice or necessity are part of a subculture that is often hidden from view and requires openness and understanding from health professionals.

RELIGION AND SPIRITUALITY

Religious beliefs are another feature of culture that influences your relationship with patients. Religion gives meaning to illness, pain, and suffering. Religious beliefs often become most apparent when a patient is seriously injured, critically ill, or dying. For example, the Christian faith, with its valuing of human life and belief in eternal life, states that a struggle for health can be meaningful. In contrast, a struggle against death at all costs to the point that the effort becomes a torment may be antithetical to their beliefs.[48] The Christian cultural view of the dying process and death itself influences treatment decisions and may promote requests for symbolically meaningful activities such as receiving rituals in the form of sacraments.

A different view of illness is evident with believers in Islam. The word *Islam* means to submit; that is, to submit their lives to the will of God (Allah). A practicing Muslim may attribute the incidence and outcome of a health condition to "inshallah" or, to put another way, to leave it in God's hands. This belief may make preventive health behaviors or self-care programs difficult to institute. Because God is perceived to be in control of the outcome, what can humans do?[49] However, what may appear to be "fatalistic" could also be shaped by another Muslim duty regarding stewardship of one's body and health. This duty prescribes clear responsibility for one's health. Thus highlighting, once again, there is more to culture and beliefs than appears on the surface.

Christianity, Hinduism, Judaism, and Islamism are widespread established religions in Western societies and relatively well known; therefore health professionals may not find much difficulty recognizing and respecting them even with minimal understanding of underlying beliefs and rituals. Regardless if one's religion is mainstream or not, patients feel respected when health professionals seek to understand and honor their religious and spiritual traditions.

CULTURAL HUMILITY AND COMPETENCE

The overall lesson to be gleaned from the brief preceding descriptions of various primary and secondary cultural characteristics is that the atmosphere in health care must rest on fully appreciating what each culture brings to the richness of our society and on acceptance rather than on fear and misunderstanding. What is needed is an approach to each patient, family, and colleague that takes into account cultural differences and appreciating that you are a multicultural being, as are others. *Cultural competence* is "an ongoing process in which the health care professional continually strives to achieve the ability and availability to work effectively within the cultural context of the patient (individual, family, and community)."[50] Part of cultural competence involves understanding your values and culture and valuing your patients' diversity. It is helpful to think about a continuum that starts at cultural destructiveness and ends at cultural proficiency. We may never feel culturally proficient given the vast number and complexities of cultural traditions; however, we can continually strive toward that.

Along these same lines, *cultural humility* should be factored into understanding culturally appropriate care and requires more than knowledge about cultural practices. Cultural humility, a prerequisite to cultural competence, requires a commitment to ongoing self-reflection and self-critique, particularly identifying and examining one's own patterns of unintentional and intentional prejudices and negative attitudes and practices. Cultural humility also includes acknowledging and attempting to mitigate the power imbalance between patient and provider and a commitment to being a lifelong learner and reflective practitioner,[51] again recognizing that cultural competence is a journey, not a destination. An essential component of becoming culturally competent is the ability to conduct a cultural assessment when interacting with patients. Among numerous cultural assessment tools in the literature, one set of questions developed by Kleinman stands out because the questions focus on the patient's perspective regarding illness, as follows:

1. What do you call your problem? What name does it have?
2. What do you think has caused your problem? Why do you think it started when it did?
3. What do you think your sickness does to you? How does it work?
4. How severe is it? Will it have a short or long course?
5. What do you fear the most about your sickness?
6. What are the chief problems your sickness has caused for you?
7. What kind of treatment do you think you should receive? What are the most important results you hope to receive from this treatment?[52]

Regardless of the patient's cultural background, the preceding questions are a logical and respectful place to start in trying to understand what brought the patient to the health care encounter. Note the open-ended nature of the questions, which allow the patient to tell you their illness or wellness story. The patient is, after all, the expert on themselves. However, we should also accept that the patient may be taken aback by the health professional asking what they think caused their illness. After all, this is why the patient came to see you! A patient who ascribes to Western medicine may expect you to have these answers. It may be helpful to preface these questions with: "For me to fully appreciate what you are going through, I am going to ask you a series of questions about what you think is going on."

Additionally, beyond individual patient encounters, health professionals should consider solutions that let go of traditional approaches to patients in general that focus only on problem identification and methods to bridge divides. Put simply, the traditional approach looks at patients, particularly patients from diverse cultural backgrounds, and asks, "What does this patient need, and how are they different so I know what to do to compensate for these differences in providing care?" It is essential to acknowledge that a focus on good communication and culturally responsive care can shore up these deficits or problems that present barriers to quality care. Use honest questions to open conversations with patients, such as, "Many of my patients experience racism/ageism/sexism in their health care. Are there any experiences you would like to share with me?"[53] From an equity-minded standpoint, health professionals would assume diversity and approach all patients to create an environment in which everyone will receive the best care.[54] From this perspective, health professionals would ask, "Why are our practices failing to produce successful outcomes for all patients, and what do we need to change?" This perspective shifts the focus to factors within the health professionals' control.

In Chapter 1, you were charged with approaching each patient respectfully. This means, among other things, consciously avoiding unfair judgments about other people's traditions, values, and beliefs. We are much more likely to respect a patient's decision or action if we understand its rationale. Misunderstandings can harm the patient in that they may hesitate to seek medical attention or follow the advice of someone out of touch with their beliefs. One common barrier to respectful interaction is the tendency for health professionals to adopt stereotypes and expect certain behaviors from patients from a certain culture simply because they are from that culture. Avoiding scripted remarks such as "Syrian refugees all believe ..." or "All Chinese patients practice ..." is the best practice as it is impossible to generalize from one patient to an entire culture.

In the face of cultural differences, you will need basic negotiation and shared decision-making skills. This means finding a place where you can feel confident in the exercise of your professional judgment while incorporating the beliefs and values of patients into their treatment plan to achieve mutually desirable outcomes. The goal of cultural humility is to provide care characterized by respect. Such care is meaningful and fits with cultural beliefs and ways of life for those involved. Because diversity in society is likely to increase rather than decrease in the coming years, access to the most current statistics regarding demography and tools to assist in providing culturally appropriate care is vitally important. Table 4.1 provides a sampling of web resources to assist you in obtaining the most current information.

Summary

The issues relevant to showing respect for diversity must continually be examined and be a topic for reflection. The concept of culture provides an appropriate starting point for health professionals to become aware and learn to honor different characteristics among groups, remaining aware that individuals may not always fit a predictable cultural pattern. Making every effort to avoid prejudice, discrimination, bias, and other negative attitudes and conduct based on difference is part of being a health professional. The only constructive approach to evaluating human differences with the goal of providing patient-centered care is to take each experience as an opportunity to learn more about the rich diversity of the human condition and to take what one learns as a gift that will help achieve the goals of the health professional and patient relationship, as well as enrich one's own life.

References

1. Gorman A. The hill we climb. *The Hill*. January 21, 2022. Retrieved from: https://thehill.com/homenews/news/535052-read-transcript-of-amanda-gormans-inaugural-poem; Accessed March 3, 2021.
2. Yosso TJ. Whose culture has capital? A critical race theory discussion of community cultural wealth. *Race Ethn Educ*. 2005;8(1):69–91. https://doi.org/10.1080/1361332052000341006.
3. Banks JA. The dimensions of multicultural education. In: *Cultural Diversity and Education: Foundations, Curriculum, and Teaching*. 6th ed. London: Pearson; 2015.
4. National Health Service Corps. *Bridging the Cultural Divide in Health Care Settings: The Essential Role of Cultural Broker Programs*. Rockville, MD: U.S. Department of Health and Human Services; 2004.
5. Uono S, Hietanen JK. Eye contact perception in the West and East: a cross-cultural study. *PLoS ONE*. 2015;10(2):e0118094. https://doi.org/10.1371/journal.pone.0118094.
6. Allport G. *The Nature of Prejudice*. Reading, MA: Addison-Wesley; 1954.
7. *Johns Hopkins Medicine Office*. Diversity, inclusion and health equity. Fast facts definition sheet. <https://www.hopkinsmedicine.org/diversity/_documents/JHM%20Office%20of%20Diversity%20and%20Inclusion%20Fast%20Facts%20Definition%20Sheet.pdf>; 2021 Accessed March 3, 2021.
8. FitzGerald C, Hurst S. Implicit bias in healthcare professionals: a systematic review. *BMC Medical Ethics*. 2017;18(1):1–18.
9. *UNHCR The UN Refugee Agency*. Figures at a glance. <https://www.unhcr.org/en-us/figures-at-a-glance.html>; 2020 Accessed March 3, 2021.
10. US Census Bureau. QuickFacts: United States. <https://www.census.gov/quickfacts/fact/table/US/RHI825219>; 2021 Accessed March 4, 2021.
11. National Conference of State Legislatures (NCSL). *Racial and Ethnic Health Disparities: Workforce Diversity*; 2014. Retrieved from: https://www.ncsl.org/documents/health/Workforcediversity814.pdf.
12. Health Resources and Services Administration. *The Rationale for Diversity in the Health Professions: A Review of the Evidence*. Bureau of Health Professions; 2006. Retrieved from: http://bhpr.hrsa.gov/health-workforce/reports/diversityreviewevidence.pdf.

13. Goode TD, Dunne C. *Policy Brief 1: Rationale for Cultural Competence in Primary Care*. Washington, DC: National Center for Cultural Competence, Georgetown University Center for Child and Human Development; 2003. Retrieved from: https://nccc.georgetown.edu/documents/Policy_Brief_1_2003.pdf.

14. Haynes MA, Smedley BD, eds. *The Unequal Burden of Cancer: An Assessment of NIH Research and Programs for Ethnic Minorities and the Medically Underserved*. Washington, DC: Institute of Medicine. National Academies Press; 1999.

15. Editorial: Genes, drugs and race. *Nat Genet*. 2001;29:239–240. https://doi.org/10.1038/ng1101-239.

16. Liu WM. White male power and privilege: the relationship between white supremacy and social class. *J Couns Psychol*. 2017;64(4):349–358.

17. Golestaneh L, Neugarten J, Fisher M, et al. The association of race and COVID-19 mortality. *eClinicalMedicine*. 2020;25:100455. https://doi.org/10.1016/j.eclinm.2020.100455.

18. Devakumar D, Shannon G, Bhopal SS, Abubakar I. Racism and discrimination in COVID-19 responses. *Lancet*. 2020. https://doi.org/10.1016/S0140-6736(20)30792-3.

19. UNC Office of the Provost Diversity and Inclusion. *Racism as a Determinant of Health Webinar*. Retrieved from: https://diversity.unc.edu/event/racism-as-a-determinant-of-health-webinar/; 2020.

20. Freeman L, Stewart H. Microaggressions in clinical medicine. *Kennedy Inst Ethics J*. 2018;28(4):411–449.

21. Smedley B, Stith A, Nelson A. *Committee on Understanding and Eliminating Racial and Ethnic Disparities in Health Care, Institutes of Medicine, Unequal Treatment: Confronting Racial and Ethnic Disparities in Healthcare*. Washington, DC: The National Academies Press; 2003:1.

22. Scharf DP, Matthews KJ, Jackson P, et al. More than Tuskegee: understanding mistrust about research participation. *J Health Care Poor Underserved*. 2010;21(3):879–897.

23. Kendi I. *How to Be an Antiracist*. London: Bodley Head; 2019.

24. Houtrow A. Becoming anti-racist for the benefit of our patients. *J Pediatr Rehabil Med*. 2020;13(1):1–2. https://doi.org/10.3233/PRM-200680.

25. Project Implicit. Harvard Implicit Association Test. https://www.projectimplicit.net/; 2011 Accessed March 4, 2021.

26. Jain SH. The racist patient. *Ann Intern Med*. 2013;158(8):632.

27. Chandrashekar P, Jain SH. Addressing patient bias and discrimination against clinicians of diverse backgrounds. *Acad Med*. 2020;95(12):S33–S43. https://doi.org/10.1097/ACM.0000000000003682.

28. Campbell A.F. Why violence against nurses has spiked in the last decade. *The Atlantic*. December 1, 2016. Retrieved from: https://www.theatlantic.com/business/archive/2016/12/violence-againstnurses/509309.

29. Speroni KG, Fitch T, Dawson E, Dugan L, Atherton M. Incidence and cost of nurse workplace violence perpetrated by hospital patients or patient visitors. *J Emerg Nurs*. 2014;40(3):218–228. https://doi.org/10.1016/j.jen.2013.05.014.

30. The Macy Foundation. *Racist Patients: Taking Action on Harmful Bias and Discrimination in Clinical Learning Environments*. Retrieved from: https://www.youtube.com/watch?utm_source=YouTube&utm_medium=Email&utm_campaign=Racist+Patients+Webinar&v=28SEAx0o8JQ&feature=youtu.be; 2021.

31. Fadiman A. *The Spirit Catches You and You Fall Down*. New York: The Noon Day Press; 1997.

32. Fulford KWM. Values-based practice: a new partner to evidence-based practice and a first for psychiatry? *Mens Sana Monogr*. 2008;6(1):10–21.

33. Dolan IJ, Strauss P, Winter S, Lin A. Misgendering and experiences of stigma in health care settings for transgender people. *Med J Aust*. 2020;212:150.

34. Association of American Medical Colleges. *Implementing Curricular and Institutional Climate Changes to Improve Health Care of Individuals Who Are LGBT, Gender Non-Conforming, or Born With DSD*; 2014. Retrieved from: https://store.aamc.org/downloadable/download/sample/sample_id/129/.

35. Konsenko K, Rintamaki L, Raney S, et al. Transgender patient perceptions of stigma in health care contexts. *Med Care*. 2013;51(9):819–822.

36. Conway-Turner K. Older women of color: a feminist exploration of the intersections of personal, familial and community life. *J Women Aging*. 1999;11(2/3):115–130.

37. Cho S, Crenshaw KW, McCall L. Toward a field of intersectionality studies: theory, applications, and praxis. *Signs: J Women Cult Soc*. 2013;38(4):785–810.

38. Crenshaw K. Demarginalizing the intersection of race and sex: a black feminist critique of antidiscrimination doctrine, feminist theory and antiracist politics. *Univ Chic Leg Forum*. 1989:139–167.

39. Janssen SM, Lagro-Janssen AL. Physician's gender, communication style, patient preferences and patient satisfaction in gynecology and obstetrics: a systematic review. *Patient Educ Couns.* 2012;89(2):221–226.
40. Mavis B, Vasilenko P, Schnuth R Female patients' preferences related to interpersonal communications, clinical competence, and gender when selecting a physician. *Acad Med.* 2005;80(12):1159–1165.
41. Andrews C. Modesty and health care for women: understanding cultural sensitivities. *Comm Oncol.* 2006;3(7):443–446.
42. Fredriksen-Goldsen KI. Promoting health equity among LGBT mid-life and older adults: revealing how LGBT mid-life and older adults can attain their full health potential. *Generations.* 2014;38(4):86–92.
43. World Health Organization. Social Determinants of Health. Retrieved from: https://www.who.int/health-topics/social-determinants-of-health#tab=tab_1; 2022.
44. Robert Wood Johnson Foundation. *Overcoming Obstacles to Health.* Retrieved from: https://www.rwjf.org/en/library/research/2008/02/overcoming-obstacles-to-health.html; 2008.
45. Williams DR, Mohammed SA, Leavell J, Collins C. Race, socioeconomic status and health: complexities, ongoing challenges and research opportunities. *Ann N Y Acad Sci.* 2010;1186:69–101. https://doi.org/10.1111/j.1749-6632.2009.05339.x.
46. Nelson JA, Gingerich BS. Rural health: access to care and services. *Home Health Care Manage Pract.* 2010;22(3):339–343.
47. Zeng D, You W, Mills B, Alwang J, Royster M, Anson-Dwamena R. A closer look at the rural-urban health disparities: insights from four major diseases in the Commonwealth of Virginia. *Soc Sci Med.* 2015;140:62–68.
48. The Catholic Health Association of the United States. *Care of the Dying. A Catholic Perspective.* St. Louis, MO; 1993.
49. Haddad LG, Hoeman SP. Home healthcare and the Arab-American client. *Home Healthc Nurse.* 2000; 18(3):189–197.
50. Campinha-Bacote J. Patient-centered care in the midst of a cultural conflict: the role of cultural competence. *Online J Issues Nursing.* 2011;16(2):1.
51. Tervalon M, Murray-Garcia J. Cultural humility versus cultural competence: a critical distinction in defining physician training outcomes in multicultural education. *J Health Care Poor Underserved.* 1998; 9(2):117–125.
52. Kleinman A. *Patients and Healers in the Context of Culture.* Berkeley, CA: University of California Press; 1981.
53. Endo JA. *Addressing Race in Practice.* Institute for Health Care Improvement; 2016. Retrieved from: http://www.ihi.org/communities/blogs/_layouts/15/ihi/community/blog/itemview.aspx?List=7d1126ec-8f63-4a3b-9926-c44ea3036813&ID=308. Accessed March 11, 2022.
54. Bensimon EM, Dowd AC, Witham K. Five principles of enacting equity by design. *Assoc Am Coll Univ.* 2016;19(1):1–8.

CHAPTER 5

Respect in Care Delivery Systems

OBJECTIVES

The reader will be able to

- Compare the perspectives of a patient's view of health care with the institutional or societal level view;
- Consider the impact of workplace culture and climate on the health professionals employed by health care institutions and the patients who seek services there;
- Identify two aspects of administration that are likely to have a direct impact on the organizational environment;
- List several types of laws, regulations, and policies that influence the practice of health professionals and what they should be able to expect from the institution in which they work; and
- Discuss the idea of regulations and guidelines to protect patients and the purposes they are designed to serve.

Prelude

If you are in the ER waiting room at around like 9 AM or 10 AM, you will see an influx of patients with the buses that sort of hit the front door and so the buses will unload, and an exodus of patients will come and register and that's sort of their project for the day to make it to Highland and out. Almost anyone in our system comes through the ED.

THE WAITING ROOM[1]

Health care is often referred to as a social institution as it exists within institutions, a larger system of institutions, and within society at large. Like a set of Russian nesting dolls (matryoshka dolls), with each larger doll holding a smaller and smaller one until we reach the tiniest doll, a doll that could represent the patient surrounded by family and intimate friends, then surrounded by acquaintances, neighbors, and perhaps health professionals, in hospitals or clinics, in a neighborhood or city, each level encompassing more people and challenges. In a nutshell, health care delivery in the United States is inherently interdependent and increasingly complex.[2] This chapter focuses on some key insights regarding the make-up of the health care system where you will exercise your professional skills. You will almost inevitably work in an institutional environment, which exists to coordinate and provide health care services to the general population or specific subgroups within the population such as a hospital dedicated to the care of children or a clinic for adults with orthopedic health issues. Your ability to understand and respect the basic structure, operations, and aims of health care institutions is essential to patient outcomes, and your professional success and satisfaction in your work. Understanding the culture and climate in which you work will contribute to how you are viewed by patients, colleagues, and the wider community.

It follows that readers of this book will be influenced by their work environment, as well as influence that environment by participating in its everyday activities. A good starting place for respectful interaction is to become familiar with the basic characteristics of such institutions and then address key characteristics of institutional relationships within them. It will also benefit you to become aware of some critical policies and practices designed to command respect from all who engage with the institution, whether employees or those seeking goods and services, so we introduce them in a general way in the final sections of this chapter.

Characteristics of Institutions

Glaser describes three realms of social activity—individual, institutional, and societal—each having an impact on the health professional's effectiveness and sense of well-being. Institutions sit at the interface between the individual and the larger society (Fig. 5.1).[3] All institutions comprise individuals and groups. A health care institution is affected by several external factors that impact the entire industry such as "health policy, federal/state/local regulations governing practice, accrediting agency standards, healthcare financing systems that document care and serve as sources of quality monitoring and reporting."[4]

Internal factors such as the unique culture and climate of a health care institution have a substantial impact on staff and patient well-being. Recall the exploration of culture in Chapter 4 and here apply the basic definition of culture to an institutional setting. An institution's *culture* can be defined as the basic assumptions about the world and the values that guide life in organizations.[5] Institutional culture is conveyed to newcomers to an institution by sharing the history of the organization, its mission, strategic aims, etc. Furthermore, there are levels of culture that reflect

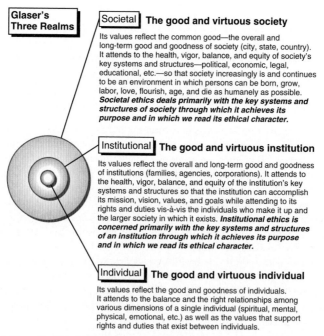

Glaser's Three Realms

Societal — **The good and virtuous society**

Its values reflect the common good—the overall and long-term good and goodness of society (city, state, country). It attends to the health, vigor, balance, and equity of society's key systems and structures—political, economic, legal, educational, etc.—so that society increasingly is and continues to be an environment in which persons can be born, grow, labor, love, flourish, age, and die as humanely as possible. *Societal ethics deals primarily with the key systems and structures of society through which it achieves its purpose and in which we read its ethical character.*

Institutional — **The good and virtuous institution**

Its values reflect the overall and long-term good and goodness of institutions (families, agencies, corporations). It attends to the health, vigor, balance, and equity of the institution's key systems and structures so that the institution can accomplish its mission, vision, values, and goals while attending to its rights and duties vis-à-vis the individuals who make it up and the larger society in which it exists. *Institutional ethics is concerned primarily with the key systems and structures of an institution through which it achieves its purpose and in which we read its ethical character.*

Individual — **The good and virtuous individual**

Its values reflect the good and goodness of individuals. It attends to the balance and the right relationships among various dimensions of a single individual (spiritual, mental, physical, emotional, etc.) as well as the values that support rights and duties that exist between individuals.

Fig. 5.1 Glaser's Three Realms of Ethics. Glaser J. *Three Realms of Ethics.* Kansas City, MO: Sheed and Ward; 1994:12.

the culture in context. The first level is the visible manifestations of health care culture such as "accepted care pathways, clinical practices and communication patterns, sometimes referred to as 'the way things are done around here.'"[6] The second level is the shared ways of thinking used to justify the visible manifestations of care. For example, in a study in which employees on a maternity unit were asked to describe their coworkers and their working relationships, most of the staff replied, "we are a family, a work family," reflecting the way the staff work together and mutually support each other.[7] In other words, this is the way staff talk about and justify their culture. Finally, the third level, unspoken and unconscious, encompasses the expectations and shared assumptions that underpin day-to-day practice that might include understanding role delineations and responsibilities for example.[6]

An institution's *climate* is the shared perceptions of and meaning attached to the policies, practices, and procedures employees experience and the behaviors they observe are being rewarded and that are supported and expected.[5] These two terms, culture and climate, are complementary ways of looking at life within institutions for those working there and patients who visit. If a culture is "toxic" or unhealthy, it can harm the individuals who work there and those they serve. Workplace culture matters particularly in health care because it has a direct impact on patient and staff outcomes.[8]

Ideally, institutional policies and practices not only reflect a deep respect for values that guide individual health professionals personally and professionally but also encourage them to be responsive to the basic societal expectation that patients should be the top priority. In turn, health professionals should not only engage in respectful interpersonal relationships with patients and families but also be respectful and loyal to management and administrative policies that guide actions within institutions.

Additionally, institutions have obligations to society, not just to the well-being of the institution and the individuals who reside within them. As Glaser argues,

> [Hospitals] need to become a more vigorous part of the community of concern shaping our health care system and less an agent of special interest pressure. They need to invest time in understanding health issues from the perspective of community good, not merely from the viewpoint of the organizational benefit.[3]

There are a variety of institutions in health care besides those that provide direct care to patients. For example, professional associations like the American Occupational Therapy Association or the American Medical Association influence professionals within the association and interact outside the association with the public. Other institutions in health care that have a major influence on health professionals and patients are educational institutions such as community colleges and universities that prepare health professionals for their roles in health care, insurance providers, information technology vendors, and pharmaceutical and device manufacturers, to name a few.

Glaser's model diagrams the interacting social activity among institutions that have a role in health care. The model highlights that the overall health of a community depends on different competing goods such as education, housing, and a healthy environment.

Organization of Health Care

The institutional realm of health care is a web of practice, ideas, and values expressed in numerous types of health care facilities. When we think of a health care institution that provides care to patients, often an image of a building such as a hospital comes to mind, but hospitals are not the only kind of institutions that exist in health care. In fact, increasingly more health care is delivered in some type of ambulatory or community-based setting such as free-standing clinics, physician-group practices, infusion centers, nursing clinics, surgical procedure centers, telehealth centers, case/disease management and care coordination organizations, hospices, rehabilitation clinics, schools, industrial settings, grocery and retail stores, and military systems that differ in a variety of ways from the traditional acute care structure of most hospitals.[9]

What is fitting for one type of facility may look quite different in another. For example, care delivery in a hospital for seriously ill patients is more controlled and predictable than in outpatient settings. In ambulatory care, one finds "multiple agents (patient, family, friends, physician, office staff) interacting with the patient's multiple, less-defined illnesses, which display the unpredictability of chaotic or random dynamics, less-specific diagnostic tests, and variable patient behavior."[10] Moreover, the organization of health care is not completely a *rational system*. Rational systems are oriented expressly to pursue one specific goal and have a highly formalized social structure designed to meet that goal.[11] An example is an airport, where the single goal is to move people and goods from place to place. The institutions of health care can be more illustrative of an *open system* in which shifting and sometimes competing interest groups negotiate for their goals to be met. In summary, "health care systems exemplify complex organizations operating under high stakes in dynamic policy and regulatory environments."[2]

There are numerous entries and exits in the health care system, which makes it an "open" system in that sense as well. For example, a patient who is elderly and suffers from a fractured hip can travel the range of institutions along the health care continuum of services. Patients often arrive in an ambulance through the emergency department (ED) (which is a common entry point to contemporary health care, as noted in the prelude quotation from an ED physician at the outset of this chapter). A patient with a fractured hip would likely move on to the operating room, then a general medical floor, before discharge to rehabilitation in a skilled nursing facility (that may or may not be part of the same health system as the hospital). Some patients return home to live independently or move into an assisted living facility with visiting therapists, nurses, and aides from another agency in the community, and often the support of family and friends.

When you enter a program of professional preparation, the basic type of institutional setting where you will work may be determined in part by the focus of your profession. For example, a focus on maintenance and health promotion may mean you will practice in a school, occupational health setting, or free-standing clinic that provides wellness education. If you are drawn to acute care, rehabilitation, chronic health, or end-of-life care needs, it is likely you will find work in a hospital, rehabilitation center, skilled nursing facility, hospice, or home care setting.

REFLECTIONS

- In what type of health care setting can you see yourself working? Why? What are the attractions—for example, the patient population, type of care delivery such as fast-paced or extended time with patients, or the type of community in which the health care institution resides such as urban or rural?
- Think of the health care settings you have experienced as a patient, employee, or student. Which ones made you want to spend time there? Why?

Institutional environments have changed and will continue to do so during your professional career. Attention to where you find the best fit for your practice will require attentiveness to the evolving styles and designs of institutional environments. The very structure of hospitals and clinics reflects these changes, with primarily private rooms in modern hospitals and consultation rooms in clinics designed to accommodate members of the interprofessional team, the patient, and the patient's extended support system. The actual design of health care buildings can have negative effects on patients and the rates of adverse events like patient falls, medication errors, and iatrogenic infections.[12] Consider the design of older, long-term care facilities with double occupancy rooms and the impact that physical space could have on the transference of an infectious disease like COVID-19.

The types of services that specific institutions within health care systems provide are often highly regulated. For example, let us take a closer look at one hospital, Highland Hospital, which is the subject of the documentary film *The Waiting Room* from which the prelude to this chapter was taken. Highland Hospital is part of the Alameda Health System, which is "an integrated public health care system of five hospitals and four wellness centers with over 800 beds and 1,000 physicians."[13] There are five hospitals, a psychiatric pavilion, and many ambulatory clinics within this particular health system. Highland Hospital has a Level I Trauma Center and the ED referred to in the opening quote of the chapter. To achieve the Level I designation, the hospital voluntarily agrees to meet specific state-developed standards that the American College of Surgeons then verifies. These standards often include comprehensive trauma care and 24-hour availability of specific medical specialties and support personnel, as well as other supportive services. Highland Hospital's ED is highly trafficked because of the elevated levels of violent crime and the socioeconomic status of many of the ED's patients who come to Highland to get primary care. This is a mere snapshot of one hospital in one health system out of the 427 licensed general acute care hospitals in the state of California where there are over 11,000 licensed health facilities of diverse types.[14] The complexity within one health system can be overwhelming. Navigating between systems can be complex for you as a health professional but even more daunting for patients.

Characteristics of Institutional Relationships

The ability to show and receive respect in the work environment requires an understanding of several characteristics of relationships that take place in health care institutions compared with other types of relationships. To highlight this point, we examine an important characteristic of health care institutions that distinguish them from others you participate in—namely, their public rather than private nature.

PUBLIC-SECTOR AND PRIVATE-SECTOR RELATIONSHIPS

Public-sector relationships are interactions reserved for engagements within institutions of public life, whereas private-sector relationships are reserved for the world of family, friends, and other intimates.[11] Individuals separate their lives into these two worlds of relationship. Public-sector relationships are designed to serve a useful purpose and then dissolve, whereas private-sector ones are more likely to continue. Student and professor or patient and health professional relationships belong to the world of public-sector relationships. Social boundaries that are maintained in a public-sector relationship permit a rapid introduction and rapid separation, promoting cooperation around a common goal. All public-sector relationships are characterized by abrupt changes from extreme remoteness to extreme nearness with the expectation that the relationship will be temporary. For example, students who become close during their years of formal preparation often go their separate ways upon graduation. Professionals in attendance at a conference of their professional organization come from different worksites to learn, share their own research or expertise, enjoy socializing, and then depart to their practice settings. Such is the nature of public-sector relationships. However, there are gray areas between the public and private sectors. Refer to the example of attending a professional meeting. It is possible and likely that deep and enduring friendships can be established at such professional meetings mingling the public-sector and private-sector aspects of our lives.

Opportunities for involvement in each other's lives and well-being and the boundaries of respect that must be honored with patients, families, and peers are addressed throughout this book, especially in Section 1.

The physical structure of an institution helps enable an effective private-sector or public-sector relationship. Hospitals, clinics, or schools, for instance, unmistakably are public buildings. What are some of the clues for this conclusion? Sometimes, the environment where health care is provided combines private-sector and public-sector environments. For instance, there are private spaces in health care for examinations or procedures and public lobbies and waiting areas. On a different scale, a home visit to a patient requires that you go to their residence, be welcomed in as a guest would be, make your way across the living room among discarded pages of the morning paper, trip over the sleeping dog, and move a bathrobe from an overstuffed chair to sit down. In a patient's home, you have entered a profoundly private-sector environment. However, your presence and professional conduct represent the type of public-sector relationship that takes place within health care institutions, and this usually suffices to set the tone for a public-sector interaction.

Patients and families lose some freedom when entering a health institution such as where they should wait, what they must wear, or how long they can visit. Even within one's own home, the presence of health professionals limits freedom in some ways. The underlying question about any infringement on a patient's freedom should be the reasonableness of the limitation. In other words, are the restrictions there to protect the well-being of patients, or are the rules in an institution there to make the staff's work easier?

These concerns will vary based on the type of condition and the value system of the individual. However, the critical point is that the patient will have concerns about what restrictions the institution will impose. Also, restrictions can change as was evident during the COVID-19 pandemic. For example, strict restrictions were put in place regarding visitors in both inpatient and outpatient settings.

Your own autonomy as a health professional in an institution where you work will also be shaped by the structure and how authority is divided. They may include policies for securing employment, regulations regarding employee conduct, expectations regarding the number of people in your care, and other institutional guidelines. These will either enable or inhibit your ability to satisfy your professional and personal goals. A crucial component of your professional choices is to find an institution that is consistent with your personality and value system. However, health professionals may still find themselves having to make compromises based on their value system with their employer. It is important to be clear about what values are nonnegotiable. As you consider an institutional environment, paying attention to Glaser's three realms should help you identify areas where individual, institutional, and societal values overlap and where they may create potential conflicts.[3]

Health professionals are also key sources of institutional change who can help create ways that respect can be expressed in humane and person-centered environments such as these strategies that were developed during the COVID-19 pandemic: improving the work schedule, encouraging self-management, and providing personal resilience opportunities, such as mindfulness-based stress reduction and mental health awareness.[15] You will recall how these opportunities contribute to respect for self in the professional role from Chapter 3. As people talk about how their well-being, autonomy, and other values can better be honored within the confines of health care institutions, you can collaborate with colleagues to think of ways to help bring about those changes.

WORKING WITH HEALTH CARE ADMINISTRATION

All employees in institutions have the opportunity and obligation to work well with their team members and administrators. The administration's role is to safeguard the interests of the institution and the individuals that comprise it and lead the effort to establish a positive workplace culture. In health care institutions, the administration includes a wide range of groups and individuals, including institutional trustees, boards of directors, and the central administration (including a chief executive officer and chief financial officer, chief diversity officer, human resources director, and departmental and unit supervisors responsible for operations or services). The range and duties of the administration should reflect the needs of the institution as determined by its mission, goals, and functions. Health care institutions will include at least the following administrative areas:
1. quality care mechanisms to ensure that patient and family rights are respected
2. officers for enforcing legal compliance with federal, state, and other policies and regulations
3. accountability mechanisms ensuring qualifications of professional employees
4. risk management personnel regarding concerns of liability and malpractice
5. means of ensuring that employees get due payment for their services

Like other well-working institutions, there will be personnel and other mechanisms devoted to care delivery oversight, quality assurance, financial solvency, public relations, legal compliance, and assurances that legal rights are honored, and overall efficiency maintained. These administrative supports should always be designed to allow for the constructive participation of professionals who work there to ensure their mutually shared goal of good health care. For example, general goals or aims of health care institutions have been widely adopted and focus on optimizing four dimensions of performance, sometimes referred to as the "quadruple aim," as follows: (1) improving the health of populations, (2) enhancing the patient experience of care, (3) reducing the per capita cost of health care, and (4) improving care team experience/well-being.[16] All four of these goals are necessary for a health care institution to achieve quality health care as they contribute to each other in direct and reinforcing ways (Fig. 5.2).

At the same time, differences in the scope of accountabilities determined by their respective roles, administrator or health professional who provides direct care to patients, could lead to understandable conflicts. The following case study outlines the different approaches of a health professional whose primary responsibility is patient-centered with those of a health care administrator, in this case a supervisor at an outpatient clinic, to the same clinical problem.

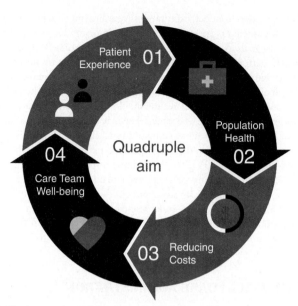

Fig. 5.2   Quadruple Aim Image—https://digital.ahrq.gov/acts/quadruple-aim.

CASE STUDY

The number of clients referred to the outpatient clinic of the Centerview Medical Center seemed to increase every week. Peter Redding, a registered and licensed occupational therapist (OTR/L), enjoyed the busy pace and the variety of clients he saw in the clinic. Peter was assigned a new client, Yongyue Wang, a 28-year-old automobile manufacturing worker who sustained a severe crush injury of his hand on the job. Peter noted that there were orders to evaluate and begin intervention. As Peter read further in Mr. Wang's medical record, he saw that the physician specifically requested a certified hand therapist (CHT) services. Peter was not a CHT, so he approached his supervisor, Vivian Gabriel, to discuss the referral. Peter explained that the physician's orders specified a CHT.

"How soon can Mr. Wang see the CHT?" Peter asked Vivian. "She's just too busy to take any new clients," Vivian responded. "I'll tell you what to do. I would hate to lose this case. It looks like it will take months of treatment to rehabilitate Mr. Wang. Why don't you just go ahead and provide services to him and have the CHT sign the notes? Who will know the difference?" Vivian then walked away.[17]

REFLECTIONS

- Rather than focusing on what Peter should do next, contrast the values underlying Peter's action, that is, refer Mr. Wang to a CHT as the physician ordered, and Vivian's alternative?
- What sort of workplace culture is Vivian encouraging or condoning through her action? In other words, what does Peter now know about his supervisor and how will that knowledge affect his relationship with her?
- What might be some possible ethically supported practical solutions for Peter and Vivian to consider?

This case is just one type of situation in which health professionals and administrators may have to negotiate decisions that are not 100% acceptable to either party. Refer to the elements of the quadruple aim and how they apply to the alternative proposed by Vivian, the supervisor. The action of encouraging Peter to treat Mr. Wang when he is not qualified to do so does not enhance the patient's experience, does not improve population health, and does not reduce cost if services are falsely charged for a CHT which Peter is not. Most importantly, this last action is insurance fraud that is illegal and unethical. Furthermore, asking a subordinate to lie and placing a patient at risk of harm from not receiving the level of care he needs could cause a great deal of stress for Peter perhaps resulting in burnout.[16] Thus none of the quadruple aims are achieved through Vivian's suggestion to deceive the patient and physician. Even if this were just a short-term remedy for the overloaded CHT situation, Vivian's action has a negative impact on the organization's culture heightened by her role as an administrator and leader within the organization. The better the communication channels and the more transparent and inclusive the development of the policies and processes for mediating tough decisions, the more likely it is that the highest possible level of mutual acceptance will be reached.

Respecting the Interface of Institutions and Society

In addition to the constraints and opportunities you, your colleagues, and your patients will experience from the design of the institution and its administrative practices and policies, your daily professional relationships in that institution also will be affected by laws and regulations that govern health care settings. The following pages illustrate some of the most widespread and important categories. They are examples only and are not intended to be up to date in all cases because the details may change at any time. For example, many states implemented different deadlines, often extending deadlines, to renew professional licenses during the COVID-19 pandemic. This sort of regulatory action and others were put in place by governors to relieve health professionals of the task of renewing their licenses during a public health emergency and retain as many professionals in the workforce as possible to deal with the increased need for their services during the pandemic. As a professional, you are responsible for keeping current with all laws and regulations regarding your profession.

LAWS AND REGULATIONS REQUIRING PROFESSIONAL COMPETENCE

To protect society from incompetent practitioners, all health care institutions that want to remain accredited by national and regional accrediting boards must take steps to ensure that their professional staff is qualified to do the work they say they can do. In the United States, laws of every state include professional licensing, certification, and registration mechanisms, whereby a person must pass a national certifying or board examination and meet other qualifying criteria to practice in that state. In other countries, provincial or national laws may be the rule. Some institutions go beyond the minimum requirements established by their government bodies by adding continuing education requirements for their professional employees. Also, national certifying bodies (e.g., specialty boards in medicine, nursing, physical therapy, occupational therapy, and other health professions) have requirements about specialized and continued competence. Today, many health professionals are personally responsible for negligence and other types of conduct that lead to malpractice claims, so institutions increasingly are requiring individuals to maintain personal malpractice insurance. These requirements should not have a negative impact on your work. They may even have a positive effect because they have been developed over the years to help ensure that the basic tenets of professional respect are maintained for all who require your services.

LAWS AND REGULATIONS TO PREVENT DISCRIMINATION

Several nondiscrimination laws developed in the second half of the 20th century continue to have a direct bearing on health care institutions in the United States, and similar ones have been crafted in other countries as well. Consider a few key historical examples:

1. *Title VII of the Civil Rights Act* (1964) prohibits employers from refusing to hire an employee based on race, color, sex, religion, or national origin. *The Equal Opportunity Act* buttressed

and expanded Title VII in 1972. The Civil Rights Act of 1991 (Pub. L. 102-166) (CRA) and the Lily Ledbetter Fair Pay Act of 2009 (Pub. L. 111-2) amend several sections of Title VII. The Employment Equal Opportunity Commission determined that transgender employees were protected under Title VII in 2012 and extended the protection to encompass sexual orientation in 2015. In addition, section 102 of the Civil Rights Act amends the Revised Statutes by adding a new section following section 1977 (42 U.S.C. 1981), to provide for the recovery of compensatory and punitive damages in cases of intentional violations of Title VII, the Americans with Disabilities Act of 1990, and section 501 of the Rehabilitation Act of 1973.[18]

2. *The Equal Pay Act of 1963* required that men and women receive equal pay for performing similar work.

3. *The Age Discrimination and Employment Act* (1967) prohibits discrimination against persons 40–70 years old.

4. *The Rehabilitation Act (Section 504) of 1973* required all employers to have an affirmative action plan that prevents discrimination based on ability. Superseding this act was the Americans with Disabilities Act of 1990, which states that institutions with more than 25 employees cannot use a physical examination to deny employment.

Understandably, laws of all types, including Executive Orders from the US President, that carry the weight of law, and policies continue to be introduced all the time; and older ones are amended and evolve. Associations for various health professions strive to keep their members up to date on new laws and policies that will impact their members' practice which is a significant help to staying current in this key area.

OTHER LAWS AND REGULATIONS THAT IMPACT HEALTH CARE SETTINGS

In addition to laws ensuring your professional competence to practice and prohibiting discrimination, others have a direct bearing on your relationship with patients. As Chapter 2 emphasized, prohibitions against some types of conduct such as touching a patient in ways not consistent with what your practice requires for diagnostic and treatment purposes, sexual intercourse with or sexual harassment of patients are often written into licensing laws, as well as reiterated in institutional policies and the ethical codes of professional organizations.

With the advent of the AIDS epidemic, numerous laws and policies were implemented nationally and within institutions to try to decrease the accidental transmittal of infections through body substances to health professionals, among patients, or to others. The most notable of these in the United States was the *universal precautions*, a federal mandate introduced in 1985 and later adjusted to be known as *standard precautions* by 1996. They require all health professionals to protect themselves and others by wearing certain types of protective clothing in treating any patient, including gowns and gloves. Goggles or other personal protective equipment (PPE) may have to be added while treating patients with infectious diseases and by adhering to strict methods for handling and disposing of body fluids, bandages, and needles. The requirements for the amounts and types of protective devices vary by the mode of transmission of the organism as was evident in the COVID-19 pandemic that required PPE to prevent airborne transmission. Of course, the obligation to follow infectious disease protocols is dependent on the availability of appropriate equipment to do so. The shortage of PPE during the COVID-19 pandemic was seen by many as society's failure of duty to care and a failure to reciprocate for the personal risk that health professionals were taking which is sometimes referred to as the fairness principle. This principle argues, "society, employers and hospitals have an obligation to keep employees safe and ensure that they are fairly treated, whether they live, get sick, or die."[19]

Depending on your area of service as a health professional, you may be regulated by other additional laws and regulations. If you work with patients or clients who have sexually transmitted or other communicable infectious diseases, you will be required to report this information to your state's department of health or a similar governing body. In the United States, if your patient population falls within reimbursement guidelines established by Medicare and Medicaid regulations, what you may offer in reimbursable services will be governed by those regulations. Private insurance also includes specific guidelines for what services are reimbursable under the benefits of a patient's policy.

Additionally, there have been dramatic changes in the number of individuals covered by health insurance since the passage of the Patient Protection and Affordable Care Act [often referred to as the Affordable Care Act (ACA)] in 2014. Before the passage of the ACA, large numbers of people—around 49.9 million in the United States in 2010—went without health insurance. The increase in coverage occurred both with private insurance (mandated by the ACA) and Medicaid (for which coverage increased in states choosing to expand coverage). As millions of people enrolled in ACA coverage, the uninsured rate dropped to historic lows in just a few years.[20]

Like many laws, the ACA faced possible changes under a new administration and presidential leadership in 2017. Proposed changes included eliminating the act all together and starting anew to other less dramatic revisions to parts of the regulations associated with the ACA. Despite the efforts to undermine the ACA, an additional 20 million Americans have health insurance largely because of the ACA. Under current law, nearly half (45%) of the remaining uninsured are outside the reach of the ACA either because they live in one of 12 states that did not expand Medicaid, they are subject to immigrant eligibility restrictions, or their income makes them ineligible for financial assistance.[20] The topic of health care as a right versus a privilege, and access to all types of health care will surely continue to be a political priority in the United States.

Laws and regulations regarding the documentation of patient status, patient progress, and other patient health information will affect the everyday practice of your profession. The medical record (whether electronic or hard copy) is a legal document, as are many other types of reports, care plans, and statements you prepare for billing, quality assurance reviews, and other activities requiring data about patients and clients. Sometimes, professionals treat documentation as a means of protecting their interests legally. However, self-interest should not be a priority when documenting a clinical encounter. Instead, think of your documentation as an accurate accounting of interactions between you and the patient. Preparation of clinical documentation, like all other aspects of your interaction within the institution, should be undertaken first with respect for the patient's dignity and rights and then with respect for the type of professional you want the world to know you are.

Although this sampling of regulations and policies is not intended to be exhaustive and focuses on the present situation in the United States, it illustrates that your relationship with society and the institution within which you practice is part of what you can do in your role as an employee and health professional.

LAWS, REGULATIONS, AND CHANGE

We conclude this section with a short reminder that laws and regulations are always in a state of flux. They deserve to be followed if you judge them to enhance your capacity to be respected and show respect in all your professional interactions. If they present significant difficulties for you practically or ethically, you should reflect seriously on how you can help bring about their change. Like every generation of health professionals before you, you have an opportunity throughout your career to help shape a better environment for the health professions by working to change unworkable, unfair, or otherwise inadequate laws, regulations, and other policies. As we introduced in Chapter 1, the professional's freedom to initiate and carry out a person-centered course for each patient is the ultimate expression of respect. All institutional activities must reflect that goal.

The process of changing unacceptable laws, regulations, and policy requires willingness, persistence, and courage. Some steps toward that end include the following:

1. Document problems diligently, both individually and as a unified interprofessional care team.
2. Gain an understanding of the informal opinion leaders and formal authorities in the type of situation you want to change within your institution or at the state or national levels.
3. Identify interprofessional colleagues and lay organizations with whom you can link arms to develop effective strategies for addressing your issue.
4. Be flexible and prepare to negotiate anew as added information comes your way.
5. Stay with the project until a change is accomplished, or you understand why it cannot be at this time.

Patients' Rights Documents

In health care institutions, patients, too, have rights and incur responsibilities. Some that are protected by law have been mentioned. However, the rights and responsibilities of patients, not addressed by legal guidelines, have been developed within health care organizations and made available to patients and families upon admission to a health facility or enrollment as a patient in an ambulatory clinic. Although such documents differ according to the mission and sponsorship of different health care entities, there is a great deal of similarity in such documents.

Rights of patients often named include the right to

1. safe, considerate, and respectful care;
2. accurate and complete information explained in a preferred language;
3. participation (directly or through a legally appointed spokesperson) in health care decisions, including the ability to ask questions and receive a timely response; and
4. privacy and confidentiality (within constraints of the law). There are also rights to information about the institution itself (e.g., who owns it and what its overall services are) and the right to have continuity of care.

Patient responsibilities often include

1. providing as complete a medical history as they can,
2. following facility rules and regulations,
3. showing respect through actions and words,
4. meeting financial commitments, and
5. working with health professionals on agreed-upon treatment plans.

Taken together, the American Hospital Association views the rights and responsibilities of patients along with expectations as the patient care partnership.[21]

All US readers of this book should also be aware of the *Health Insurance Portability and Accountability Act* (*HIPAA*) regulations, which originally went into effect in 2003. The regulations, called the *New Federal Medical-Privacy Rule*, were designed to help protect patient privacy. They have had a profound impact on health professionals and health care institutions regarding the type of confidential information that can be transmitted into medical records and other information systems. The rule also contains requirements regarding information about research subjects. The following types of details are among the most important that may *not* be photocopied or faxed without specific authorization to do so by the patient: psychotherapy records, counseling about domestic violence, sexual assault counseling, HIV test results, records regarding sexually transmitted diseases, and social work records.[22] Moreover, as a health professional you are not allowed to provide current medical status and information about a patient to third parties, even family members, without the patient's explicit consent.

The Health Information Technology for Economic and Clinical Health Act (HITECH) of 2009 expanded and strengthened these privacy laws and went into full effect in 2013. This law stipulated new obligations on covered entities, business associates, and subcontractors. The act also designated funding to expand national electronic patient records with measures.[23] The recent COVID-19 pandemic spurred the Office of Civil Rights and the US Department of Health and Human Services to issue a bulletin to ensure that HIPAA-covered entities were aware that the protection of patient privacy was still important during a pandemic. The ways patient information could be shared during such a public health emergency are as follows: "The HIPAA Privacy Rule protects the privacy of patients' health information (protected health information) but is balanced to ensure that appropriate uses and disclosures of the information still may be made when necessary to treat a patient, to protect the nation's public health, and for other critical purposes."[24]

REFLECTIONS

- Do you think the rights and responsibilities of patients should be included in nationally binding documents in your country of employment? If so, what should those rights and responsibilities include?
- What do you see as strengths and challenges with the HIPAA regulations?

Grievance Mechanisms

In recent years, several professional organizations and institutions have created grievance mechanisms to assist patients who believe their rights or other reasonable expectations are not being honored. Some institutions employ patient representatives, or ombudspersons, whose job is to listen to patients' problems and try to help solve them. Another mechanism to deal with complex decisions is institutional ethics committees that bring together health professionals and patients and their families as they try to determine what to do next in life-and-death decisions or to help resolve conflicts among various members of the group. The following case illustrates the types of differences that can arise around seemingly straightforward health policy decisions within an institution and the negative impact of such decisions on patients.

CASE STUDY

You work in a long-term care facility that recently experienced an outbreak of scabies (a highly communicable skin disease caused by an arachnid, *Sarcoptes scabiei*, the itch mite). When the usual public health measures fail to prevent new and recurring cases, the decision is made by a committee of senior health professionals in the facility to treat all patients and staff with permethrin. One patient, Cora Grosklaus, who is 82 years old, alert, and oriented, has refused the treatment. She understood the treatment process to kill the mites—that is, the permethrin cream would be applied from the neck down, left on overnight, and then washed off. This application would have to be repeated in 7 days. This treatment is the safest and most effective treatment for scabies. The scabies mite is resistant to hot water and soap. Without effective treatment, the lifecycle of the scabies mite can continue indefinitely. Regardless of the explanations, the staff has provided about the importance of the treatment for her well-being and that of others, Mrs. Grosklaus will have none of it, stating, "I will not submit to such humiliating treatment." The health professionals involved believe the measure being undertaken is to benefit Mrs. Grosklaus, as well as an important public health measure to protect others within the long-term care facility including residents and staff.[25]

Sometimes, health care institutions feel trapped by patients (or, in this case, long-term care facility residents) who refuse treatments that health professionals think are necessary for the patients' well-being. Sometimes, individuals do just the opposite of Mrs. Grosklaus and insist on treatments that health professionals believe will not benefit them or will harm them. At other times, patients insist on leaving the hospital before the treating physician thinks they are ready. In the latter case, they are said to have left "AMA"—against medical advice. They may be asked to sign a document confirming they have been informed of the physician's judgment but are choosing to act contrary to such advice. About 1.5% of patients are discharged AMA annually. These patients are often considered a vulnerable population and may have a higher risk of readmission.[26]

The good news is that great strides have been made toward recognizing and respecting patients' preferences as an integral aspect of patient-centered decision-making in health care institutions. At the same time, problems do remain. A part of the process of preparing to be a professional is to learn how to recognize, analyze, and help patients move toward an acceptable decision when differences create distress for the parties involved.

Grievance mechanisms for employees are also available. Disputes about policies or practices, salary increases, work hours, and termination of employment are frequent reasons employees seek recourse through institutional processes designed for airing their disapproval and coming to resolution.

A key area of employee protection has been implemented in recent years for personnel whose grievance involves their perception of wrongdoing by others in their institution. *Whistleblowers* disclose to a person or public body, outside the usual channels and management structure, information concerning unsafe, unethical, or illegal practices.[27] In the past, the necessity of "blowing the whistle" on an incompetent, unethical, or unsafe practice was often suppressed by the realistic fear of reprisal by the institution. If institutions develop processes and policies to protect the interests of everyone involved until the matter is investigated and resolved rather than threaten employees, there would be no need to whistle blow.[28] This is consistent with Glaser's statement in the graphic of the three realms that the good and virtuous institution "attends to the health, vigor, balance, and equity of the institution's key systems."[3] To uphold this goal, adequate mechanisms must be in place to help ensure that an employee who documents the misconduct of another employee or unsafe practices that affect the safety of patients and staff is protected.

Summary

Respect within health care institutional environments requires the cooperation and responsible participation of individuals, institutional leaders, and society. Professionals' efforts at providing high-quality care in a well-working setting will be fruitless without support from institutional leaders. At the same time, respect is so fundamental that you have an opportunity and duty to exercise it at all levels: as an individual professional, as an employee of the institution, and as a citizen. Today, numerous legal regulations and guidelines help shape health care institutions in ways that protect and honor the interests of everyone involved. When institutional policies, practices, or processes threaten to diminish or destroy a respectful environment, a professional's obligation extends to help constructively change the situation.

References

1. *In The Waiting Room, "Exodus." A Project of Open'Hood*; 2012. Retrieved from: www.whatruwaitingfor.com/2010/03/exodus.
2. Rosen MA, DiazGranados D, Dietz AS et al. Teamwork in healthcare: key discoveries enabling safer, high-quality care. *Am Psychol*. 2018;73(4):433–450. http://doi.org/10.1037/amp0000298.
3. Glaser J. *Three Realms of Ethics*. Kansas City, MO: Sheed and Ward; 1994:12.
4. Mastal M. Evolution of a conceptual model: ambulatory nursing care. *Nurs Econ*. 2018;36(6):296–299. p. 298, 300, 303.
5. Schneider B, Ehrhart MG, Macey WH. Organizational climate and culture. *Annu Rev Psych*. 2013;64:361–388, p. 361. http://doi.org/10.1146/annurev-pych-113011-143809.
6. Mannion R, Davies H. Understanding organisational culture for quality improvement. *Br Med J*. 2018;363:k4907, p. 2. http://doi.org/10.1136/bmj.k4907; published November 2018.
7. Ali E, White D, Bouchal SR, Tough S. Single room maternity care model: unit culture and healthcare team practices. *Int J Stud Nurs Sch*. 2019; 6, p. 3 Article #33. ISSN 2291-6679.
8. Braithwaite J, Herkes J, Ludlow K, et al. Association between organizational and workplace cultures and patient outcomes: systematic review. *BMJ Open*. 2017;7:e0177708.
9. Mastal M. Ambulatory care nursing: growth as a professional specialty. *Nurs Econ*. 2010;28(4):267–269. 275.
10. Kanterdahl D, Wood R, Jaén C. A method for estimating the relative complexity of ambulatory care. *Ann Fam Med*. 2010;8(4):341–347, p. 341.
11. Scott WR. *Organizations: Rational, Natural and Open Systems*. Englewood Cliffs, NJ: Prentice Hall; 1981.
12. *The Hastings Center*. The bioethics of built health care spaces. <http://www.thehastingscenter.org/the-bioethics-of-built-health-care-spaces>; 2020 Accessed February 25, 2021.
13. *Alameda Health System*. <https://www.alamedahealthsystem.org/about-us/history>; Accessed February 25, 2021.
14. *California Department of Public Health, Center for Health Care Quality*. Licensed and certified health care facilities. <https://datavisualization.cdph.ca.gov/t/LNC/views/OpenDataFacility-FacilityCounts/FacilityCounts>; 2020 Accessed February 25, 2021.
15. Fessell D, Chermiss C. Coronavirus disease 2019 (COVID-1) and beyond: micropractices for burnout prevention and emotional wellness. *J Am Coll Radiol*. 2020;17(6):746–748. [epub ahead of print]. https://doi.org/10.1016/j.jacr.2020.03.013.
16. Barnett KA. In pursuit of the fourth aim in health care: the joy of practice. *Med Clin North Am*. 2017;101:1031–1040. http://doi.org/10.1016/jmcna.2017.04.014.
17. Haddad A. Ethical issues related to orthotic provision. In: Coppard BM, Lohman H, eds. *Introduction to Orthotics: A Clinical Reasoning and Problem-Solving Approach*. 4th ed. St. Louis, MO: Mosby; 2015:440–449.
18. *U.S. Equal Employment Opportunity Commission, Title VII of the Civil Rights Act of 1964*. <https://www.eeoc.gov/statutes/title-vii-civil-rights-act-1964>; Accessed February 25, 2021.
19. Kirsch T. What happens if health-care workers stop showing up? *The Atlantic*. https://www.theatlantic.com/ideas/archive/2020/03/were-failing-doctors/608662/; 2020 Accessed February 24, 2021.
20. Garfield R, Orgera K, Damico A. *The Uninsured and the ACA: A Primer – Key Facts About Health Insurance and the Uninsured Amidst Affordable Care Act*; 2019:1. <https://www.kff.org/uninsured/report/the-uninsured-and-the-aca-a-primer-key-facts-about-health-insurance-and-the-uninsured-amidst-changes-to-the-affordable-care-act-view>; Accessed February 24, 2021.
21. *American Hospital Association*. The patient care partnership: understanding expectations, rights and responsibilities. <https://www.aha.org/other-resources/patient-care-partnership>; Accessed February 25, 2021.
22. Federal Register: 67:53182–53273, 2002 https://www.federalregister.gov/documents/2002/08/14/02-20554/standards-for-privacy-of-individually-identifiable-health-information.
23. Salz T. HIPAA: training critical to protect patient practice. *Medical Econ*. 2013;25:43–47.
24. Office for Civil Rights, U.S. Department of Health and Human Services. *BULLETIN. HIPAA Privacy and Novel Coronavirus*. Washington, DC. <https://www.hhs.gov/sites/default/files/february-2020-hipaa-and-novel-coronavirus.pdf>; 2020 Accessed February 24, 2021.

25. Smith M, Strauss S, Baldwin HJ. *Pharmacy Ethics*. Binghamton, NY: Pharmautical Products Press; 1991:534. Case adapted from p. 534.

26. Tan S, Feng J, Joyce C, Fisher J, Mostaghimi A. Association of hospital discharge against medical advice with readmission and in-hospital mortality. *JAMA Network Open*. 2020;3(6):e206009. http://doi.org/10.1001/jamanetworkopen.2020.6009.

27. Mannion R, Davies HT. Cultures of silence and cultures of voice: the role of whistleblowing in healthcare organisations. *Int J Health Policy Manag*. 2015;4(3):503–505.

28. Blair W. Supporting whistleblowers. *Kai Tiaki Nurs New Zealand*. 2019;25(8):42.

Respect for the Patient's Situation

Introduction

Section 3 examines closely the person who seeks professional services—the patient—and does so in two different but connected ways. Just as history does not exist in nature, but is created in the telling, so, too, autobiography and the patient's history emerge out of interactions, which means that they are at the same time both less and more than the "facts" of the case.[1] Chapter 6 focuses on how we understand our patients by examining the ways the patients' stories are created. Illness and injury are major events in patients' lives; at times life-altering. "Patients tell a story about a symptom or concern, its context, how it is affecting them, and why they came to the doctor."[2] Every patient shares their perspective on their illness journey in a different way. In other words, the patient's story, at least initially, belongs entirely to them.[3]

The clinical record is one place where the experience of the patient is set into words by individuals other than the patient, words that are shared with the interprofessional care team. The format, syntax, perspective, and language we use to tell the patient's story deserve your attention as much as the content. It becomes apparent that it is not enough to merely describe the chronology of events that bring patients to us.

You will want to understand why things happened the way they did, what meaning the patient gives to the experience, and what the patient expects from you. To come closer to understanding the meaning your patients give to their life experiences, you will depend on your ability to relate and communicate, which is explored in Section 4.

Chapter 7 examines the patient regarding how their intimate and close personal relationships are affected, specifically the role of traditional and contemporary families as collaborators in the patient's care. In this chapter, you will gain a better understanding of how families define themselves, how they function, and how to best interact with them across care delivery systems.

We also explore how a family's health and functioning are affected by the uncertainties of illness or injury of one of its members. Alterations in roles and responsibilities are common in close relationships, and health professionals must partner with patients and family caregivers to optimize health outcomes within the context of each family culture. Health professionals are in a unique position to help patients, families, and friends express their stressors, fears, needs, and concerns related to care, finances, and social burdens of health care.

Ask yourself the following questions as you read about the patient's story and the various relationships that make up a patient's life:

- How do my attitudes and conduct convey respect toward a patient?
- What do I need to know about patients to effectively work with them and the significant people in their lives to set reasonable patient and family-centered goals consistent with their deepest values?
- How can I best honor and support the patient in the context of their intimate and close personal relationships, their changing life roles, their culture, and their community?

References

1. Greenhalgh T, Hurwitz B. Why study narrative?. In: Greenhalgh T, Hurwirtz B, eds. *Narrative Based Medicine: Dialogue and Discourse in Clinical Practice*. London: BMJ Books; 1998.
2. Zahariais G. What is narrative-based medicine? *Can Fam Phys*. 2018;64(3):2/9. https://www.ncbi.nlm. nih.gov/pmc/articles/PMC5851389/.
3. DasGupta S. Narrative humility. *Lancet*. 2008;317(9617):980–981.

Respecting the Patient's Story

The reader will be able to

- Distinguish between the different "voices" encountered in the telling of a patient's story;
- Identify the use of narrative in health care communications to elicit the patient's perspective;
- Describe two of the contributions of narrative to respectful health professional and patient interaction;
- Discuss what a health professional can learn from a patient's account of illness or injury using a variety of literary forms;
- Relate a patient's narrative to his or her own experiences, values, beliefs, and meaning making; and
- Discuss how literary narratives about patients' and health professionals' experiences apply to improving patient-centered care.

Prelude

I flipped through the CT scan images, the diagnosis obvious: the lungs were matted with unnumerable tumors, the spine deformed, a full lobe of the liver obliterated. Cancer, widely disseminated. I was a neurosurgical resident entering my final year of training. Over the last six years, I'd examined scores of such scans, on the off chance that some procedure might benefit the patient. But this scan was different: it was my own.

I wasn't in the radiology suite, wearing my scrubs and white coat. I was dressed in a patient's gown, tethered to an IV pole, using the computer the nurse had left in my hospital room, with my wife, Lucy, an internist, at my side. I went through each sequence again: the lung window, the bond window, the liver window, scrolling from top to bottom, then left to right, then front to back, just as I had been trained to do, as if I might find something that would change the diagnosis.

We lay together on the hospital bed.

Lucy, quietly, as if reading from a script: "Do you think there's any possibility that it's something else?"

"No," I said.

P. KALANITHI[1]

For many decades, most health professionals believed that if they carefully observed a patient and listened to the patient's responses to the numerous routine questions they posed, they could arrive at an accurate clinical diagnosis and treatment plan. However, this approach to understanding the patient's experience or story to lead to effective interventions is not sufficient for several reasons. First, asking an established list of questions to arrive at a diagnosis of any type shapes the story along health care lines, not the lived experience of the patient.

Second, the patient's role is passive in this traditional model of interviewing and ignores the fact that a "new" story of what is wrong, what needs to be fixed, or what needs attention is being unilaterally created by the health professional. This chapter offers a different way of viewing what happens during interactions between health professionals and patients, as well as an understanding of the roles both play in framing the patient's story. The terms *story* and *narrative* will be used interchangeably throughout the chapter to encompass the functions of storytelling. In the health care encounter, the stories patients tell serve a special purpose, that is to share not only the facts of their illness or injury as they understand them but to also share the accompanying emotions and underlying fears and concerns that are distinct to them.

Human beings experience illness, injury, pain, suffering, and loss within a narrative, or story, which shapes and gives meaning to what they are feeling moment to moment.[2] In other words, "storytelling is a way of working out attitudes toward whom the story is about; it is a way of establishing relationship with those to whom the story is told; and storytelling is a way of learning about yourself, because you hear the story you tell."[3]

One may say that our whole lives are enacted narratives. Another way to understand this is to think about life as an unfolding story. *Narration* is the forward movement of the description of actions and events that makes it possible to later look back on what happened. And it is through that backward action that we can engage in self-reflection and self-understanding.[4] Illness and injury are often referred to as milestones in a person's life story. "The practice of medicine is lived in stories: 'I was well until . . .' 'It all started when I was doing . . .' are common openings of the medical encounter."[5]

REFLECTIONS

Think about an illness or injury "story" from your own life.
- How does your story begin?
- Is your story a tragedy or a comedy?
- Who has a starring role?
- Who has a supporting role?

All these elements of an illness or injury story tell us a lot about who you are as a person, how you see the world, and what is important to you. The same is also true of the patients you encounter in professional practice.

Much of this book has emphasized that health professionals are called into a particular relationship with patients because of the importance of an illness experience or serious injury. The setting of that relationship is the patient's story. This chapter will help you grasp the importance of paying attention to the unique and personal story of a particular patient's life beyond the more general suggestions we have offered so far. Because the final focus of all our efforts in health care is the patient, the insights that arise from listening to the patient's account of what is meaningful about an illness or injury experience are essential to delivering high-quality, compassionate care. Furthermore, narrative analysis or narrative theory can offer ways for health professionals to understand the stories that patients tell from a variety of perspectives. We highlight how different voices offer different stories of the patient's predicament. We briefly explore some of the basics of narrative theory and apply it to health care communications, such as textbooks, scientific journal articles, and the medical record. We go beyond professional, scholarly literature to the humanities to include some examples of literature such as poetry and short stories to give you an opportunity to read and think in different terms about patients' and health professionals' experiences.

Who's Telling the Story?

When a patient enters the health care system, regardless of the place of entry, an exchange of stories begins. It might be hard for you to consider the patient's "history" portion of a traditional history and physical examination to be a kind of story, but it is. So are the entries in a medical record and the scientific explanation of a particular pathological condition in a textbook. Even within the health record, for example, many individuals who are members of the health care team contribute their voices and perspectives to the single entity of the patient's health record.

Montgomery has convincingly argued that all knowledge is narrative in structure.[6] Although her work focuses on the physician and patient encounter as a story, her insights apply to all health professional and patient encounters. In these encounters, patients tell the story of an illness or injury, which Montgomery notes is an interpretive act in that the patient chooses certain words and not others and reports some incidents and not others. The health professional then interprets the story and translates it into a list of possible diagnoses. Interpretation can be influenced by many factors, including the social and scientific metaphors such as the body as "machine" metaphor. "The story's insistence on being literally true is part of that metaphor: machines are unequivocal, unevocative, reducible to components, every part accessible, parts interchangeable, tended by experts who are adjunct parts, themselves interchangeable."[7] Think about how often hearts are referred to as pumps, muscles as pistons, or the function of nerves like electrical wiring and you get the idea.

Another factor that can influence the patient's story is suggested by Frank in that the story is often guided by the health professional's notion of "getting it right." He further comments, "Diagnostic stories are about getting patients to the appropriate treatment as quickly as possible."[8] From the patient's perspective, however, getting it right may not carry the same meaning as the professionals about what is most important. For example, a patient who has a chronic illness such as multiple sclerosis might have a story that is guided by figuring out how to cope with the unpredictable nature of the disease, or a dying patient might want to address challenges to their faith. Getting to a correct diagnosis does not seem like the appropriate response to either of these patients' stories. The act of interpretation begins by really listening to what the patient is trying to say. The health professional must listen with a narrative ear.

Narrative theory helps us understand what patients are experiencing and to appreciate or adopt others' perspectives.[9,10] Narratives pull elements such as events, characters, and setting(s) together in a meaningful way. If we think about a novel as one type of narrative, the preceding explanation makes sense in that we expect that every novel will include events, characters, and setting(s) arranged in some manner. The novel will also include a plot, point of view, and motivation so we can understand why the characters act the way they do. It is only when we apply these components of narrative theory to verbal and written communication within the health care setting that things get confusing because the genres are so different. One way to help clarify the application of narrative theory to clinical practice is to begin with the narrator, or the person who tells the story. You will see that when the narrator shifts, so do the content of the story and the arrangement or prioritization of the various elements of the story.

From the Patient's Perspective

One way to highlight the different ways that the same story can be viewed is to look at it from various perspectives. For example, how is a cerebral vascular accident (CVA) seen from the perspective of the patient, written about in the medical record, and described on rounds or in a health care textbook? Before we look at these different "stories" about a CVA, consider the most basic differences in language here regarding what we call the neurovascular injury in question, a *cerebral vascular accident*, or, in common language, a *stroke*. Think of all the metaphoric meanings of the word "stroke" that are stripped away using the clinically sterile term *cerebral vascular accident*. Even this technical term uses a word that leaves room for interpretation because an accident connotes a variety of meanings. An accident is unintended, not foreseen. Think about how we would view this diagnosis if the term were cerebral vascular *event* rather than *accident*. What is the difference between an event and an accident? Next consider how health professionals distance themselves even further from the patient's experience by replacing "cerebral vascular accident" with the acronym "CVA," a shorthand that only people who speak the complex language of health care would comprehend. We will now return to the patient's perspective with a personal written account from a woman who had a stroke. She recounts her experience in the past tense. This is common because most patient stories are recollections.[11] Also, some illnesses or injuries remove or inhibit the patient's ability to speak or make sense out of what is happening at the time of the event and so they piece together a coherent story from what others provide who were witnesses to the event. The following is an excerpt from a much longer account of the stroke that changed this person's life:

> *It was an unseasonably chilly August night in 2013 around 10 p.m. and I was making a grilled cheese for my son. "That's the way this story always starts," he says now. As if he is the cause of the tale that follows. The light shining in the kitchen made the night feel closer, deeper. I was happy—the kind of dumb happiness I feel whenever Saul, who is now 29, comes to visit.*

> *The dizziness, when it hit, was brief and breathtaking, like cresting a hill on a roller coaster and surrendering to the near vertical fall. I put my head down on the counter and, before I could straighten up, the right side of my body started tingling. I felt a thousand pinpricks—as if slivers of light from a hand-held sparkler were falling on my skin. For a second, the song Needles and Pins, sung by the Searchers in 1964 flashed through my brain with the emphasis on pins just the way they sang it.*

> *As the weekend crisis counsellor at the largest trauma hospital on Vancouver Island, I know how denial functions. Still, when I called the nurse's helpline and was told to "hang up and call 9-1-1," I refused. "What's the big deal?" I thought to myself, before suggesting to my husband, Patrick, that perhaps we should go to the hospital to see if I had somehow pinched a nerve.[12]*

The description is written in the first-person voice. *Voice* is the personality of the writer coming through the words on the page. Voice can give the reader an indication of the uniqueness of the person who is speaking in the text. When a writer uses the first-person voice, it feels as if the writer is talking directly to the reader. The story begins with what could appear to be an unnecessary detail in that the patient tells us that she was making a grilled cheese sandwich for her son. Although we do not need to know this, the information gives us some insight into how the patient marked the moment the stroke began and a bit about how important her son is to her.

REFLECTIONS

- What did you notice first about the patient's story? What does the patient's choice of words (e.g., "the dizziness was like cresting a hill on a roller coaster" or "I know how denial functions") tell you about her?
- The patient is a writer. She also shares that she is a crisis counselor at a trauma hospital. What do these bits of information about who the patient is as a person mean to how you read her story?
- What sorts of emotional reactions, if any, did you have to the patient's story?
- Consider another story, this time a verbal account from a Ted Talk, from Jill Bolte Taylor, a neuroanatomist who also suffered a stroke (http://www.ted.com/jill_bolte_taylor_my_stroke_of_insight). How are these two stories about the experience of having a stroke similar or different?

We know this is not the first time the patient told the story of her stroke, because of the son's comment about how the story "always starts." However, it could be the first time that she wrote about her experience. In the telling and retelling of landmark experiences such as the trauma associated with a stroke, the story gives the reader context and meaning from the patient's unique perspective. When patients begin to tell you their story of illness, you might be able to discern whether this is a familiar, often told story or if the patient is still trying to figure out what happened and make sense of the experience. Clearly, only in retrospect could the patient know that she was in denial when she refused to call 9-1-1. She includes this information in her written account to help make sense out of her illness experiences.

The Story the Health Record Tells

Beginning with the patient's direct experience of the trauma that she has undergone, let us move forward in time to a different setting and interpretation of the story of her CVA and what is happening to her. The patient reports that when she arrived at the hospital, a CAT scan was immediately performed, then repeated later that same night with contrast dye. The admitting physician confessed that nothing showed up on the scans. Two days later, an MRI revealed that she had an acute infarct in the thalamus region of the brain or in simpler language, a stroke in a part of the brain that acts like a switchboard for movement and sensory information. In a hospital, one of the vehicles for communication between health professionals who care for a specific patient is the health record. The health record might be handwritten but is today more commonly an electronic health record (EHR). Here are three hypothetical but typical EHR entries from the first 3 days immediately following the patient's stroke: the first from the medical progress notes, the second from physical therapy, and the third from occupational therapy. Assume that the notes were written on the third day of hospitalization.

> Physician's Progress Note–7/18/20__ Dx: L ischemic infarct thalamus; Pt. stable; echo, CXR, repeat MRI; continue OT/PT for rehabilitative care.
>
> Physical Therapy Notes–7/18/20__:
>> S: Pt reports that she is feeling overwhelmed but is looking forward to walking today. "I need to get out of this bed!"
>> O: Pt. alert, oriented to person, place and time.
>> Vital signs: BP 118/76, HR 72, RR 16, O2 sat 98% on room air.
>> Bed mobility: Independent with bed mobility with use of the bed rail and v/c to use the R UE
>> Transfers:
>>> Supine to sit with min A and able to sit at edge of bed independently with CTG – Vital signs in sitting 112/72, HR 80. No reports of dizziness in sitting.
>>> Sit to stand with mod A. Manual cues to facilitate weight shift over the R LE and equal weight bearing through LEs in standing. Pt unable to tolerate standing >1 min due to reports of dizziness and lightheadedness. Standing to sitting with Mod A. Seated vitals: 102/66, HR 88. Performed bilateral ankle pumps and long arc quads in sitting. Vital signs stabilized after 2 minutes in sitting. Patient requested to return to bed. Positioned in supine with head of bed elevated.
>> A: The patient was seen today for 30 minutes to continue to address functional mobility. Progress towards balance assessment in standing and gait training was limited by symptoms associated with orthostatic hypotension although unable to obtain vital signs in standing to confirm. Pt continues to be motivated to participate in PT.
>> P: Continue progress towards STG to address identified impairments within limits of hemodynamic response.

Occupational Therapy Notes–7/18/20__:

S: "I never thought this would happen to me"

O: Pt seen this am for 30 minutes for ADL and sensory training. Pt required min A and min v/c to complete grooming and hygiene tasks (hair care, oral care, facial care) at the sink side. Pt. required min tactile cues for integration of R UE into bilateral fine motor tasks. Educated pt. in sensory protection strategies.

A: Pt is making steady progress toward functional goals. She is motivated and expressing appropriate post-CVA emotions. Insight is emerging. Excellent candidate for inpatient rehab.

P: Continue daily OT until transfer to rehab for STGs as outlined in care plan.

REFLECTIONS

- What do you notice first about these versions of the patient's story?
- Do you understand all the terms, acronyms, and language?
- Do these more objective, clinical renderings of the patient's illness give you different insights into what you can do to help the patient?
- How do these clinical narratives compare to the patient's accounts in content and tone?

Clearly, there is a difference in how the patient and health professionals describe what is going on. In Chapter 9, we discuss the use of jargon in health care and how it serves a useful purpose of facilitating communication between the interprofessional care team but can also distance patients from providers. The jargon in these sample entries from a fictitious medical record almost becomes impenetrable to a novice in the official language of health care. Did you understand the terms and abbreviations? Did you know that "echo" is shorthand for "echocardiogram" and that "CXR" is an acronym for "chest X-ray"?

Although the patient describes her experience of having a stroke in the first-person voice, the EHR refers to her in the third person. She is now "Pt.," which is shorthand for "Patient." In the assessment notes from the physical therapist, the patient is almost completely invisible in the account. We will discuss the point of view in more detail later in this chapter. It is sufficient here to note the type of voice used in writing and the implications of using a particular voice. The third-person voice distances us from what is going on in the narrative. In some ways, the EHR is an improvement over the older, paper version in that it is more accessible to health care professionals and past records can be easily retrieved. However, the EHR moves us farther away from textual accounts to drop boxes that merely require a check or click to categorize the diagnosis or problem and the plan of care from a range of standardized choices. "With the increasingly prominent role that technology and big data play in clinical interactions, the risk is that less attention will be paid to the singularity and significance of each patient's illness narrative."[13]

The fact that a patient is upset and "teary" may not be captured in a health care record that is largely based on billable categories of care. And as a result, the care of the whole patient may be overlooked as health professionals rely on prepopulated data. All health records, whether written or electronic, are essentially monologues, with each member of the health care team entering information from their individual encounters. This offers little opportunity for collaborative narrative interaction, emphasizing the importance of interprofessional teaming at the bedside.

Consider one more version of the patient's story, this one even further removed from the personal experience of a CVA. In a current medical diagnosis textbook, the clinical signs and symptoms of a cerebral vascular disease are described as follows:

Rapid evaluation is essential for use of acute treatments such as thrombolysis or thrombectomy. However, patients with acute stroke often do not seek medical assistance on their own because they may lose the appreciation that something is wrong (anosognosia) or lack the knowledge that acute treatment is beneficial; it is often a family member or a bystander who calls for help. Therefore, patients and their family members should be counseled to call emergency medical services immediately if they experience or witness the sudden onset of any of the following: loss of sensory and/or motor function on one side of the body (nearly 85% of ischemic stroke patients have hemiparesis); change in vision, gait, or ability to speak or understand; or a sudden, severe headache. The acronym FAST (Facial weakness, Arm weakness, Speech abnormality and Time) is simple and helpful to teach to the lay public about the common physical symptoms of stroke and to underscore that treatments are highly time-sensitive.[14]

What does this final version of the experience of a CVA tell you? How does this technical version mesh with the patient's account and the language in the EHR poststroke? The authors of the medical text are not concerned with a specific patient who has a stroke but write in more general terms about the critical signs and symptoms of a stroke. The description is objective, one written for health professionals—hence the use of abstract terms—and one that can be applied to all patients who suffer a stroke before moving on to a differential diagnosis of the exact kind of stroke it is, its location in the brain, etc. The symptoms are described as a matter of clinical, scientific fact, not of personal experience. You might be thinking, "Perhaps this is not all bad. A general description helps a health professional learn what to expect when a patient has had a cerebral hemorrhage." The danger lies in accepting the textbook description as "fact" or the truth as opposed to just one more interpretation of what a CVA is and means to individual patients. To assist you in scrutinizing the narratives you encounter in clinical practice, turn now to some basic concepts from narrative theory.

Awareness of Literary Form in Your Communication

When you see a poem on a page, even if you do not know anything about poetry, you recognize it as a poem because of its form and structure (i.e., the way it looks on the page). Because it is a poem, you also know that the words the poet chose are important. In poetry, every word matters. It is unlikely that you look at the writing in your textbooks, even this one, in the same way. Yet any type of written communication (whether on paper or digital) has a form and structure, subtle, or obvious. By paying attention to these aspects of the various types of written communication you encounter in clinical practice, you can develop an appreciation for how language is used and its impact on your thinking and behavior. Two assumptions from narrative theory applicable to narratives encountered in health care are that (1) language is not transparent and (2) language does not reflect the whole reality of what is going on.

LANGUAGE IS NOT TRANSPARENT

The language of narrative does not function like a clear glass that lets messages pass between sender and receiver. In other words, it is not transparent.[15] No language is neutral or "colorless." This is true of any narrative, whether it is a story, a case study, or an article in a scholarly, professional journal. Scientific writing does not call attention to itself the way language does in a poem, play, or novel. As you saw in the sample clinical documentation entries for the patient who had the CVA, there were no metaphors, similes, or figures of speech. The physical therapist didn't note, "The patient is as helpless as a newborn kitten." Yet if the therapist used this type of language, we would understand in a different way what they meant regarding the patient's vulnerability. Professional writing in health care is devoid of this kind of richer description, but it is based on and created in a particular context for a particular purpose.

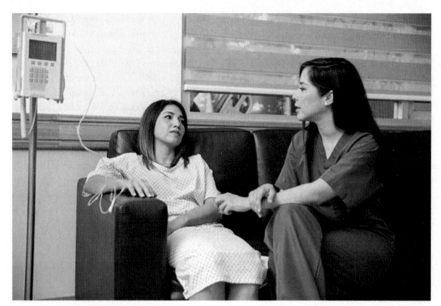

Fig. 6.1   A health professional listening while a patient shares his story. © JackF/iStock/Thinkstock.com.

In Chapter 9, you will discover that one skill you must learn in your professional preparation is to write in a technical, objective manner to communicate with other professionals.
Robert Coles describes an interaction with one of his teachers during his training as a health
professional.

> *He remarked that first-year medical students often obtain textured and subtle autobiographical
> accounts from patients and offer them to others with enthusiasm and pleasure, whereas fourth-year
> medical students or house officers are apt to present cryptic, dryly condensed, and, yes, all too 'struc-
> tured' presentations, full of abbreviations, not to mention medical or psychiatric jargon. No question:
> The farther one climbs the ladder of medical education, the less time one has for relaxed, storytelling
> reflection.*[16]

How and what one writes or conveys verbally about the patient's story of illness or injury is a
choice and should be a conscious one. Although you need to learn enough jargon to know what
colleagues are saying, you do not have to be limited by it. Rita Charon, a general internist trained
in literary theory, does not begin patient interactions with a battery of questions. Instead, she
begins her interactions this way (Fig. 6.1):

> *I find that I have changed my routines on meeting with new patients. I simply say, "I'm going to
> be your doctor. I need to know a lot about your body and your health and your life. Please tell me
> what you think I should know about your situation." And patients do exactly that—in extensive
> monologues, during which I sit on my hands so as not to write or reflexively call up their medical
> record on the computer. I sit and pay attention to what they say and how they say it: the forms, the
> metaphors, the gaps, and silences. Where will be the beginning? How will symptoms intercalate
> with life events?*[17]

REFLECTIONS

- Why do you think Charon states she has to "sit on her hands" while patients tell their stories?
- Charon uses a somewhat unusual word, "intercalate" in the last sentence of the preceding quote rather than a more familiar synonym such as "interact." How does that single word choice change the meaning of that sentence?
- What is the hardest part of listening to a patient's story for you? Why?
- What mindfulness and gratitude practices introduced in Chapter 3 might you integrate to assist you in listening with a narrative ear during your patient encounters?

There is a long-term, positive impact on sitting on one's hands and listening to patients noted in a recent study that paired medical students with volunteer patients and families over the course of the first two years of their training. Students in the study were strictly prohibited from attempting to provide medical advice or medical care to the volunteers to avoid approaching them only to obtain information for the history or to develop skills in the physical exam. Rather, the students were instructed to be fully present to hear the stories the volunteers would tell about their illness and their care. Outcomes of these interactions between student and patient were evident several years later including (1) awareness of the patient's perspective; (2) impact on how they approached patients; (3) influenced how they taught; and (4) insight into the big picture of how patients live their lives. This reinforces the quality outcomes that can result when the story is regarded as the central feature of patient-centered care.[18]

LANGUAGE CREATES REALITY

Rather than reflecting reality, language creates reality.[19] For example, without thinking much about it, most health professionals would say that a patient's history in a medical record states the case as it is. In other words, the history is simply recorded observation. Yet the language used creates the reality of the case insofar as it frames the kinds of questions, we ask about it, how we seek answers, and how we interpret what we find. It also sets limits on what we observe or even consider. Refer to the structure of the therapist's notes earlier in the chapter. Did you know what the letters S, O, A, and P that preceded the entries meant? The SOAP charting method is one way to record information in clinical records. The words being abbreviated by SOAP are *subjective* (usually a direct quotation from the patient), *objective* (the health professional's observations or description of the situation), *assessment* (the health professional's interpretation of the situation), and *plan* (actions to be taken to solve the problem presented).[20] The opening step in SOAP charting, subjective, involves interpretation on the part of the health professional because a choice is made about which quote to include among the many things patients might say if they are able to talk. If not, descriptions of gestures or other attempts at nonverbal communication might be noted in the subjective part of the SOAP notes. The quote is an important choice because it is a springboard for the rest of the entry. Furthermore, the whole structure of SOAP charting requires one to think of patients as individuals with problems that need professional resolution, which shapes our thinking about the patient and what we attend to in our interactions.

Language also can be used to exclude others. A clinical ethicist noted this manipulation of language on medical rounds:

> *As I began to watch this process more carefully, it became apparent that the physicians spoke a language which was quite understandable when they thought the ethical issues were fairly clear and where there would probably be some consensus but resorted to high code when they felt uncomfortable with the decision(s) before them or when there was dissent in the group.[21]*

So, when things were easy and comfortable within the group, everyone spoke the same language. When things get tough, providers can switch to a technical language that allows them to distance themselves from the discussion and enables them to dominate it as well.

The use of extremely technical language, or "high code," creates an atmosphere that prevents people who do not understand the key to the code from participating in the conversation. In addition, scientific language and technical information are more often highly valued than what the patient has to say, as poet and physician Jack Coulehan notes:

> *Witness the time devoted on rounds to discussing serum magnesium levels as compared to the time spent discussing the patient's experiences. When the patient's narrative (variously called "subjective," "qualitative," or "soft" data) conflicts with laboratory or radiographic findings (considered "objective," "quantitative," "hard" data), the narrative is usually given the lesser weight; it might well be ignored or minimized and the patient attacked for being a "poor historian."[22]*

Although the language may vary from profession to profession the health professional's language often tends to prevail over that of the patient.

Contributions of Literature to Respectful Interaction

Health care practice is a rich metaphor for so many archetypal human dramas, featuring such riveting themes as life and death, love and loss, and ability and disability. All these human experiences and emotions play out in different scripts, some meaningful and others trivial, each experience providing its own opportunity for wonder at the infinite capacity for human invention. There is an increasing emphasis on the use of literature, a specific type of narrative, in health professions education. A recent study by Doherty, Chan, and Knab[23] evaluated students' attitudes about a literary account of an illness experience and if they applied lessons from a common fictional reading to the delivery of patient-centered care. Several themes emerged from this narrative learning experience. Those with significance to the health professional and patient interaction include seeing family members as stakeholders, applying lessons to clinical practice to better see the patient as a person, and taking alternative perspectives to step into the shoes of the patient.[24] The premise is that studying literature about illness, death, or caregiving will help you, the student, relate more personally to patients, hear patients' stories more clearly, and make decisions that reflect a humane appreciation of patients' situations.[24] Reading novels, stories, plays, and poetry is a means of participating imaginatively in other lives; it encourages you to construct your own stories in relation to the ones you are reading. Consequently, you will come to know yourself better, too.

LITERARY TOOLS

Narrative literature, and by this we mean language used in an intensified, artistic manner, can be used to offer a fresh way for you to understand the encounter between health professional and patient. You can use some simple literary tools such as point of view, characterization, plot, and motivation to examine narrative literature and, as you have seen, the usual types of narrative writing in health care communication, such as the patient's medical record, consultants' reports, informal shift-change sharing of information and even more formal interprofessional clinical rounds in the hospital.

Point of View

Point of view is a good place to begin when reading any type of literature because it gives you an immediate sense of who is speaking to you through the poem or story. As you think about point of view, here is a simple question to get you started: Who is the narrator of the piece? Put more simply, who is telling the story? In a health record, the point of view is always third person. Health professionals commonly talk about the patient in the third person, even avoiding pronouns whenever possible; that is, the patient is referred to as "Pt." and not as "him," "her," or "them". In the excerpt from *Harrison's Principles of Internal Medicine*, 20th edition, that described the signs and symptoms of a CVA earlier in this chapter, the point of view is that of an omniscient, authoritative narrator but one who is almost invisible. The personal voice is deeply hidden in scientific and professional writing, yet it is always there and exudes authority.

Characterization

In stories that engage us, characters bring their whole intricate selves to the story. For instance, if the character in a story or a drama is a social worker, you will also learn that he is a son, maybe a husband and father, a friend, and a softball coach. You may also learn that he smokes and has tried to quit many times, cheats at cards, and loves pizza. As the narrative unfolds, you appreciate how multiple, often conflicting, interests and identities figure in the twists and turns of his motivations and decisions. You follow along, getting the feel of his prejudices, fears, passions, and pains. Then, if you are lucky, the magic of transference will take you on a journey into the story and eventually into the byways of your own life, but from some new and different angle. The lived quality of narrative is what makes it plausible. "I could be them," feels the reader. "I've been there, too." On the other hand, some characterizations can cause discomfort, which can teach us about our "unspoken, unacknowledged, and often unknown fears, biases and prejudices."[23] As you studied in the discussion of transference in Chapter 2, learning about what makes you uncomfortable is equally valuable as the characters or principles that you identify with when reading a novel, short story, or watching a play. All this knowledge has implications for your interactions with patients who may be like you or very different from you.

Plot and Motivation

Narratives of clinical interest tend toward plot in their structure rather than the more basic narrative of a simple story. In his oft-cited work, *Aspects of the Novel*, E.M. Forster explains the difference between a simple story and a plot: "in a story we say 'and then—and then'... in a plot we say 'why'?"[25] Why do the people in a clinical narrative make certain choices and act in specific ways? You can examine the motives of the individuals in clinical narratives in the same way you can those of characters in a short story or novel. Once again, you may have to try harder to find motivation in clinical narratives because so much work goes into hiding the feelings or emotional reactions of health professionals. Even emotional outbursts by patients are written to appear objective and "clinical."

POETRY

Literature written from the patient's perspective is particularly helpful to health professionals as it allows them to gain insights into the illness or disability experience. Poetry is one form of literature that deliberately calls attention to the specific words in the poem, as well as how the words are placed on the page. There are many definitions of poetry, but the following basic description of poetry perhaps captures it best: "Poetry is a type of literature based on the interplay of words and rhythm."[26] The following poem explores the poet's experiences as a patient with a colostomy. We suggest that you read the poem at least twice before reading the questions to help you appreciate it. After you have read through the poem, you should be able to recognize who is speaking, what his situation is, and to whom he is speaking. These are just a few questions to help you begin to understand the poem and find meaning to take away to help you in clinical practice.

A RARE AND STILL SCANDALOUS SUBJECT
From Susan Sontag's *Illness as Metaphor*

The title of my confession
is "Colostomy." The word,
cured and salted,
sizzles on my tongue.

This is shame:
standing naked at the sink,
unsnapping the adhesive flange
from my abdomen.

I couldn't have imagined
the stoma, the opening,
red glistening intestine.
Peristalsis moves it like a caterpillar, hatched
from a visceral cocoon.

My life depends on the stoma,
which insists on gratitude,
gurgling, "Listen to me,"
but I place my hand over it,
even now when I am alone.

R. SOLLY[27]

REFLECTIONS

- Before reading on, take each stanza in turn. What mood is the author trying to convey?
- Refer to the poem's title, "A Rare and Still Scandalous Subject." The title is taken from the book, *Illness as Metaphor* by Susan Sontag. What is the "subject" in the title the poet is talking about?
- What is it like for the narrator of the poem to live with a colostomy?
- Why is the poem a "confession"?
- How does the poem inform you as a health professional?

SHORT STORIES

A short story should be complete, which means it should have a beginning, a middle, and an ending. Stories should also have proportion (i.e., the parts of the story should be in proportion to one another). Generally, more time is devoted to the beginning than the ending. Every incident in a story must point to a solution, favorable or unfavorable, to the problem introduced at the beginning of the story.[28] However, if there is too little time dedicated to the ending, the reader may feel cheated and complain that the story was tied up too quickly at the end. The ending of story in literature diverges from real-life endings. No one can tell with complete accuracy how a patient's story will end. Although everyone knows that health professionals cannot predict the future, that doesn't stop patients from asking questions about how their story will turn out such as "Will I recover?" or "What's in store for me?" Literary stories and their endings can offer the reader insights into how others deal with loss, adversity, or uncertainty in their lives.

The same literary tools that apply to poetry also apply to fiction. It is important to understand that the narrator or voice in both poetry and a work of fiction is not necessarily the author. Authors can create reliable narrators who are involved in the story, that is, narrators who can be trusted. Of course, the opposite is also true, in which the authors can create narrators who are unreliable. Consider the following short story about a mother and daughter and a trip to the oncologist's office.

Lights Out

Rain hits the car window like paint pellets, sharp splats followed by fat circles of water that distort and gray the lines on the pavement in front of me. I've been traveling this road weekly for the last two months, and each time the stretch seems longer.

"Watch the road! My God!" my mother says. "Do you have your lights on?"

"Yes, Mom, they're on."

I hear her mumble something about not feeling safe in my car, and I cut her short. "We're almost there," I say.

"When we get to the doctor's, make sure you tuck in your shirt and put on some lipstick." She emphasizes the word lipstick by puckering her mouth and puffing her cheeks.

I focus on my breathing and keeping the car at maximum speed without hydroplaning into a ditch. My mother, Veronica, is sitting next to me, in the passenger seat. She's short of breath from her brief exchange with me. She sniffs in oxygen from the tube that connects her to the cylinder behind the seat.

That, along with her wheelchair, takes up all the space in the back of my Volvo. Every time I shift the gears, the soft spot of my elbow hits the pressure valve on the tank propped behind me. I grip the steering wheel and keep my foot firm on the accelerator until I see the green roof of the doctor's office. Then I turn onto the side street fast enough to make my mother slide over towards the door. But after I brake and twist to unbuckle my seatbelt, I feel a twinge of guilt for my speedway exit into the parking lot. My mother is looking at me with a soft gaze, the first sign that her memory has lapsed again.

"Who are you again?" she says. "Where are we?" It's barely a whisper.

"Mom, it's me, your daughter. You live with me."

This woman, my mother, whose chronically impaired lungs are now invaded by cancerous cells, pats my arm with affection. It was only yesterday that she let out a long series of expletives and pushed over the aluminum walker I asked her to use in the house. She ended her tantrum by telling me what a piss poor housekeeper I was.

I get out of the car and walk to her side with an umbrella in hand and help her out. The steps she takes from the car door to the wheelchair leave her winded. Her chest heaves up and down. I step in closer to offer my arm, and she clutches it as she pivots and sits.

"Remember, Mom? Your doctor's appointment. That's why we're here." When I squat down to put her feet on the pedals, her pupils brighten and her brow relaxes.

"Oh, that's right," she says.

"Here, let me button your coat." After getting her comfortable, I roll her into the office and with a nod from the receptionist, right into an exam room. After the doctor scans his eyes back and forth at x-rays, he confirms what I suspect, the cancer has spread. My mother's clothes hang loose, her skin has become oddly colored, and when I look in on her at night, sometimes seconds go by before I see her chest rise.

I am trying to focus on what the doctor is saying, but it's difficult to listen. She is pulling on the edge of my frayed sweater, fingering the places that have begun to pill. "Mother!" I push her hand away, but she tugs at my shirt again.

With the tip of her tongue behind her teeth, she makes the sucking sounds I've heard since my teen years when I carried an extra ten pounds of baby fat and failed to make the cheerleading squad. I put her wrinkled hand back in her lap and speak in the modulated voice I reserve for these visits. "Mom, please, the doctor is talking." I turn my attention back to him.

"Aggressive treatment for your mother would be risky at this point. Her lung capacity and tidal volume would . . ."

While he talks, my eyes dart around the room. It's the same one we were in the last time; the lilac painted walls, the plastic flowers crammed into the ceramic vase by the sink. I remember thinking how cheap they looked and wondering why the town's only oncologist couldn't afford anything better. But I can't complain. Last October he removed a tumor from her lung and got her out of the nursing home in six weeks. Today he is not speaking as confidently. He's using phrases like "in the case of an emergency" and "comfort measures."

"It's up to you to decide how to proceed. I see from our records that you have power of attorney." While handing me a stack of papers and forms, he explains options in a practiced, impartial tone. Chemotherapy. Radiation. Parenteral nutrition. Resuscitative efforts. The last paper has large type across the top, Do Not Resuscitate, with the first letter of each word bolded and underlined. I know what it means without having to read the content.

Do nothing.

I pull the DNR paper to the top and look at the doctor through narrowed eyes. Doing nothing has never been considered good enough by my mother. Crap, what I have done has never been good enough.

He gives me a pat on the shoulder and an almost sincere smile. Kneeling low so he is eye to eye with her, he praises her efforts and pats her on the hand. "You're a sweet lady, Veronica."

If he only knew.

When we leave, the rain has stopped, and I push her wheelchair through a shallow puddle.

"That man," she says, "he looked like Tyrone Powers."

I murmur absentmindedly. "Yeah, he's handsome."

She is quiet on the way back, only fidgets with her limp curls and slaps my hand when I reach to turn on the radio. Once home, I help her change into night clothes and place a heated dinner at her bedside. I get the standard wrist flick, my mother's signal for me to leave her alone. The running oxygen hisses in the background of the game show Wheel of Fortune. I am almost out the door when she clears her throat and calls me in a scratchy voice. "That man we saw."

"Yes, Mom."

"He's out of your league." She frowns. "You'll never get a man, with the way you look." She lets out a snort and turns her attention back to the contestant picking out vowels.

I shut her door and walk toward my bedroom on the other side of the house. As I pass through the kitchen, I stop to sign the DNR forms on the counter. Then I turn off the lights.[29]

REFLECTIONS

- Recall the concept of characterization in stories. As the story unfolds, how do multiple, often conflicting, interests and identities figure in the twists and turns of the daughter's motivations and decisions?
- Who is the narrator in the story and what does that perspective offer in the telling of the story?
- How did the ending of the story impact you, if at all? Were you surprised, sad, angry? Explain your reaction.
- How might this story impact your future patient/caregiver interactions?

The story form of narrative expands beyond the basic facts of most health care interactions into the experience of the event, creating an opportunity for reflection on your reaction to challenging patients and families.

ILLNESS STORIES/PATHOGRAPHIES

A third type of literary narrative is the *pathography*, a form of autobiography or biography that describes personal experiences of illness, treatment, and sometimes death. "What it is like to have prostate cancer," or "How I live with multiple sclerosis," or "What it means to have AIDS" are examples of the typical subjects of pathography that help us understand the experience of illness and endow it with meaning.[30] Pathographies are commonly of the testimonial type in which the author offers uplifting advice and guidance to others who are faced with the same disorder or problem that they, seemingly, have conquered or have come to peace with.

A particularly interesting form of pathography is those written by health professionals who become patients. The insights gained by health professionals who are patients are often dramatic. For example, the prelude that opened this chapter was written by Paul Kalanithi, a neurosurgeon who was diagnosed with stage IV lung cancer in 2013. Despite his illness, he completed his residency and continued to care for patients. He had a passion for literature and writing and contributed several essays to the New York Times and Washington Post about his illness journey and mortality that reached a very wide readership. His memoir published after his death in 2015 at the age of 37, *When Breath Becomes Air*, became a nonfiction best-seller.

The Internet allows for, and perhaps encourages, an interactive and public form of pathography in the form of blogs and websites. For example, shortly after Stephanie Chuang, a 31-year-old reporter in San Francisco learned that she had stage 3 non-Hodgkin's lymphoma, she founded a website called The Patient Story (www.ThePatientStory.com/founder-story). The purpose of the website was not to offer uplifting testimonies but to provide patients with a similar diagnosis "insider" information about the patient experience and the opportunity to share their experiences. www.thepatientstory.com/patient-stories[31]

Pathographies offer you yet another type of narrative to provide you with insights into the experiences of patients in their everyday lives without being prestructured by other actors in health care.[32]

Where Stories Intersect

After exploring all the various ways a story can be told, you might wonder: "What is the true story?" The health professional must listen carefully to the patient's story but also understand that the patient does not know the "whole truth" either. There are clearly differences between the patient's experience and the health care professional's explanation of the experience. So how do we get coherence, if not the true story? The first step to a coherent, richer account could be to recognize the dialogical nature of narrative that includes the exchange of ideas and opinions as Frank affirms:

> We tell stories that sound like our own, but we do not make up or tell our stories by ourselves; they are always co-constructions. Stories we call our own draw variously on cultural narratives and on other people's stories; these stories are then reshaped through multiple retellings. The responses to these retellings further mold the story until its shape is a history of the relationships in which it has been told.[8]

The kind of exchange described by Frank among a patient, health professionals, and family members produces a fuller interpretation of the patient's story than any one person could produce, including the richest account a patient could offer.[33-35] Viewing the interview process as "building" a history rather than "taking" a history from a patient is a step in the right direction. Building suggests collaboration and the positive outcome of mutual work rather than taking something from the patient and making it your own.[36]

Summary

Literary explorations of the subjective and interpersonal responses of patients, family members, and health professionals to the tensions encountered in health care settings can engage you in your own personal questions and reflections about your response to similar situations in professional practice. Narrative, in all its forms, offers a way of seeing the deeper, subtle nuances involved in your interactions with patients, families, and peers, thereby improving the chances that the opportunities for showing them due respect are not missed or behaviors misguided.

Your role in your patients' stories will vary from assisting them to recover to witnessing their deaths. Whatever roles you take, recall that you also bring your own unfolding story to the relationship. You will build a story with each patient you encounter that becomes another part of the unfolding narrative of both of your lives.

References

1. Kalanithi P. *When Breath Becomes Air*. New York: Random House; 2016:3–4.
2. Donald A. The words we live in. In: Greenhalgh T, Hurwirtz B, eds. *Narrative Based Medicine: Dialogue and Discourse in Clinical Practice*. London: BMJ Books; 1998.
3. Frank A. Not *whether* but *how:* considerations on the ethics of telling patients' stories. *Hastings Cent Rep.* 2019;49(6):13–19, p. 13.
4. Churchill LR, Churchill SW. Storytelling in the medical arenas: the art of self-determination. *Lit Med.* 1982;1:73–79.
5. Hatem D, Rider EA. Sharing stories: narrative medicine in an evidence-based world. *Patient Educ Couns.* 2004;54:251–253.

6. Hunter KM. *Doctors' Stories: The Narrative Structure of Medical Knowledge*. Princeton, NJ: Princeton University Press; 1991.

7. Gadow S. Whose body? Whose story? The question about narrative in women's health care. *Soundings: An Interdisciplinary Journal, Fall/Winter* 1994;77(3-4):295-397, p. 298.

8. Frank AW. From suspicion to dialogue: relations of storytelling in clinical encounters. *Med Humanit Rev.* 2000;14(1):24–34.

9. Bruner J. *Acts of Meaning*. Cambridge, MA: Harvard University Press; 1990.

10. Charon R. *Narrative Medicine: Honoring Stories of Illness*. New York: Oxford University Press; 2008.

11. Robinson JA, Hawpe L. Narrative thinking as a heuristic process. In: Sarbin TR, ed. *Narrative Psychology: The Storied Nature of Human Conduct*. New York: Praeger; 1986.

12. Joseph E. How a stroke changed how writer Eve Joseph views herself. *The Globe and Mail*. January 9, 2015.

13. Milota MM, van Thiel GJMW, van Delden JJM. Narrative medicine as a medical education tool: a systematic review. *Medical Teacher.* 2019;41(7):802–810, p. 810. https://doi.org/10.1080/01421 59X.2019.1584274.

14. Smith W.S., Johnston S., Hemphill III J. Cerebrovascular diseases. In: Jameson J, Fauci AS, Kasper DL, Hauser SL, Longo DL, Loscalzo J, eds. *Harrison's Principles of Internal Medicine, 20e*. McGraw-Hill; 2018. https://accessmedicine-mhmedical-com.cuhsl.creighton.edu/content.aspx?bookid=2129&section id=192531947; Accessed March 19, 2021.

15. Donley C. Whose story is it anyway? The roles of narratives in health care. *Trends Health Care Law Ethics.* 1995;10(4):27–31.

16. Coles R. *The Call of Stories: Teaching and the Moral Imagination*. Boston, MA: Houghton Mifflin; 1989.

17. Charon R. Narrative medicine: attention, representation, affiliation. *Narrative.* 2005;13:261–270.

18. Stojan JN, Sun EY, Kumagai AK. Persistent influence of a narrative educational program on physician attitudes regarding patient care. *Medical Teacher.* 2019;41(1):53–60. p. 54.

19. Weed LL. Medical records that guide and teach. *N Engl J Med.* 1998;278:593–600.

20. Rogers J. Being skeptical about medical humanities. *J Med Humanit.* 1995;16(4):265–277.

21. Coulehan J. Pearls, pith, and provocation: teaching the patient's story. *Qual Health Res.* 1992;2(3):358–366.

22. Doherty RF, Chan P, Knab M. Getting on the same page: an interprofessional common reading program as foundation for patient-centered care. *J Interprof Care.* 2018;20:1–8.

23. Davis C. Poetry about patients: hearing the nurse's voice. *J Med Humanit.* 1997;18(2):111–125.

24. Wear D, Aultman JM. The limits of narrative: medical student resistance to confronting inequality and oppression in literature and beyond. *Med Educ.* 2005;39:1056–1065.

25. Forster EM. *Aspects of the Novel*. New York: Harcourt, Brace; 1927.

26. Literary Terms. Literary terms. https://literaryterms.net/; 2015 Accessed March 24, 2021.

27. Solly R. *A rare and still scandalous subject*. (Unpublished. Reprinted with permission of the author's daughter.)

28. Mueller L, Reynolds JD. *Creative Writing: Forms and Techniques*. Lincolnwood, IL: National Textbook; 1992.

29. Bartlett S. Lights out. *Bellevue Literary Rev.* 2014;14(36, Number 1); New York: 2014:146–149.

30. Hawkins AH. *Reconstructing Illness: Studies in Pathography*. West Lafayette, IN: Purdue University Press; 1993.

31. The Patient Story: Human Answers to Your Questions About Cancer. www.thepatientstory.com/patient-stories. Accessed October 13, 2022.

32. van de Bovenkamp HM. Understanding patient experiences: the powerful source of written patient stories. *Health Expect.* 2020;23:716–717.

33. Poirier S, Rosenblum L, Ayres L, et al. Charting the chart—an exercise in interpretation(s). *Lit Med.* 1992;11(1):1–22.

34. Brody H. "My story is broken, can you help me fix it?" Medical ethics and the joint construction of narrative. *Lit Med.* 1994;13:85–87.

35. Manoogian MM, Harter LM, Denham SA. The storied nature of health legacies in the familial experience of type 2 diabetes. *J Fam Commun.* 2010;10:40–56.

36. Haidet P, Paterniti DA. "Building" a history rather than "taking" one: a perspective on information sharing during the medical interview. *Arch Intern Med.* 2003;163:1134–1140.

Respect for the Patient's Family and Significant Relationships

OBJECTIVES

The reader will be able to

- Define family and discuss the role of the family as collaborators in care delivery;
- Identify five realms of family health that can lend insight into family and patient dynamics;
- Make several suggestions that will help support healthy functioning in families experiencing illness or disability;
- Identify three major stressors patients and their loved ones may encounter as they experience possible alterations in their close relationships during illness or injury;
- Understand the role of family and friends as informal caregivers, including the benefits and burdens of this role;
- Distinguish the role of health care professionals as advocates for patients and families faced with the social and financial burdens related to health care; and
- Describe opportunities to assist patients in their attempts to strengthen and revitalize their significant relationships.

Prelude

A special pattern of communication developed between Robin and Mark (her father) during his hospitalization. Each morning Mark phoned home to tell her about the animal picture on the sugar packet that he had saved from his breakfast tray. One morning Robin explained to Mark that she had a cold, and then, with 3-year-old directness, asked, "What do you have, Daddy?"

After a pause he replied, "I have cancer."

She handed the phone to me and said, "I think Daddy's crying." Though he had never hesitated to discuss his illness with others who asked, he was deeply shaken by the weight of Robin's question and the implications of his answer.

S.A. ALBERTSON[1]

In this excerpt from a book portraying a young family coping with the fatal illness of a father and husband, we suddenly see a moment when the patient breaks down unexpectedly, touched deeply by the implications of his beloved young daughter's innocent question. The personal life of a patient exists in a web of activities and intimate or close personal relationships that help provide status, meaning, support, and belonging. Respect for this fact is immensely important if you are to reach the goal of maintaining the patient's dignity and achieving a truly caring response during your professional interactions with patients and families.

This chapter focuses attention on patient relationships and family. In today's society, the patient identifies who "family" is and determines how they will participate in their care and decision-making. In times of illness or injury, a patient's relationships with family, close friends, business associates, neighbors, and others who are important to the patient are greatly affected. Special attention in this chapter is devoted to family members or other persons who become caregivers for the patient because their relationship is often dramatically challenged by illness or injury. We offer suggestions about how and when you can become a source of support and encouragement to a patient and those close to them as they go through stressful and often difficult times.

Family: An Evolving Concept

Mainstream health care in the United States has evolved from a system focused primarily on the patient as the sole recipient of care to attending to the entire family as the focus of care. Today we know how important it is to care for patients, especially youth and elders, in the context of their families. The family is implicitly and explicitly recognized as a critical context surrounding and influencing its members and, in turn, being influenced by its members. Care can best be accomplished if it is considered a collaborative venture between the family and the interprofessional care team. Patient- and family-centered care is "an approach to the planning, delivery, and evaluation of health care that is grounded in mutually beneficial partnerships among health care providers, patients, and families."[2] This approach leads to better health outcomes, improved patient and family care experiences, increased patient satisfaction, decreased clinician burnout, and wiser allocation of resources.[3-5] The components of patient- and family-centered care in Box 7.1 provide a context for recognizing the family's central role. If you are to work with families as collaborators in maintaining the health of family members who are injured or are experiencing acute or chronic illness, you must understand how families define themselves, how they function, and how best to interact with them.

Family Defined

The term *family* has been defined in a variety of ways. One notion of what constitutes a family is influenced by values, culture, upbringing, and occupations or professional perspectives. The most common type of familial bond is traditionally through spousal and blood relationships. Families may include several generations of blood kin, a mix of stepparents and children, or a combination

---

BOX 7.1 ■ Core Concepts of Patient- and Family-Centered Care

1. *Dignity and Respect.* Health care practitioners listen to and honor patient and family perspectives and choices. Patient and family knowledge, values, beliefs, and cultural backgrounds are incorporated into the planning and care delivery.
2. *Information Sharing.* Health care practitioners communicate and share complete and unbiased information with patients and families in ways that are affirming and useful. Patients and families receive timely, complete, and accurate information to effectively participate in care and decision-making.
3. *Participation.* Patients and families are encouraged and supported in participation in care and decision-making at the level they choose.
4. *Collaboration.* Patients and families are also included on an institution-wide basis. Health care leaders collaborate with patients and families in policy and program development, implementation, and evaluation; in health care facility design; and in professional education, as well as in the delivery of care.

Reprinted with permission from the Institute for Patient- and Family-Centered Care: http://www.ipfcc.org.

of friends who share in household responsibilities and childrearing. An area of growth in family units over the last decade is same-gendered parents, and the shift from nuclear to extended families.

As society evolves through scientific and social advances, it must redefine what is meant by "family." New Mexico's Memorial Task Force on Children and Families and the Coalition for Children offers the following definition:

> We all come from families. Families are big, small, extended, nuclear, multigenerational, with one parent, two parents and grandparents. We live under one roof or many. A family can be as temporary as a few weeks, as permanent as forever. We become part of a family by birth, adoption, marriage, or from a desire for mutual support. As family members, we nurture, protect, and influence one another. Families are dynamic and are cultures unto themselves, with different values and unique ways of realizing dreams. Together, our families become the source of our rich cultural heritage and spiritual diversity. Each family has strengths and qualities that flow from individual members and from the family as a unit. Our families create neighborhoods, communities, states, and nations.[6]

REFLECTIONS

- Who do you consider to be the members of your family?
- Name two ways your family contributes to your health and two ways your family distracts from your health.
- If you were acutely ill, which member of your family would you call first and why? How does this family member support you in your day-to-day life?

A definition of family should be inclusive and allow the members to define themselves as a family unit, acknowledging the variety of cultural styles, values, and alternative structures that are part of contemporary family life. In fact, families define a unique culture—that is, a unique behavioral complex that is socially created, readily transmitted to family members, and potentially maintained through generations.[7]

Family Structure and Function

Family structure and function have important influences on health. Family structure involves the characteristics that make a family distinct. This includes family composition and household roles. According to the latest US Census, the average household size was 2.53. Of the households, 39% included people under 18 years, and 29% included people 65 years and over. Multigenerational family households (three generations of relatives or more living together) are on the rise, as are unmarried partner households.[8]

To work with families, you also must understand how families function. An individual's physical and emotional health and cognitive/social functioning are strongly influenced by how well the family functions.[9,10] There are numerous family theories describing how families operate and how they respond to events both internal and external. Most health professionals use a combination of family theories in their work with families, but all have in common the fact that the focus of health care shifts from the individual member who is ill, injured, or disabled to the family as a unit of care. In this chapter, we focus on a particular method of viewing the family—the family health system approach.[11] According to this approach, care is directed toward five processes: (1) interactive, (2) developmental, (3) coping, (4) integrity, and (5) health. The Case Study of Ian will help show how the family health system model applies to a particular child and his family.

Ian is a low-birth-weight infant with short bowel syndrome (SBS). SBS is characterized by maldigestion, malabsorption, dehydration, electrolyte abnormalities, and both macronutrient and micronutrient deficiencies. Owing to new interprofessional approaches and advances in medical and surgical treatments, the SBS survival rate has improved from an average of 70%, to as high as 90% in recent studies.[12] Ian will require long-term parenteral nutrition (PN); that is, he will not be able to take food orally and will be dependent on intravenous solution to provide the bulk of his nutritional needs. Ian is the first child of Dylan and Adrianna Chapel, both in their early 30s. After a stay in the neonatal intensive care unit, Ian was sent home with his parents, who have provided care since that time with the help of a home care agency and a nutritional support company. The Chapels do not have other family members nearby. Most of Ian's care falls to them.

Ian is now an active 2-year-old. Mrs. Chapel is the primary caregiver during the day and most evenings. She works weekends as a nursing assistant at a local assisted living center to supplement their family income. Mr. Chapel works as a paralegal in a law firm and attends law school at night. The Chapels' insurance coverage is through a group plan at the law firm where Mr. Chapel works.

Assume you are assigned to work with the Chapel family during an on-site educational experience with the home care agency providing primary care. The goal of your interaction with Ian and his family is to help promote family adaptation to his chronic condition (SBS) and empower the Chapels to develop and maintain healthy lifestyles. By reviewing the five processes listed earlier, you can get a picture of the family's functioning and possible areas for intervention.

INTERACTIVE PROCESS

The *interactive* process of the family is composed of communication, family relationship, and social supports.[10] In your assessment of the interactive process of the Chapel family, you will explore the types of communication patterns they use; the effect of Ian's illness on the communication of the family both internally and externally; the types of relationships within the family; and the quality, timing, amount, and nature of social support they receive. Open communication should be encouraged. One aspect of care could be to assist the Chapels in mobilizing the informational and emotional support they need to cope with Ian's illness. Because the Chapels do not have family support in the immediate community, they may have to rely on informal support systems, such as friends, members of their faith community and coworkers, and formal support systems, such as respite care agencies, to assist them in the care of their child. Perhaps, there are other children who have SBS or who must rely on PN in the community. The caregivers of such children may have or could form a support group to help troubleshoot common problems and offer advice, including online and telehealth groups which provide support across a variety of geographic areas and time zones.

DEVELOPMENTAL PROCESS

Assessment of the developmental process includes the family developmental stage and individual developmental stages. The Chapels, as a family, are in the second stage of family development as described by Duvall in his classic work.[13] Stage II of the family life cycle involves integrating an infant into the family unit, accommodating new parenting roles, and maintaining the marital bond. Ian is moving from infancy to becoming a toddler, and soon he will be increasingly interested in his environment and want to explore it. Ian will become increasingly mobile and develop language during this stage. (You will be introduced to basic development needs of toddlers later in Chapter 10.) All of this is influenced by the presence of his chronic condition.

It is appropriate for you as a member of the interprofessional care team to assess how well developmental tasks are being achieved. You will educate the Chapels in the developmental milestones Ian should achieve and the tasks involved. For example, Ian needs freedom of mobility to explore objects in his environment and learn to walk, so his nutritional solution could be placed in a backpack to allow him to move more freely. Children with SBS also may require frequent visits to the bathroom throughout the day when the time comes for toilet training. To decrease the Chapels' frustrations, you could plan for this next developmental milestone and work with them to plan a structured routine that is consistently implemented and results in success for all involved, especially the child. There is some evidence that children with SBS experience lower health-related quality of life and neurological or developmental delays.[14,15] Thus you will also want to watch for possible developmental delays to plan for early therapeutic interventions.

COPING PROCESS

Coping has been identified as problem-solving, adaptation to stress and crisis, and management of resources.[11] Coping helps us lower our anxiety so that we can meet the demands of the day. Each person has a different coping style when dealing with uncertainty. Coping styles can be both problem focused and emotion focused. In general, coping styles depend on what a person is like as a person and their role in the family.[16] The uncertainty of illness presents a variety of stressors for families. In your work with the Chapels, you should assess their ability to handle stress and the impact that Ian's illness has on everyday activities while reinforcing a coping style fitting for them.

REFLECTIONS

Which of these questions would most help you show respect for the Chapel family?
1. How do the Chapels conceptualize and manage Ian's diagnosis as a family? What meaning does it have?
2. Has Ian's illness caused a change in the family's life plans? For example, did Mrs. Chapel plan on returning to full-time work outside the home after the birth of her son?
3. If the family planned on Mrs. Chapel returning to work, can the family adapt to the loss of income, or are support services available to allow Ian to be cared for during the day so that Mrs. Chapel can work?
4. Were the Chapels intending to have several children? Have Ian's care needs changed their family planning?
5. What else do you need to know to care for the Chapel family?

Overall, you would want to assess how the family deals with crises in general. You can support the Chapels' coping processes by
   1. offering advice on the progression of the illness;
   2. discussing the normal feelings of frustration and guilt that accompany the care of a chronically ill or disabled family member; and
   3. offering resources to help the family cope more effectively, such as respite care and other support groups.

The Chapels will also have to cope with financial stressors. Even with the best health insurance, there are lifetime limits on coverage; in addition, there are many out-of-pocket expenses related to the care of a child with this diagnosis. Although most children experience small bowel adaptation over time and can be weaned from PN, some children suffer liver dysfunction, and many require extensive intestinal rehabilitation, including intestinal lengthening procedures and transplantation.[12,17] Thus the Chapels may be facing years of out-of-pocket expenses and expensive hospital stays, procedures, and medications. This kind of financial pressure can be stressful for any family.

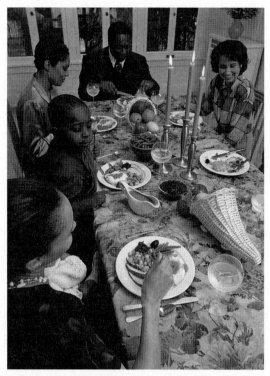

Fig. 7.1 The process of family life involves family values, rituals, history, and identity. © Ryan McVay/Photodisc/Thinkstock.com.

INTEGRITY PROCESS

The integrity process of family life involves family values, rituals, history, and identity.[11] These aspects of the family process greatly affect its behavior. Family rituals, one facet of the *integrity* process, provide a useful framework for building a family's resilience and integrity.[18] Family rituals include celebrations and traditions such as activities surrounding birthdays, religious holidays, or bedtime routines for children (Fig. 7.1). Suggestions for evaluating family rituals include assessment of the following[19]:

1. *Does the family underuse rituals?* Families who do not celebrate or mark family changes such as birthdays, deaths, anniversaries, and so forth may be left without some of the benefits that accompany rituals, such as bringing the family together or marking changes in life and family roles.
2. *Does the family follow rigid patterns of rituals?* In families who are inflexible, things are always done the same way, at the same time, and with the same people. Families who are rigid may have difficulty responding to changes that disrupt routines and rituals occasioned by illness and injury.
3. *Are family rituals skewed?* A family with skewed rituals tends to emphasize only one aspect of family life (e.g., religion) and ignore others. For example, a family might spend all its time celebrating with one side of the family on religious holidays and ignore the different rituals cherished by the patterns practiced on the other parent's side.
4. *Has the ritual process been interrupted?* For example, a child born with a physical or cognitive impairment or congenital condition may threaten family identity and permanently

disrupt family rituals. In the case of the Chapels, they have elected to stay home for traditional family holidays because almost all holidays involve a focus on food. For the foreseeable future, Ian cannot tolerate most food orally, so the Chapels should consider what this interruption in ritual means to their life together and may have to develop other rituals at holiday time that do not focus so prominently on food.

5. *Are the rituals hollow?* Rituals performed just for the sake of performing them have lost their lives and may be stressful for the family rather than a source of joy and strength.

In addition to changes in ritual that occur over time in families, many role changes also occur, particularly when chronic illness or impairment is involved. For example, Mrs. Chapel has become the primary caregiver. She may or may not have expected to take on this role. Essential interventions include helping the Chapels redefine major family roles and maintain their new responsibilities.

HEALTH PROCESS

The final process of family experience is related to health. This process includes health status, health beliefs and practices, and lifestyle practices.[11] Assessing a family's definition of health and how they define the health of the individual members is a key step in this process.

REFLECTIONS

- Given the responsibilities involved in caring for a child who requires parenteral feedings, what might the Chapels do to maintain their own health?
- In what ways could the Chapels deal with health problems? To whom might they turn?

Interventions in the health process include education, encouragement, and counseling regarding the short- and long-term aspects of Ian's care. The situation of Ian and his parents illustrates the family health system as one useful approach to the care of patients and families. The family health system applies to all families, whatever the composition and stage of familial development as one of its primary goals is to improve health outcomes. This approach, along with patient and family engagement strategies to support patient self-management, patient–provider communication using shared decision-making, and mobile health and electronic health record tools to improve collaboration have strong evidence linked to health outcomes in the care of chronic conditions.[20] You are encouraged to explore other models of working with a family and their effectiveness in achieving optimal family health. Regardless of the model you choose, it is clear that family relationships are an important consideration in understanding the conduct of any patient and for developing an effective mode for respectful interaction with that patient.

Facing the Fragility of Relationships

At this point in your training, you are acutely aware that living with illness or disability is not just an individual journey but one that has a profound impact on a patient's friends and family. Families are deeply influenced by the health and wellness of each member of the familial unit, so any significant change in a person has the power to alter their status and roles in various relationships. When one person in a relationship changes, everyone must pull together to adapt and balance family functioning. As patients become aware of changes, they often express concerns of abandonment or fears that they will be unable to contribute to their key relationships in meaningful ways. Whatever else characterizes close relationships during times of illness or injury, one sure thing is that there will be stress. *Stress* usually conjures up only negative feelings, and dictionary definitions support this meaning. But psychologists and others have probed the dynamics of what happens when the stakes are high or the chips are down: Stress is, at its core, a psychological motivator. Stress can have results that are destructive or that enhance individuals and relationships. Rambur and colleagues[21] divide stressful experiences and conditions into negative outcomes of *distress* and positive ones of *eustress*. In this section, we ask you to consider some areas of potential distress with some suggestions for helping all involved to realize eustress opportunities as well.

Concern That Others Will Lose Interest

The social functions and activities that partners, families, and friends enjoy with others can dwindle with illness, isolating the patient and caregivers from familiar sources of enjoyment and their feeling of belonging within their larger communities. Most hope that our families, friends, and associates will take our problems to heart—fortunately, they usually do. However, sometimes patients are unpleasantly surprised by the degree of indifference they feel many people show to the struggle they went—or are going—through. The loss of a job can further distance patients from longtime associates and patterns. For many, it is easier to stay away than to face the hard realities with the affected persons. Internal divisions within families also may erupt, often over differing hopes and expectations about who will take responsibility for various aspects of caregiving. The patient may begin to feel as if they have caused all the distress and withdraw further from contributing to the vitality of key relationships.

Fear and Avoidance

Unfortunately, a special burden falls on relationships when the patient has a condition that carries a social stigma of some sort. Loss of a social life may be accompanied by a loss of status. In most such cases, what appears to be a loss of interest may be an even deeper disdain and rejection. People who have a diagnosis of substance use disorder are prime examples of such a group who (by virtue of their illness) may lose their social life or job security. Although great strides have been made in the United States and elsewhere to educate about recovery, and laws and policies have been put in place to prevent discrimination against the person and family, this disease still has the power to marginalize patients and their loved ones from their communities and important relationships.

Social stigma toward individuals with substance use disorders exceeds stigma toward those with mental illnesses or physical disabilities across cultural contexts.[22] Unfortunately, it is also common for health professionals to have negative attitudes toward individuals with substance use disorders, contributing to suboptimal health care.[23] Sometimes, people close to the patient are also expected to feel ashamed for accusations that they had a role in allowing, causing, or worsening a patient's predicament. An example was relayed to us by a colleague who was traveling in another city when her adult son overdosed. She recalls the following conversation on hearing the news that her son was in the intensive care unit:

Hospitalist: Your son has overdosed and is in the intensive care unit.

Woman: Oh my, no! What happened?

Hospitalist: [Explains some medical details.] Was he well when you left?

Woman: He seemed fine! We know he struggled with abstinence in the past, but thought it was under control since he has been under the care of the addictions team. [More questions about his condition.]

Hospitalist: His primary care doctor has told me that he has had trouble staying on his treatment program in the past. Has he been attending his check-ins and support group?

Woman (still shaken): I think so! I've been traveling for a week but . . ..

Hospitalist: Oh, yes. Young adults often fall off the wagon when their parents are away.

The woman said that, whether or not the doctor was intentionally trying to shame her for not being there when her son overdosed, just by that conversation she was afraid she would be shunned by his professional caregivers.

What can you do in your role to help decrease the deleterious effects of others' loss of interest or shunning of the patient or loved one? Some straightforward suggestions include the following:

1. Listen to your own comments with a reflective third ear to think about how they might be coming across to the patient or caregivers. Do they sound off-putting? Blaming?
2. Facilitate contact with patient and/or family support groups of similarly affected persons.
3. Be prospective as a resource, suggesting additional supports available at your worksite such as religious counselors, psychologists, or social workers who are skilled in dealing with the negative stresses caused by the situation.
4. Speak up to counter destructive shame-inducing attitudes and behaviors in the larger society.

You may think of other ways to decrease the distress related to both patients and their loved ones who are concerned about real or imagined loss of interest by others or who are feeling shunned and therefore increasingly isolated.

Weathering the Winds of Change

Patients also justifiably worry about other relationship-related effects of serious illness or impairment from injury. Unfortunately, the change a person undergoes during illness or injury may in some cases cause them to become almost a stranger to loved ones.[24] In extreme cases, the established patterns of old relationships become unrecognizable in the present situation. For example, a spouse who sustains a traumatic brain injury may act like a child; a longtime business partner with bipolar disorder may become suspicious toward trusted associates, or clients; or a young firefighter known for his bravado may become fearful of hanging out with the guys after a heart attack, convinced they will see him as a has-been.[25]

REFLECTIONS

Think about a relationship you hold dear—and would count on the most—if you were to become a patient with a serious illness or injury.
- What do you think would be your greatest worry in terms of the changes you knew your condition could impose on your loved one?
- List one or two people you could call on to help you and the other person make it through the hard times of such a change.

Now put yourself in the position of a family caregiver for your loved one.
- What type of condition might be the greatest challenge to your relationship as it now stands? Why (i.e., what values and behaviors have seemed to sustain the "core" of the relationship during other stressors)?
- How might you build your resilience in coping with these relationship stressors?

These types of exercises can help you imagine the challenges and concerns patients and their closest resources are facing and sympathetically acknowledge that most people must navigate stresses in their intimate relationships when one person in it is changed by illness or injury. This recognition is extremely important because all too often the health of family or other caregivers has been ignored to the detriment of everyone involved, especially when the new situation requires an intense, long-term (or even lifelong) commitment. You may ask how important it is for you in your professional caregiver role to gain an understanding of the family or close friend caregiver's situation. The answer is extremely important. The US Department of Health and Human

Services estimates that family and friend (called *informal*) caregiver services will be one of the biggest changes this society will see as the baby boomer generation ages. Informal caregivers provide assistance with a variety of health-related tasks, including assisting family and friends with self-care and other activities of daily living, cooking and home management tasks, transportation, medication management, medical encounters, and financial activities such as bill paying. In 2019 alone, more than 1 in 5 Americans (21.3%) provided care to an adult or child with special needs at some time in the past 12 months.[26] Recent data on informal caregivers reveal that 34 billion hours of care were provided to adults with limitations in daily activities. The estimated economic value of their unpaid contributions was approximately $470 billion.[27]

The majority of informal caregivers provide care for a relative or loved one. Although most caregivers are adults there are increasing numbers of teenagers who serve in this role. Most family caregivers rise to the occasion with remarkable courage, good spiritedness, and, if all else fails, resignation. Despite this, physical, emotional, and financial demands of caregiving can be high.

Positive outcomes of caregiving include a sense of meaning, the confidence that one's loved one is well cared for and feeling closer to the recipient.[28,29] Negative outcomes include consequences to mental, physical, and financial health, including[26,29,30]

1. a frequent occurrence of negative stress-related disorders, including increased rates of depression and anxiety;
2. serious physical injury from lifting or lack of good judgment due to exhaustion;
3. emotional hardships on relationships and social isolation;
4. financial hardships as a result of giving up paid work to care give or high out-of-pocket care expenses; and
5. increased risk factor for death (especially among older caregivers).

The importance of family caregivers in society has been highlighted by the COVID-19 pandemic; however, the negative effects and challenges of caregiving have also been exacerbated by this recent public health emergency.[31] The combination of social distancing, quarantine, and lockdown resulted in many caregivers experiencing a break in available care support for their loved ones. Caregiver burdens were high and bore at increasing percentages by women. This has raised increased attention to the need for systematic societal and individual resources to support caregiver reslience.[32] A burgeoning new industry of caregiver supports and technologies, as well as other professional services, is popping up everywhere to provide respite and help build resilience in caregivers for these uncompensated roles.

Enduring the Uncertainties

The issues facing close relationships we have been discussing all contain elements of uncertainty. This theme is so fundamental that we now turn to uncertainty to consider it directly. At some time in every recovery or adjustment process, a patient's uncertainties loom before them (Fig. 7.2). Whenever that happens, the reverberations race through intimate and close personal relationships. As a young child put it to one of the authors, "My sickness is like a ghost that hangs around our house. I'm doing OK, then it can creep up on me and 'Pow!' because I can't see it coming. When that happens everybody in my family has to change their plans." His condition was characterized by roller coaster–like exacerbations and remissions, keeping everyone in suspense about what would be possible for all of them from day to day.

One persistent theme is uncertainty about the unsettling effect of illness on the patient's close personal relationships. This manifests itself in many ways that health professionals must be prepared to interpret and try to respond to respectfully. Behavior changes or comments by the patient will often give you clues.

Patients who have dark doubts about what lies ahead may be asking a deeper question, although not always directly: "Will you stay with me through this situation, whatever the outcome?" You

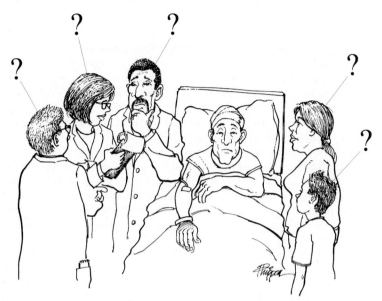

Fig. 7.2 Varying degrees of uncertainty is a problem patients face during recovery or adjustment, and negative stress reverberates into his or her significant relationships, as well as presenting challenges to professional caregivers.

can respond by assuring the person that you and your colleagues will do everything you can for them within your role. Such a question should also be an opportunity for you to gently explore whether this qualm is coming from uncertainty about whether persons important to the patient will be there at some critical juncture or whether they all will be able to make it through their ordeal without your skilled assistance. What can you do then and there to make a sincere effort to decrease their distress? You can:

1. Make time to provide them with as much certainty about their condition and its future course as your own information and role allow.
2. Collaborate with members of the interprofessional care team and refer to others who are more qualified to respond to questions.
3. Exercise restraint by not giving questionable information, instilling false hope around areas of your own uncertainty. The truth will do. The desire to comfort patients by providing false certainty will lead to their feeling of distrust or betrayal in the long run.
4. Assure the patient that although the patient's condition may not improve, you will always care for them. When goals of care shift from cure to comfort, patients and families need to know that you will be by their side. Uncertainty can arise around longstanding habits of who makes decisions between a couple or among family members.

A variety of family decision-making dynamics can be observed across cultures and generations. For those in marital relationships, convictions surrounding the decision-making authority role may be challenging to both parties when one is left out of the information loop. This dynamic is rarely static and can be difficult to unravel. Uncertainty complicates these dynamics, and today's family caregivers have an array of responsibilities, including advocating for their relatives' preferences and interests, dealing with health insurance claims, and communicating and coordinating care with various health care providers and settings. As the care demands increase, it is essential that each member of the interprofessional team, including professional staff, paraprofessional staff, the client, family, and caregivers value the other's opinion, feel respected and heard.[33]

What else can health professionals do to decrease the negative stress of their own uncertainties when concerns arise over who will speak or decision make for the patient?

1. Family meetings approved by the patient can become an avenue of fact finding and clarification for all involved. When health professionals commit to the power of listening, they give families the space to reflect on their views and demonstrate respect and care.[34]

2. Ethics committees or ethics consultants are a mechanism to help navigate situations that the professional caregivers find unethical or illegal and therefore cannot accept.

3. Documenting patient requests in the electronic medical record signals to other members of the health care team why you may be relying on someone other than the patient themself to make decisions about their health care regimen.

4. The help of professionals qualified to detect unhealthful relational dynamics should be sought for the benefit of all involved.

5. Keep the patient in the forefront. Remind the interprofessional care team that the goal of any such discussion and discernment is not ultimately to decrease your own distress but to do so only when the patient's distress has been fully addressed.

Having reviewed some important uncertainties patients and their loved ones' face, as well as the ripple effect of uncertainties you face in such situations, we turn in the next section to economic challenges and how these challenges affect the patient's personal relationships.

Close Relationships and Health Care Costs

In today's health care arena, at least in the United States, health care expenditures are largely affected by current law and existing regulatory environments. The Patient Protection and Affordable Care Act's expansions of eligibility for Medicaid and the creation of state Marketplaces (in which people can purchase health care coverage) represented some of the largest expansions of health insurance in the United States since the establishment of Medicare and Medicaid in 1965.[35] Despite this, 30 million US residents lacked health insurance in the first half of 2020 and the uninsured are disproportionately likely to be Black or Latino; be young adults; have low incomes; or live in states that have not expanded Medicaid.[36] Many patients struggle to afford health care, and many of their significant relationships are dramatically affected by costs associated with health care–related expenses.

Since cost and coverage are intertwined, persons in relationships touched by serious illness or injury are more vulnerable to financial duress.[37] This may come about by the cost of the initial health care episode, the necessary changes in employment made by the person or family caregiver, or the decreased likelihood of being able to find health insurance coverage for future conditions and ongoing maintenance. An adult's values may include that of being a good provider for those that depend on them, but the loss of opportunity to earn money for a time (or permanently) may be compounded by the high cost of medical and other health care bills. Patients who decide to make a highly desirable change in life direction or lifestyle with a loved one may feel prohibited from doing so by the reality of the desperate financial distress the illness or injury has caused.

Their distress may express itself in depression or cause patients to make health care choices you do not understand. It is well known that many instances of so-called nonadherence on the part of patients are occasioned by the cost of medications, treatments, devices, or services. High deductibles and copays often present financial challenges. Patients need to weigh those goods against that same money being spent for food, housing, or other necessities for themselves and their children or others dependent on those resources.

As a health professional, you are in a good position to be an advocate on behalf of patients and their families or other caregivers. Fortunately, many health care educational programs include courses designed to help you understand the financial mechanisms supporting or constraining what you can offer in the way of services and assurances. This can give you some certainty about how, and if, to talk realistically about what is available. Beyond that, what does advocacy entail in such a situation?

1. Inform patients and their caregivers of available institutional resources (e.g., social workers and case managers) who can help them maneuver through the confusing web of bureaucratic procedures they must traverse to receive essential services.

2. Be attuned to community services that patients, families, and others in caregiver relationships with the patient may be able to access.

3. Educate yourself regarding the basic language and concepts of health care financing and how it operates in your area of expertise so you can contribute to discussions and strategies about it in areas relevant to your role. Attend educational conferences or in-service sessions addressing these areas of your professional practice.

4. Document instances in which you are forced by inadequate or unjust policies to say "no" to interventions or services you know will strengthen the relationships most critical to the patient's quality of life. For example, in the United States, Medicaid, Medicare, or private insurance reimbursement practices often control the number of days the patient is eligible for treatment, placing both professional and family caregivers in an untenable position.

5. Judiciously gather empirical data regarding treatment effectiveness and patient outcomes to assist policy-makers in creating cost-effective approaches to care.

6. Work directly with your colleagues and professional organizations to influence legislation or other policy in your institution, state, or province and nationally.

7. Implement innovations in your workplace to address the strengths and weaknesses of cost-containment policies and value-based payments linked to quality patient outcomes.

In short, although many of the family's financial burdens will remain outside of your sphere of responsibility or influence, these steps can be taken for you to advocate for them and for all coming down the road in similar situations.

Revaluing Significant Relationships

Bookstores brim with titles such as *Ten (or a Hundred) Places to Visit Before You Die*. On the scale of opportunities for deep human flourishing, an even more compelling book should be *Ten People to Spend More Time with Whether or Not You Are Dying*. Having reviewed some questions and problems patients and their loved ones' face, this final section of the chapter ends on a positive note, turning to the enrichment that can be realized in relationships touched by adversity. Although families and health professionals often focus on the negative effects of stress related to illness or injury, there are, gratefully, some positive aspects that can sometimes motivate, leading to "eustress."[21] "*Eu*" is a Greek prefix meaning "good" or "positive" or "beauty."

A stressor can shock one into putting priorities in order and focus on what is important. In his poignant novel, *When Breath Becomes Air*, neurosurgeon and author Paul Kalanithi illustrates this point, stating "The tricky part of illness is that, as you go through it, your values are constantly changing. You try to figure out what matters to you, and then you keep figuring it out."[38]

Many people faced with illness or injury discover that it prods them to reflect on the value of significant relationships, past and present. In the epilogue to the abovementioned book, Paul's wife, Lucy, reflects on their relationship and the marital trouble they experienced before Paul's diagnosis. Knowing that most of her family and friends were unaware of that trouble before the publication of the book she reflects on their relationship, writing "We each joked to our close friends that the secret to saving a relationship is for one person to become terminally ill. Conversely, we knew that the trick to managing a terminal illness is to be deeply in love—to be vulnerable, kind, generous, and grateful."[39]

This reflection may give you a glimpse of the urgency with which you might invoke the help of others if you thought they were a resource for fulfilling one or more of your relationship-related goals. As a health professional, you will sometimes be brought into the patient's thoughts or plans as the person reflects about things done and left undone regarding his or her relationships.

Longstanding breaches with a friend or loved ones are the biggest challenge for most patients. We have noted that sometimes a patient is surprised to feel a stirring to make amends. Of course, sometimes a past trauma weighs so heavily on a patient or family member that they never fully recover from it and their relationship remains mired in anger or grief. At other times, the illness or injury highlights a deeper burden of estrangement the person has been carrying.

The good news is that most people do recover or adjust sufficiently to take stock of what is important in their lives. A young couple may decide their differences are not that important after all and try to make a new life together. A man who felt he was too busy golfing may decide to take the opportunity to resume regular golf games with his longtime buddies and the camaraderie that they enjoy. An older woman may decide to move out of a secure but highly competitive job environment to find a new position where she believes she will find more work–life balance and support. Religious and spiritual beliefs can also help provide meaning to the patient's experience and aid in the healing or adjustment of intimate and close personal relationships.

Sometimes, patients will ask your advice or even intervention, and at times you may feel you are faced with a dilemma about what to say or how much to get involved. A good general rule is to be mindful of the nature of respectful health care provider and patient relationships. You have been gaining some ideas about that as you have read and reflected on the chapters in this book. The result is that often you will have the satisfaction of watching patients or former patients use their conditions, however unwelcome illness and injury is, as opportunities to think things over and start afresh, and in the process rejuvenating or bringing new perspectives to their personal relationships.

Summary

The personal life of the patient involves a web of activities, roles, and relationships that help provide status, meaning, support, and a sense of belonging. Today, the term *family* is defined in a variety of ways. Guided by the principles of patient- and family-centered care, health professionals must understand how families function and how to best interact within the context of each family culture. The family health systems approach offers one such method to optimize health outcomes for the delivery of efficient, effective, and compassionate care. The most immediate intimate relationship for most people is their family; therefore showing respect for the patient and assessing the stressors facing the patient mean thinking about how one's health status affects the family and vice versa. Shifting the focus of health care from the individual member who is ill, injured, or disabled to the family as a unit of care is key to compassionate care. Despite this shift, the fragility of relationships is often increased by the fears and realities facing patients, their loved ones, and other supporters. Sometimes, they see interest and support falling away; they may suffer from the changes that are taking place and from the uncertainties that lie ahead. Financial burdens are almost always an added stress. In all instances, the patient's responses are influenced by those closest to them. In turn, those near the patient become enmeshed in the concerns, new responsibilities, and changes. Those who become family or other "informal" caregivers represent a growing group of persons who can be at risk for injuries, burnout, and other debilitating conditions. They require the health professional's respect and considered attention to help nurture their most treasured relationships. The good news is that illness or injury also may become an opportunity for relationships to draw on their past strengths and find renewed vitality and vision. One of the most critical and ultimately satisfying contributions you can make in your professional capacity is to engage in behaviors that express genuine care for everyone in the patient's circle of key relationships.

References

1. Albertson SA. *Endings and Beginnings: A Young Family's Experience With Death and Renewal*. New York: Random House; 1980.
2. *Institute for Patient- and Family-Centered Care*. What is patient and family-centered care. n.d. http://www.ipfcc.org/about/pfcc.html. Accessed September 25, 2021.
3. Hsu C, Gray MF, Murray L, et al. Actions and processes that patients, family members, and physicians associate with patient- and family-centered care. *BMC Fam Pract*. 2019;20:35. https://doi.org/10.1186/s12875-019-0918-7.
4. Lv B, Gao X-r, Sun J, et al. Family-centered care improves clinical outcomes of very-low-birth-weight infants: a quasi-experimental study. *Front Pediatr*. 2019:7. https://doi.org/10.3389/fped.2019.00138.
5. Kaslow NJ, Dunn SE, Henry T, Partin C, Newsome J, O'Donnell C, Wierson M, Schwartz AC. Collaborative patient- and family-centered care for hospitalized individuals: Best practices for hospitalist care teams. *Fam Syst Health*. 2020;38(2):200–208. https://doi.org/10.1037/fsh0000479.
6. Developed and adopted by the Young Children's Continuum of the New Mexico State Legislature, June 20, 1990; contributed by Polly Arango, Family Voices founder.
7. Sparling JW. The cultural definition of family. *Phys Occup Ther Pediatr*. 1991;11(4):17–28.
8. U.S. Census Bureau. America's families and living arrangements: 2020. In: *Current Population Survey, 2020 Annual Social and Economic Supplement*; 2021. Available from: https://www.census.gov/data/tables/2020/demo/families/cps-2020.html.
9. Schor E. Family pediatrics: report of the Task Force on the Family. *Pediatrics*. 2003;111:S1541–S1571.
10. Tramonti F, Petrozzi A, Burgalassi A, et al. Family functioning and psychological distress in a sample of mental health outpatients: implications for routine examination and screening. *J Eval Clin Pract*. 2020;26(3):1042–1047.
11. Anderson KH. The family health system approach to family systems nursing. *J Fam Nurs*. 2000;6(2):103–119.
12. Duggan C, Stamm D. In: Hoppin, AG, ed. *Management of Short Bowel Syndrome in Children*. Waltham, MA: UpToDate Inc. Topic 5894 Version 36.0. May, 13 2021. http://www.uptodate.com; Accessed September 30, 2021.
13. Duvall EM. *Family Development*. 5th ed. Philadelphia, PA: Lippincott; 1977.
14. Neam VC, Oron AP, Nair D, Edwards T, Horslen SP, Javid PJ. Factors associated with health-related quality of life in children with intestinal failure. *J Pediatr*. 2020;216:13. https://doi.org/10.1016/j.jpeds.2019.08.049.
15. Gunnar RJ, Kanerva K, Salmi S, et al. Neonatal intestinal failure is independently associated with impaired cognitive development later in childhood. *J Pediatr Gastroenterol Nutr*. 2020;70(1):64–71.
16. Doherty RF, Kwo J, Montgomery P, et al. *Maintaining Compassionate Care: A Companion Guide for Families Experiencing the Uncertainty of a Serious and Prolonged Illness*. Boston, MA: MGH Institute of Health Professions; 2008.
17. Flahive CB, Goldschmidt M, Mezoff EA. A review of short bowel syndrome including current and emerging management strategies. *Curr Treat Options Pediatr*. 2021;7(1):1–16.
18. Harrist AW, Henry CS, Liu C, Morris AS. Family resilience: the power of rituals and routines in family adaptive systems. In: Fiese BH, Celano M, Deater-Deckard K, eds. *APA Handbook of Contemporary Family Psychology: Foundations, Methods, and Contemporary Issues Across the Lifespan*. In: APA Handbooks in Psychology Series. American Psychological Association; 2019:223–239.

19. Imber-Black E, Roberts J, Whiting R. *Rituals in Families and Family Therapy*. New York: Norton; 1988.
20. Bennett WL, Pitts S, Aboumatar H, Sharma R, Smith BM, Das A, Day J, Holzhauer K, Bass EB. *Strategies for Patient, Family and Caregiver Engagement. Technical Brief (Prepared by the Johns Hopkins University Evidence-Based Practice Center Under Contract No. 290-2015-00006-I.) AHRQ Publication No. 20-EHC017*. Rockville, MD: Agency for Healthcare Research and Quality; 2020. https://doi.org/10.23970/AHRQEPCTB36.
21. Rambur B, Vallett C, Cohen JA. The moral cascade: distress, eustress and the virtuous organization. *J Organ Moral Psychol*. 2010;1(1):41–54.
22. Kennedy-Hendricks A, Barry CL, Gollust SE, et al. Social stigma toward persons with prescription opioid use disorder: associations with public support for private and public health–oriented policies. *Psychiatr Serv*. 2017;68:462–469.
23. Franz B, Dhanani LY, Brook DL. Physician blame and vulnerability: novel predictors of physician willingness to work with patients who misuse opioids. *Addict Sci Clin Pract*. 2021;16(1):33. https://doi.org/10.1186/s13722-021-00242-w.
24. Zuckerman C. 'Til death do us part: family caregiving at the end of life. In: Levine C, ed. *Always on Call: When Illness Turns Family Into Caregivers*. New York: United Hospital Fund of New York; 2000.
25. Akin C. *The Long Road Called Goodbye: Tracing the Course of Alzheimer's*. Omaha, NE: Creighton University Press; 2000.
26. AARP and National Alliance for Caregiving. *Caregiving in the United States 2020*. Washington, DC: AARP; 2020. https://doi.org/10.26419/ppi.00103.001.
27. Reinhard SC, Feinberg LF, Houser A, Choula R, Evans M. *Valuing the Invaluable: 2019 Update Charting a Path Forward*. AARP Public Policy Institute; 2019. https://www.aarp.org/content/dam/aarp/ppi/2019/11/valuing-the-invaluable-2019-update-charting-a-path-forward.doi.10.26419-2Fppi.00082.001.pdf; Accessed September 30, 2021.
28. Freedman VA, Skehan ME, Hu M, Wolff J, Kasper JD. *National Study of Caregiving I-III User Guide*. Baltimore, MD: Johns Hopkins Bloomberg School of Public Health; 2019. Available from: http://www.nhats.org.
29. *Family Caregiver Alliance*. Caregiver statistics: health, technology, and caregiving resources. https://www.caregiver.org/caregiver-statistics-health-technology-and-caregiving-resources; https://www.caregiver.org/resource/caregiver-statistics-demographics/; 2021 Accessed September 25, 2021.
30. *Center for Disease Control and Prevention*. Caregiving for family and friends—a public health issue. July, 30, 2019. https://www.cdc.gov/aging/caregiving/caregiver-brief.html; Accessed September 25, 2021.
31. Lorenz-Dant K, Comas-Herrera A. The impacts of COVID-19 on unpaid carers of adults with long-term care need and measures to address these impacts: a rapid review of evidence up to November 2020. *J Long-Term Care*. 2021;2021:124–153.
32. Geschke K, Palm S, Fellgiebel A, Wuttke-Linnemann A. *Resilience in Informal Caregivers of People Living with Dementia in the Face of COVID-19 Pandemic-Related Changes to Daily Life: A Narrative Review*. GeroPsych; 2021. Advance online publication. https://doi.org/10.1024/1662-9647/a000273.
33. Schell BAS, Doherty RF, Thomas A, Knab M. Clinical and professional reasoning in community oriented practice. In: Pizzi MA, Amir M, eds. *Interprofessional Perspectives on Community-Oriented Practice: Promoting Health, Well-Being and Quality of Life*. Slack Publishing; 2022.
34. Grant, A. *Think Again: The Power of Knowing What You Don't Know*. New York: Viking Press; 2021.
35. Decker SL, Lipton BJ. Most newly insured people in 2014 were long-term uninsured. *Health Aff*. 2017;36(1):16–20.
36. U.S. Department of Health and Human Services. *Trends in the U.S. Uninsured Population, 2010-2020. (Issue Brief No. HP-2021-02)*. Washington, DC: Office of the Assistant Secretary for Planning and Evaluation, U.S. Department of Health and Human Services; 2021.
37. Ryan C, Hilary D, Thomas GC, et al. Envisioning a better U.S. health care system for all: coverage and cost of care. *Ann Intern Med*. 2020;172:S7–S32. https://doi.org/10.7326/M19-2415. [Epub ahead of print January 21, 2020].
38. Kalanithi P. *When Breath Becomes Air*. New York: Random House; 2016:160–161.
39. Kalanithi P. *When Breath Becomes Air*. New York: Random House; 2016:216.

Respect Through Collaboration and Communication

Introduction

The most immediate "tool" you have available for respectful interaction is your own communication, whether that tool is used verbally or nonverbally, in interactions with colleagues or patients. Effective communication between health professionals is an integral component of interprofessional collaboration and team-based health care. Interprofessional communication is important because many patients have complex health issues that require the involvement of a variety of health care professionals. Furthermore, to reduce the risk for errors in hospitals and other health care settings, there must be a clear exchange of information by all members of the health care team. Effective communication can create a safer care delivery environment, improve patient outcomes, decrease redundancies in care, reduce patient and societal costs, and improve workforce well-being. Chapter 8 provides an overview of the Core Competencies for Interprofessional Collaborative Practice.[1] Elements of collaborative practice skills such as mutual respect and trust, communication, shared decision-making, and care planning by interprofessional teams are discussed. Barriers to effective interprofessional communication and methods to improve collaborative practice are explored.

What you say, how and when you say it, and how you communicate nonverbally through gestures and other types of physical messages will set the tone for everything that happens in the health professional and patient relationship. Chapter 9 focuses on components of respectful interaction in verbal and nonverbal aspects of communication. As you read and reflect on all the types of messages you give and receive, think back to Sections 1 and 2, especially to the parts of those chapters addressing values and culture. It is almost certain that you will work with colleagues and patients from countries and backgrounds different from your own. There also will be differences in levels of health literacy and basic literacy, as well as facility with the various technological tools for communication and engagement such as the Internet, smart phone applications, digital patient portals, and social media tools. These differences in culture, language, literacy, and understanding are evident as we attend to patients and listen to or read what they choose to include in their stories and what is left unsaid. Consider how the challenge of communicating both verbally and nonverbally, face-to-face or from a distance, is enhanced and influenced by these factors.

Reference

1. Interprofessional Education Collaborative. *Core Competencies for Interprofessional Collaborative Practice: 2016 Update.* Washington, DC: Interprofessional Education Collaborative; 2016.

CHAPTER 8

Respectful Interprofessional and Intraprofessional Communication and Collaboration

OBJECTIVES

The reader will be able to

- Describe the purpose of core competencies for interprofessional collaboration;
- Delineate individual and team attributes for interprofessional collaboration that ensure respect for the patient will be honored;
- Explain the impact of interprofessional communication and collaboration on patient safety, quality of care, and workplace enhancement;
- Describe barriers to optimal interprofessional communication;
- Enumerate essential elements of care collaboration and coordination for successful personal goal setting and interprofessional collaborative practice; and
- Use the skills of effective interprofessional teamwork to develop shared goals and treatment plans.

Prelude

One of the things the PT did very well was making it crystal clear that there was a dramatic and unsatisfactory change in the patient. I wonder if for efficiency, if she could have led with that and the concern that she [the patient] is not safe alone. And I wonder and I am thinking she needs further evaluation today to keep her [the patient] safe. And that may have led to a more efficient exchange.

CUNNINGHAM, MUSICK, AND TRINKLE[1]

In previous chapters, you were introduced to some basic components of respectful interaction with patients, families, and others. Often, the discussion focused on you as an individual professional. Still, you could observe from our examples—and likely from your own experience—that much interaction between professionals and patients today does not occur between a sole health care provider and a patient. In contrast, your interventions often are one of several provided by a group working together on the patient's behalf. In this situation, we have referred to you as a member of an interprofessional care team. In the following pages, we examine in more depth the concepts, dynamics, and processes of care provided by multiple professionals working together to care for a patient and your role as an effective member of such teams bonded by common goals and purpose.

Begin by examining the medical student's comments about his interaction with a physical therapy student in a telephone consultation in the prelude at the opening of this chapter. The medical student is reflecting on the telephone interaction and begins by complimenting the PT student and her emphasis on a disturbing change in the patient's status. The medical student goes on to say that it might have been better, for the patient, if the PT student had opened up with this concern rather than waiting to bring it up later. We assume both students are motivated by the common goal of delivering quality care and ensuring the safety of their patients and that working together is necessary to achieve such ultimate goals. However, they may differ on the best way to work together to accomplish such goals. Reflective thinking about one's performance and those of one's colleagues and ways to improve communication, listening skills, and other competencies are essential for providing high-quality care and ensuring safety.

Focus on Interprofessional Collaboration

Attention to the importance of health care teams working together effectively took root because of the increasingly complex needs of patients along with an emphasis on reducing errors in a fragmented health care delivery system. These problems led to the call for *interprofessional collaboration*. In 2001, the Institute of Medicine (IOM; renamed the National Academy of Medicine) recommended that health professionals who worked together in interprofessional care teams be better equipped to address the challenging needs of contemporary patients.[2] The next year, the IOM specifically called for greater focus on interprofessional education in their report *Who Will Keep the Public Healthy? Educating Public Health Professionals for the 21st Century* and repeated this appeal in a 2010 report.[3,4] Later, the IOM published a report on measuring the impact of interprofessional education.[5] Likewise, The Joint Commission, an independent, not-for-profit organization that accredits and certifies health care organizations and programs in the United States, noted the damaging effects that poor workplace communication can have on patient care and the need to improve interprofessional communication because of the increasing number of errors in health care.[6,7]

The term *interprofessional collaborative practice* brought these ideas into further usage. The World Health Organization defined it accordingly: "When multiple health workers from different professional backgrounds work together with patients, families, carers, and communities to deliver the highest quality of care."[8] Initially, this formal, intentional "working together" was thought to be necessary mostly for specific, complex patient care situations, and indeed, there are some practice environments in which interprofessional care teams have been the norm since their inception. Examples are rehabilitation, hospice, geriatric care, and mental/behavioral health settings.[9] Perhaps because of the multifaceted and often chronic nature of the health problems experienced by patients cared for in these specialties, as well as the focus of care on common goals, interprofessional care teams were more prepared to share their expertise and perspectives to work toward achieving the patient's maximum level of independence and recovery from an injury or live with a chronic illness. Interprofessional collaboration is now widely recognized as the basis for all effective care delivery. Collaborative efforts to develop best practice models for training of health professionals in interprofessional collaboration are ongoing.[10] Table 8.1 provides a timeline for some of the most important educational and practice recommendations regarding interprofessional collaboration made by national and international health care organizations.

Why are interprofessional collaboration and communication so critical to the delivery of high-quality, patient-centered care? As has been mentioned several times, patients today generally have multiple health problems and therefore require the expertise and care of more than one health professional to address their needs. Research has affirmed that collaborative interprofessional practice improves efficiency, reduces errors, promotes patient satisfaction, and enhances job satisfaction among health professionals (Fig. 8.1).[12,13] Poor interprofessional collaboration has the opposite impact on patient care in a variety of ways, including errors, increased hospital costs, unnecessary readmissions, pain, and suffering and turnover among professional staff.[6,14]

TABLE 8.1 ■ Organizations and Resources Supporting Interprofessional Education and Collaborative Practice

Organization	Year	Publication
Institute of Medicine	2001	Crossing the Quality Chasm: A New Health System for the 21st Century[2]
Institute of Medicine	2002	Who Will Keep the Public Healthy? Educating Public Health Professionals for the 21st Century[3]
Joint Commission	2008	Sentinel Event Alert. Behaviors That Undermine a Culture of Safety[6]
World Health Organization	2010	Framework for Action on Interprofessional Education & Collaborative Practice[8]
Carnegie Foundation	2010	Educating Nurses and Physicians: Toward New Horizons[10]
Institute of Medicine	2010	The Future of Nursing: Leading Change, Advancing Health[4]
Joint Commission	2011	Accreditation Program Hospitals: National Patient Safety Goals[7]
Institute of Medicine	2015	Measuring the Impact of Interprofessional Education on Collaborative Practice and Patient Outcomes[5]
Interprofessional Education Collaborative	2016	Core Competencies for Interprofessional Collaborative Practice[11]
Health Professions Accreditors Collaborative	2019	Guidance on Developing Quality Interprofessional Education for the Health Professions[10]

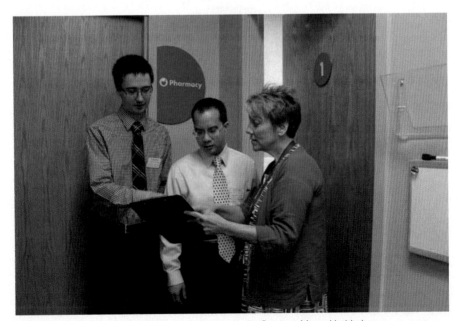

Fig. 8.1   Members of interprofessional care team on rounds. Courtesy Maren Haddad.

Core Competencies for Interprofessional Collaboration

About the same time as the call for interprofessional collaboration was being promoted from a variety of constituencies in health policy and accreditation, the Interprofessional Education Collaborative (IPEC) formed and developed core competencies for interprofessional collaborative practice specifically for the prelicensure/precredentialed future health professional.[11] Recall the professional competencies for all health professionals presented in Chapter 1. Note the differences and similarities between the individual professional competencies and the following interprofessional core competencies.

IPEC defines *interprofessional competencies* in health care as "integrated enactment of knowledge, skills, values, and attitudes that define working together across the professions with other health care workers, and with patients, along with families and communities, as appropriate to improve health outcomes in specific care contexts."[11] The four initial competency domains included interprofessional communication, values/ethics, roles and responsibilities, and teams and teamwork. IPEC updated the 2011 competencies in 2016 to integrate population health competencies and respond to the changes in the health care system, including the focus on the Quadruple Aim, presented in Chapter 5, and the implementation of the Patient Protection and Affordable Care Act in 2010.[15] The original four domains now fall under the single domain of interprofessional collaboration (Fig. 8.2).

The IPEC competencies are now incorporated into almost all health professions' accreditation standards. What began with the participation of six national associations of schools of health professions that created the core competencies expanded to 15 members in 2016. The following are a few examples of what these standards look like in physical therapy, pharmacy, and occupational

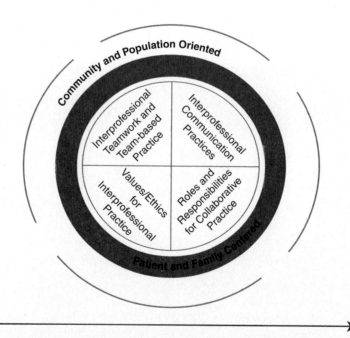

The Learning Continuum pre-licensure through practice trajectory

Fig. 8.2 Interprofessional collaboration competency domains. Copyright © 2016 IPEC Interprofessional Education Collaborative.

therapy. The following standard is from physical therapy and became effective in 2018: "The didactic and clinical curriculum includes interprofessional education; learning activities are directed toward the development of interprofessional competencies including, but not limited to, values/ethics, communication, professional roles and responsibilities, and teamwork."[16] Similarly, interprofessional education is required by the Accreditation Council for Pharmacy Education in the following standard, "The curriculum prepares all students to provide entry-level, patient-centered care in a variety of practice settings as a contributing member of an interprofessional team. In the aggregate, team exposure includes prescribers as well as other healthcare professionals."[17] The Accreditation Council of Occupational Therapy Education's most recent standards include the following competencies regarding interprofessional collaboration, "Demonstrate knowledge of the principles of interprofessional team dynamics to perform effectively in different team roles to plan, deliver, and evaluate patient- and population-centered care as well as population health programs and policies that are safe, timely, efficient, effective, and equitable."[18] Most health profession programs include a required standard on interprofessional education like these. Integrating interprofessional competencies into discipline-specific accreditation standards ensures that today's health professions student is effectively prepared to function as an entry-level member of the interprofessional care team. Furthermore, since individual accrediting agencies independently created accreditation policies, processes, or standards for interprofessional education, it is possible that such standards could create barriers to effective and quality interprofessional education.[10]

Intraprofessional Collaboration

Not only do health professionals consistently interact with colleagues from other disciplines but also they interact with members within the same broadly defined discipline but at different levels. Problems with coordination and communication can occur even among those who share a similar disciplinary perspective, understanding of their professional obligations, and shared ownership of patient care interventions. For example, an occupational therapist (OT) and occupational therapy assistant (OTA) are both part of the profession of occupational therapy, but each may not necessarily effectively draw on the other's specific contributions to increase efficiency to provide direct service to patients. Intraprofessional collaboration is so important to occupational therapy practice that an accreditation standard was developed to ensure that programs included content to achieve these competencies, "Demonstrate effective intraprofessional OT/OTA collaboration to: Identify the role of the occupational therapist and occupational therapy assistant in the screening and evaluation process. Demonstrate and identify techniques in skills of supervision and collaboration with occupational therapy assistants."[19]

An early study regarding how to improve intraprofessional collaboration within occupational therapy noted, "If team members' needs are not satisfied, dysfunctional intraprofessional teams result."[20] The needs that they identified were mutual respect, mastery or effective performance, and personal growth and professional socialization. Similar findings were the outcome of a study of licensed practical nurses (LPNs) and registered nurses (RNs). An LPN expressed the following feelings of being devalued by an RN colleague on the team: "She has more years at school than me, but I think that when we talk rationally together we can come to an agreement calmly for the sake of our patient and not to see where me or she is right."[21] The LPN seems to be asking for mutual respect and the opportunity to contribute to the care of the patient. Because many professional disciplines include members at the assistant or technical level, there is a need to strengthen these intraprofessional relationships in the same manner as interprofessional collaboration. This ensures that respect is extended to all who contribute to the care of the client, regardless of professional-level credentials. Even though they might share a common knowledge base, intraprofessional factions exist within every profession and challenge communication through contrary views and cultures.

Physicians struggle with intraprofessional tensions that are especially evident between primary care physicians and other specialty physicians who often manage the same disease state in a patient population but have very different beliefs and priorities regarding balancing health aims for patients.[22] Generally, methods to improve interprofessional interactions apply equally well to intraprofessional interactions.

REFLECTIONS

A certified nursing assistant (CNA) in a skilled nursing facility had this to say about her interactions with her nurse coworkers:

I *think* about my job and how to do it better. I try to address issues I have but most of the time it is met with resistance, and I never do it in a "complain" way. If I have a concern, I always begin with "I need some clarification," and address my concern as a question. I *am* the eyes and ears of the nurse. I see things an RN doesn't because I spend more time with each patient. While I may not be the one to call the doctor or the family about a loved one's condition you can bet it's an aide who has brought it to someone else's attention.[23]

- What unique contributions do members of the team such as a CNA bring to the care of patients?
- What actions by coworkers would send a message to this CNA that she is a valued member of the team?

Elements of Collaborative Skills

Key elements of successful collaborative interaction are built on an understanding of one's own professional identity and select dispositions or character traits. The following are essential attributes that health professionals should possess and develop to optimize interprofessional collaboration as an individual and a member of the health care team.

INDIVIDUAL ATTRIBUTES FOR SUCCESSFUL COLLABORATION

Self-Awareness

The first personal attribute for successful collaboration is the ability to reflect on personal knowledge, skills, and abilities and is built on an understanding of your personal identity based on your own value set, as introduced in Chapter 1. Self-awareness also requires the examination of biases, motivations, and emotions that have an impact on your personal and professional growth. "Each individual brings to the team a unique personality and position, which reciprocally affects team function."[24]

An important component of self-awareness for any health professional is professional identity, which is more than completing a specified course of study and passing a licensure examination. To be a full member of a profession means one must behave like a member of that profession. What does it mean to behave like a member of a profession?

First, at its most basic level, members of a profession share a language; that is, they know the way to talk in a kind of shorthand with members of that profession. As we note in Chapter 9, health professionals share a general culture of health care with its common language that is often foreign to patients. In addition, each profession has its own language that is sometimes reduced to acronyms that only full-fledged members of that profession understand. For example, the term *MTM* is common parlance in pharmacy practice, but only a member of the profession or someone who took the time to translate this acronym would know that it means "medication therapy management." MTM is at the heart of pharmacy practice and refers to a broad range of health care services provided by pharmacists.

Second, one behaves like a member of a health profession when one asks the types of questions those within that profession ask. For example, we would expect a social worker to ask questions about income, living conditions, or sources of family and community support but might be surprised if an oncologist did so. Certain questions are particularly relevant to each health profession's role, responsibilities, and scope of practice.

Third, to behave like a member of a profession one should understand and explain things the way a member of the profession does.[25] We return to these components of professional identity that profoundly affect successful collaboration when we discuss differences in communication styles among professions.

Competence

The second individual attribute necessary for collaborative work is being secure in your knowledge, skills, and abilities in your own discipline. This acts as a benchmark of respect for the patient introduced in Chapter 2. Sometimes, discussions of professional competence that emphasize individual experience and confidence overlook the fact that it also includes the ability to successfully work with others. Being competent in your field allows you to explore and appreciate the contributions of other disciplines. In fact, curiosity and a willingness to learn about the unknown or unfamiliar are assets in interprofessional collaboration.

Trust

Just as trust between professionals and patients is essential for respectful interaction, individuals also must be able to trust other members of the team. "The ability to trust originates from self-knowledge and competence."[26] Trust is often described as a prerequisite to teamwork of any type and begins with the idea that we approach other members of the team as if they are competent and have good intentions. Trust must be earned through credibility which means doing what you say you are going to do.[27] Oftentimes, health care teams comprise providers from different personal and professional backgrounds, thus starting points for trust need to be established, such as a clear understanding of the norms and expectations for the professionals on the team and a history of successful interpersonal exchanges among team members.[28] One must have the inclination to trust other members of the team and appreciate that trust continues to develop over time.

Commitment to Team Goals and Values

The fourth individual attribute is commitment to a unified set of team goals and values that provides direction and motivation for individual members.[26] Later, we discuss the importance of a shared goal or aim as part of successful collaboration. Here, we are talking about the personal sense of responsibility you feel as a member of a team. When you are committed to a commonly agreed-on cause or project, you feel responsible to the other members of the team and are thus often willing to work harder to reach a goal if that is necessary. Sometimes, commitment is expressed by the metaphor of "having each other's backs," in that we will support each other even when the going gets tough.

Flexibility

Flexibility is defined as "the ability to maintain an open attitude, accommodate different personal values, and be receptive to the ideas of others."[26] Flexibility requires you to keep an open mind and a willingness to see things in different terms often from the perspective of another member of the team. Feeling confident about one's role in a team begins with creating a flexible professional identity which means constantly questioning oneself and updating one's professional identity.[29] Also, the complexity of a patient's predicament can require a novel approach that is much more likely achieved by all members of the team contributing their various perspectives including the patient and family.

Acceptance

Finally, one must be accepting of differences among the members of the team. It is easier and more comforting to be among the familiar; however, our differences make us better. In health care, today, a health professional cannot avoid working in an interprofessional environment, so our choice really comes down to whether we want to work together well or badly. At times, territorial issues of different professions, as well as different world views, conspire to make this a difficult task.[30] All members of the interprofessional care team must move beyond tolerance to acceptance and understanding for effective collaboration. When grounded in the principles of dignity and respect, members of the team can clarify specific values that are central to one's own profession with other members of the team. It is likely that just as there is blurring across professional boundaries, there also will be blurring, or perhaps better put, sharing of core values that can help with cross-disciplinary understanding.[31]

REFLECTIONS

Consider the individual attributes for participating in successful collaboration with other members of the health care team—that is, self-awareness, competence, ability to trust, commitment, flexibility, and acceptance.
- Which of these attributes do you possess, and which do you need to develop more fully?
- Consider the following scenario: You are participating in morning rounds on an inpatient unit with an interprofessional care team. At one point, you realize that you strongly disagree with the recommendation of another member of the team. Which individual attributes would be particularly helpful in resolving the differences of professional opinion to maintain good interprofessional collaboration?
- How else might you communicate your disagreement to your teammate?

TEAM SKILLS FOR COLLABORATION

In addition to individual attributes, skills more specific to team collaboration also are essential for optimum patient-centered outcomes. A team is defined as "a small group of interdependent people who collectively have the expertise, knowledge, and skills needed for a task or ongoing work."[12] This definition of a team is particularly important for health professionals who may be used to working in a hierarchical structure because the definition emphasizes interdependency. The term *interdependency* highlights that the team does not exist to help meet the needs or aims of those at the top of the organizational hierarchy but rather to fulfill mutually agreed-on common goals for the welfare of the patient, family, or community. A team needs expertise in the following skills if it hopes to succeed in attaining such goals.

Mutual Respect

The IPEC core competencies specifically refer to mutual respect as a requirement for working with individuals of other professions.[15] As noted previously, such respect is built on the personal trust among members of the team that develops into mutual respect over time. For mutual respect to exist, there must be a culture of "status-equal" basis. All members of the team need to see each other as peers with the capacity to step into the leadership role at any time that specific expertise or skills are needed. Additionally, all members of the team must believe in the value of what the other members of the team bring to the table as differing professional perspectives can support or hinder effective decision-making as a team.

Communication Skills

All the basic verbal and nonverbal communication skills discussed in Chapter 9 come into play in interprofessional communication, with the added challenge of differing language and communication styles among health professionals. For example, nurses lean toward being very descriptive and detailed in their communication, whereas physicians are generally brief in the information they provide about the patient's situation or treatment.[32] Thus physicians might think when nurses are speaking, "I wish they would get to the point," which can be frustrating to nurses who value a fuller understanding of a patient's story that, from their perspective, is essential to planning patient care. A qualitative study of communication between physicians and other health professionals in an inpatient unit explored current patterns of communication by observing interprofessional and intraprofessional exchanges.[14] Physicians in the study exhibited a consistently terse communication style in which they offered brief reports on their patients' medical status, requested information, or informed the team of patient-related orders. Most of the deliberative communication in which a patient's case was discussed beyond basic medical issues was between members of nonmedical professions such as nursing, occupational therapy, and social work. When physicians did have more in-depth discussions about a patient, it was most often intraprofessional, that is, with another physician, not a health professional from a different discipline.

Negative communication is a problem that often reflects a lack of respect or a resistance to changing the traditional hierarchy in health care. Negative communication includes disparaging comments such as intimidating or condescending language, deliberate delays in responding to requests, reluctance to work as a team, and impatience with questions.[33] Efforts should be directed at eradicating such negative communication, which clearly affects the quality of the exchange of information across professions. Communication should be clear and precise, calm and supportive, respectful, and responsive. Members of the team can contribute to positive communication by sharing pertinent information, listening attentively, respecting others' opinions, validating concerns, using common language, and providing feedback as well as accepting feedback.[34] Two concrete ways to create a safe environment for communication from others on the interprofessional team are to (1) ask questions and (2) express gratitude for contributions both of which help establish psychological safety.[35] You can also ask "What if we . . ." or "It seems to me that….what are your thoughts?" signaling the idea that you and the topic at hand are open to discussion. This approach assures that team members are seen and heard. It invites collective imagining from all members of the team.[35]

Shared Planning

Shared planning and decision-making are essential to good teamwork. However, health professionals often get stuck in their disciplinary silos and focus on specific tasks or decisions that are important to the values of their profession and ignore or discount the larger picture. These types of isolated decisions about specific treatments or tests do little to achieve overarching goals for the patient, which should serve as a central focus of the team. Shared planning requires the integration of different perspectives and, at times, compromise. Members of the team must anticipate that there will be differing viewpoints that may lead to conflict but do not have to do so. When disagreements happen, one can respectfully disagree and work productively through shared values to reach a common plan.[26] Reasoning from alternative approaches or angles about a given situation should be encouraged initially and then ideally be part of a team's culture. The establishment of mutually understood and agreed-upon goals, even though such goals may change in the future, is necessary for all members of a team (including the patient and family).

Interprofessional Communication and Collaboration: Challenges and Opportunities

Clearly, with so many variables that affect a more collective approach to professional and patient interactions, there are barriers and opportunities to refine what an individual health professional can accomplish in providing respectful, patient-centered care.

BARRIERS TO EFFECTIVE INTERPROFESSIONAL APPROACHES

Time Constraints

One of the most prevalent barriers to interprofessional communication and collaboration is that busy health professionals do not have the time to meet with other members of the interprofessional care team, let alone really learn about the unique or special contributions of other professions. Additionally, there is often no physical space for different members of the team to meet where they can privately deliberate and think they are not being overheard or interrupted. It is common to see health professionals conduct "hallway consultations" or "corridor consults," terms applied to unplanned encounters between two or more different members of the team who stop and obtain quick, informal feedback or urgently request information to guide their decision-making. Protected time, dedicated space (literally space to meet), and support for formal discussions for shared planning and decision-making are essential for true collaboration. Although hallway consultations will not disappear, they should not be the only means for members of the team to communicate. Finally, members of the interprofessional team must learn to accept that collaboration of this type takes time and requires an active effort on everyone's part.

Lack of Shared Structures for Communication

Another barrier to interprofessional communication is a lack of an agreed-upon conceptual structure for such dialog among colleagues. As noted previously, different health professions have their distinct ways of communicating based on underlying values, understanding of their professional obligations and skills, and habits they acquire by observing the actions and conduct of other members of their specialty. A promising example is that considerable research and effort have been focused on the improvement of the *handoff* of a patient when the patient's condition warrants a change involving health disciplines because of a change in the patient's status or when one shift in an institution is ending and a new one beginning. A handoff is "the transfer of patient information and responsibility between health care providers" and is a critical point of vulnerability to communication error (Fig. 8.3).[36] As you can see, if done well, it is an excellent opportunity to ask questions and participate in shared decision-making, so the patient's high quality of care remains seamless. To provide structure and improve the transfer of information at the handoff, a variety of common mental models have been proposed and studied, such as *SBAR*, which stands for Situation, Background, Assessment, and Recommendation; *SBIRT*, which stands for Screening, Brief Intervention, and Referral to Treatment and is often used in emergency departments (EDs); and *I-PASS*, which is a mnemonic for I: Illness Severity, P: Patient Summary, A: Action List, S: Situation Awareness, and Contingency Planning and S: Synthesis by Receiver.[36–39] The last component, synthesis, is often used as a sort of closure in the feedback loop in the military and aviation industry. The person receiving the information repeats it back so that the sender can affirm that the correct message was sent.

All such mental models are an attempt to create a standard language that is not "native" for any one of the professions involved, so there is a lower risk for miscommunication and a stronger focus on the patient's situation. Although proven very useful for minimizing communication errors at handoff and clearly useful for assessment and communication of patient status

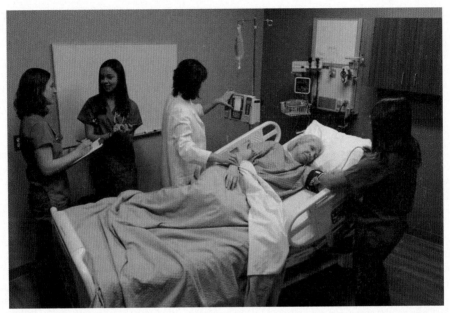

Fig. 8.3 Interprofessional communication is critical during handoffs between health professionals. Courtesy Maren Haddad.

in emergent or high-stakes situations, some have noted that these models are not very helpful for the breadth of information that composes a holistic picture of the patient such as social or psychological factors that have great potential to influence patient care.[39] Also, no one mental model for a shared language has risen to the level of best practice, so all of these acronyms and others can be in play within and between different health care institutions which can be confusing and frustrating. Despite this, handoffs and shared mental models are excellent opportunities to ask questions and participate in shared decision-making so the patient's high quality of care remains seamless.

Uncertainty

Uncertainty about one's own contributions and those of others can be a barrier to interprofessional communication. Even with competence and confidence, you also need basic knowledge of the roles and responsibilities of members of the interprofessional care team. Often members of an interprofessional care team operate on unconscious stereotypes about other professions and misunderstandings about boundaries and scopes of practice. There also can be an overlap between professions and role blurring. Additionally, some teams change every week or month. Turnover in team members can be a real challenge to all involved. It contributes to uncertainty and can lead to a lack of continuity in the delivery of safe, efficient, effective, and compassionate care.

The traditional assumption that the physician is always the designated leader of the interprofessional care team is another barrier that persists in health care. Collaborative practice works best when leadership is shared or assigned because of specialized knowledge or technical skills that are relevant to the specific decision at hand. Clearly, there is no one person on a team today who possesses all the specialized knowledge and technical skills needed in a complex case, so informed leadership should shift as the situation dictates. Even given this reality of the need to share the leadership role to best serve the patient, there are members of the team who are reluctant to give up their authority or conversely fearful of accepting the responsibility of a leadership role. For an interprofessional care team to work effectively, members of the team must be able to speak up, not just ask for permission or to give orders. It is only through the elimination of established but unnecessarily inflexible power structures and assumed roles that members of the team can see the whole picture, not just focus on what they need to get done within their individual scope of practice.

Gender and Generational Differences

Differences in *gender* and *generational differences* among health professionals are long-standing barriers to effective communication and collaboration. These differences and the stereotypes that accompany them inform role expectations that have historical and social roots. Health professionals are influenced by these abiding images of their professional roles such as the analytic, knowledgeable, objective decision-maker, which is connected to traditional masculine traits versus the caring, compassionate, hands-on traits of femininity. As was discussed in Chapter 4, such gender stereotypes as well as those connected to race, ethnicity, etc. limit the varied and complex contributions that all health professions offer to the team. For true collaboration, all members of the team must be considered equal partners who possess an array of knowledge, skills, perspectives, and abilities.

Generational differences between members of the health care team can arise in several ways that affect interprofessional collaboration because each generation has lived through different social and historical events. Individual members of a generation though will not experience the exact same events in the same manner so it is prudent not to stereotype everyone born during a certain generation assuming they will all have the same personality traits. The following cohorts have been defined as The Silent Generation (1925–45), the Baby Boomer Generation (1946–64), Generation X (1965–80), Generation Y or Millennials (1981–94), Generation Z (1995–2009), and Generation Alpha (2010–20).[40] Although it is likely that generational cohorts will exhibit varying degrees of skills and abilities with younger generational cohorts exhibiting more adept technological skills as digital natives, not every Generation Z health professional will outperform a Baby Boomer in this area. In other words, all members of the team need to be valued for the generational strengths they bring to patient care.[41]

Geographic Barriers

Finally, *geography* is a barrier to interprofessional communication. Proximity yields familiarity. When members of a team are in one place, there are greater opportunities for the development of trust and socialization. Geographic barriers can be overcome by distance technology, but more effort is required to establish relationships built on shared experiences both within and outside of the work environment. The constraints of the COVID-19 pandemic have had the positive effect of more virtual communication among team members that increased familiarity with the technology, changed communication dynamics, and allowed more members of the team and members of the patient's family to be virtually present and participate from a variety of geographically distant locations.[42]

Opportunities for Improving Interprofessional Approaches

As you read the case involving Dr. Halamek and the Collins family, note where the key elements for effective collaborative practice are present or lacking.

CASE STUDY

David Halamek, MD, is a new pediatrician in a large children's ambulatory clinic that includes the full range of health professionals among the clinic's staff. Because he just became a member of the pediatric group practice, all Dr. Halamek's patients and families are new to him. One of these families is the Collins family, who were making their first visit to Dr. Halamek. There was not much in the background information Dr. Halamek received before he saw the Collins family. He knew there were two children, ages 2 and 4, and that this was a visit for a routine physical for the 4-year-old. He also saw in their records a recent evaluation from one of the OTs at the clinic regarding the 2-year-old, Mia. The note from the OT said: "Mia has left hemiparesis resulting from an intracranial hemorrhage secondary to prematurity. She has full passive range of motion and active range of motion in her left upper extremity, but there is mild-to-moderate increased tone. She has a well-controlled reach with the left arm, but her hand goes into a flexor synergy (i.e., tends to close) before reaching the object she is trying to grasp. She likely needs orthotic intervention to improve manipulation of objects."[43] Dr. Halamek also noted that there were no records of immunizations for either child. At the outset of the visit, Dr. Halamek asked Mrs. Collins if she could remember the vaccinations her son had previously received. She told Dr. Halamek that her son had never received any vaccinations and that she did not plan on vaccinating her children because she had heard from several reliable sources that they were the cause of autism. Dr. Halamek informed Mrs. Collins that her views about the connection between autism and vaccinations were based on faulty information. He had encountered parents like Mrs. Collins before, so he had a copy of the now infamous journal article that featured a retraction of previously published false data on the alleged connection between vaccines and autism. He gave the copy of the article to Mrs. Collins. But Mrs. Collins did not want to discuss it. After moments of frustration and further attempts to convince Mrs. Collins about the importance of immunization for her children and others, Dr. Halamek told Mrs. Collins that he would not be able to treat her children if she was unwilling to agree to the approved immunization schedule. Mrs. Collins picked up Mia, grabbed Todd's hand, and left the room. One of the other pediatricians and a nurse practitioner were standing in the hallway as Mrs. Collins huffed out of the office. When Dr. Halamek stepped out of the examination room, they inquired what happened. He explained that Mrs. Collins refused to immunize her children. He then said, "I had no choice but to tell her that I couldn't care for her children under those conditions." His colleagues looked surprised at Dr. Halamek's story. The nurse stated, "There are other options to use with vaccine-hesitant or vaccine-refusing parents, the first of which is to work with the other members of the team in complicated situations like this, so we are consistent in our approach. We have been working for months with Mrs. Collins to get Mia the services she needs. I am going to worry sick about that little one." The pediatrician added, "We are all part of a team here, so no one has to or should make decisions alone. We need all the help we can get to resolve stressful situations like this." Dr. Halamek was not entirely convinced that this was a "team" decision because he felt that keeping vaccine refusers in his practice would be tantamount to approval of providing substandard care as well as imposing high risks of infection on other patients who could not receive vaccinations for various health reasons.[44]

REFLECTIONS

- What barriers to effective interpersonal collaboration were at play in the case? Consider the actions of all those involved, that is, Dr. Halamek and the other members of the team.
- Which members of the interprofessional care team should have been involved in setting goals, specifically about how to approach the subject of immunizations, for the Collins family? Why?
- What core concepts of Patient and Family Centered Care presented in Chapter 7 might serve as helpful guides to Dr. Halamek and the interprofessional care team as they seek to re-engage in follow-up care for this family?

What might have occurred in this case if Dr. Halamek had worked with other members of the team to make a collaborative decision on how best to work with the Collins family before this first interaction? Let us rewind the case, back to the beginning when Dr. Halamek looked at his new patients for the day and noticed that there were no records of the Collins children's immunizations. How might the following skills of effective teams make a difference in communicating with

Mrs. Collins about vaccinations? Note that the focus here is not which approach to working with vaccine-hesitant parents is the best in this case but on the contributions of effective interprofessional teamwork in providing quality patient-centered care.

COOPERATION

Cooperation is defined as "acknowledging and respecting other opinions and viewpoints while maintaining a willingness to examine and change personal beliefs and perspectives."[45] Starting from a place of collaborative practice means that the members of an interprofessional care team rely on the expertise and talents of each member (including the patient and family) and their contributions to the plan of care. The team participants must be able to cooperate with each other, which means that they must acknowledge and respect other opinions and viewpoints perhaps different from their own. Dr. Halamek acted independently as a solo health professional and relied on his own experience and knowledge on the topic of vaccine refusal. For him, it was a matter of lack of accurate information on the part of Mrs. Collins, and he acted to correct the problem. It appears he did not consider that others in the clinic likely have encountered vaccine-hesitant parents and may have different ideas about the reasons for Mrs. Collins's refusal and effective interventions. Nor did he know what conversations had already taken place with Mrs. Collins and the other members of the team. On the other hand, it does not appear that other members of the team made any effort to inform Dr. Halamek regarding past interactions with and plans for the Collins family.

In fact, effectively communicating with parents about vaccination is a common and sometimes challenging issue in pediatric care. By seeking the input of colleagues such as other pediatricians, the OT, the nurse practitioner, or even the clinic's legal counsel in some cases, Dr. Halamek could have discovered valuable information about how the clinic views the use of vaccines and how they routinely approach vaccine-hesitant parents. However, cooperation is more than the process of getting advice from others who have something to contribute to a decision. Cooperation means that you view the issue from the perspective of the team, mindful of what others can and should contribute that you cannot.

ASSERTIVENESS

Assertiveness is also required for effective collaboration. Individuals on the interprofessional care team not only have to speak with confidence but also make sure that their voice is heard. Dr. Halamek's colleagues demonstrated assertiveness when they told him, "There are other options, the first of which is to work with the other members of the team in complicated situations like that" and "We are all part of a team here, so no one has to or should make decisions alone. We need all the help we can get to resolve stressful situations like this." Their comments are focused and clear. They affirm values of teamwork and interdependence that undergird a philosophy of practice of which Dr. Halamek is now a part.[45] They do not tell Dr. Halamek that he was wrong in the way he handled the situation, rather they use broad statements offering him an opportunity to gain from their support, not the kind that places Dr. Halamek in a defensive position. They are not being aggressive, which could be demeaning to Dr. Halamek, who may already be frustrated and embarrassed after Mrs. Collins's exit. The power of the interprofessional team is highlighted here. As you will note, through affirming the values of teamwork, clinician well-being is supported, and the hope is that Dr. Halamek feels empowered to create positive change rather than experience the negative impact of moral distress.

RESPONSIBILITY

Each individual member of the interprofessional care team has responsibilities for certain tasks and duties related to patient care. There are also shared or mutual responsibilities that the team must fulfill. This means that individual members of the team must accept and share responsibilities and actively participate in group decision-making and support the decision approved by consensus.[45] This element of collaborative practice means that once a decision is made, all members of the team must be supportive even if it does not fully reflect that person's individual views or perspective. Getting to consensus depends on autonomy and good communication among team members, so individuals believe their input has been fairly considered in the decision-making process. It is especially important that all members of the team are supportive when a decision requires reconsideration based on new information. In the case of Dr. Halamek, there was no group decision-making involved. It is possible that there was past group decision-making and consensus on the part of the clinic personnel to follow a protocol for working with vaccine-hesitant parents depending on where the parents fell on the continuum from cautious acceptance to outright refusal.[46] This is a good example of the importance of educating new members of a team about the existing culture—that is, explaining what protocol the team follows in specific cases or about commonly occurring issues.

COMMUNICATION

Communication, which is the "effective sharing of important information and exchanging of ideas and discussion," has already been mentioned as an important individual and team skill.[45] Collaborative practice is actualized when all members of the interprofessional care team are willing to learn about, from, through, and with each other. In doing so they develop fluency in the language of each other's professions and cultures to understand their collective perspective and contributions. Being aware of what is relevant in any situation to help move the interprofessional teamwork in a positive direction is a key. In this case, where there was little communication on the part of Dr. Halamek with any other members of the interprofessional care team, it may have moved the situation along for him to have asked if there was an established protocol. At a minimum, he would know more about how situations such as this were handled, even though his view on the subject might not be shared by his new colleagues. He would also learn how his colleagues communicate about this topic and what skills they must work toward to achieve the shared goal of protecting the Collins children and other children as well. For example, the daughter Mia was previously seen by an OT. Dr. Halamek might have taken advantage of that relationship with the family to revisit the vaccine question at a later visit rather than dismissing the family.

AUTONOMY

It might not seem that autonomy, the "ability to work independently," would be a key element of effective collaborative practice.[45] Interprofessional collaboration requires interdependence. However, autonomy does play a role. Members of the interprofessional care team may have less individual autonomy, but the team is more autonomous with all the members working together. Despite the focus on collective goals, individual members of the team may continue to hold to certain interests or duties unique to their role and maintaining a certain amount of autonomy.[47] Hence, when Dr. Halamek admits that he is not entirely convinced that this was a "team" decision regarding what is the best approach for vaccine-hesitant parents, he is expressing the tension between individual autonomy and the autonomy of the team.

COORDINATION

The final element for effective collaboration is coordination, defined as the "efficient organization of group tasks and assignments."[45] All members of a team need to possess the comprehension and communication skills to deliver patient-centered care. The discussion of vaccines in the ambulatory setting is but one example of a nearly inevitable challenge in pediatric practice that requires interprofessional coordination.[48] If the members of an interprofessional care team are coordinated in their efforts, they can avoid duplication and ensure that the most qualified person or persons on the team take care of the issue or problem that moves the team toward the goals of care.

Teams also need practice to improve coordination. Different types of scheduled interprofessional collaboration that have proven to be effective are team rounding with the patient and the family at the bedside or if there are a lot of team members present, in a conference room. Shared care and discharge plans that bring together the unique perspectives of all the relevant members of the team is another way to coordinate services that might be needed in the home setting after discharge. Again, patients and family members should be included in care and discharge plans.[49]

Coordination today also requires that each member of the team be aware of guidelines, policies, and laws established by government, institutional, and professional specialty groups to further refine their individual and collective contributions. For example, referring to Dr. Halamek's situation, the American Academy of Pediatrics Clinical Report on responding to parental refusals of immunization provides useful strategies and resources pediatricians should take advantage of in situations of vaccine refusals.[50] A supportive mechanism for coordinating and addressing interventions that go awry in the clinical setting is care team rounds (or what you may have heard them referred to in the hospital setting as morbidity and mortality "m and m" rounds). Traditionally conceptualized in medicine as a way for professionals to present a case to their peers for further evaluation, rounds are now used across many interprofessional care settings. Rounds are forums for health professionals to reflect on care delivery openly and honestly through facilitated debriefing, reflection, dialog, case discussion, problem solving, and resource sharing. Outcomes of rounds include enhanced clinical decision-making, expanded perspective taking, and increased team building.[51]

Summary

As emphasized throughout this chapter, the focus of the interprofessional care team is to realize the overarching goals of patient care. Our description of major challenges and opportunities of achieving collaborative practice highlights that these goals depend in part on the individual professional's preparation discussed in previous chapters. However, given today's health care structures and the complexity of patient care, it often takes the members of a team exercising the elements of collaborative practice to fully realize the purpose of your work as a professional.

This chapter brings into center focus aspects of your professional identity and activity that so far have been addressed only in the background. Learning to be a collaborative member of an interprofessional care team relies on a solid foundation of individual preparation in your chosen field but adds components that help ensure you and others can meet the benchmarks of respect essential for high-quality care and patient safety. Specific competencies for interprofessional collaboration have been developed by professional organizations and are being implemented widely in health care. Personal attributes that are elements for ensuring your skillful participation on a team include trust, self-awareness, and flexibility. There are also several elements that the teams themselves must express, including mutual respect and strong communication skills. Our descriptions of barriers to collaboration and opportunities to successfully meet these challenges are resources that you can call on to help optimize your success.

References

1. Cunningham S, Musick DW, Trinkle DB. Evaluation of an interpersonal learning experience for telephone consultations. *Adv Med Educ Pract.* 2021;12:215–225, p. 222.
2. Institute of Medicine Committee on Quality of Care in America. *Crossing the Quality Chasm: A New Health System for the 21st Century.* Washington, DC: National Academy of Sciences; 2001.

3. Institute of Medicine. *Who Will Keep the Public Healthy? Educating Public Health Professionals for the 21st Century.* Washington, DC: National Academy of Sciences; 2002.

4. *Institute of Medicine.* The future of nursing: leading change, advancing health. http://www.nationalacademies.org/hmd/Reports/2010/The-Future-of-Nursing-Leading-Change-Advancing-Health.aspx; 2010.

5. Institute of Medicine. *Measuring the Impact of Interprofessional Education on Collaborative Practice and Patient Outcomes.* Washington, DC: The National Academies Press; 2015.

6. *Joint Commission.* Sentinel Event Alert. Behaviors that undermine a culture of safety. Issue 40. http://www.jointcommission.org/sentinel_event_alert_issue_40_behaviors_that_undermine_a_culture_of_safety/; 2008.

7. *Joint Commission.* Accreditation program hospitals: national patient safety goals. https://www.jointcommission.org/standards/national-patient-safety-goals; 2021.

8. World Health Organization. Framework for action on interprofessional education & collaborative practice. In: *WHO Reference Number: WHO/HRH/HPN/10.3*; 2010:13. http://www.who.int/hrh/resources/framework_action/en/.

9. Hall P. Interprofessional teamwork: professional cultures as barriers. *J Interprof Care.* 2016;19(suppl 1): 188–196.

10. Health Professions Accreditors Collaborative. *Guidance on Developing Quality Interprofessional Education for the Health Professions.* Chicago, IL: Health Professions Accreditors Collaborative; 2019.

11. Interprofessional Education Collaborative. *Core Competencies for Interprofessional Collaborative Practice.* Washington, DC: Interprofessional Education Collaborative; 2011.

12. *Carnegie Foundation.* Educating nurses and physicians: toward new horizons. http://www.macyfoundation.org/publications/educating-nurses-and-physicians-toward-new-horizons; 2010.

13. McCaffrey RG, Hayes R, Stuart W, et al. An education program to promote positive communication and collaboration between nurses and medical staff. *J Nurses Staff Dev.* 2011;27:121–127.

14. Zwarstein M, Rice K, Gotlib-Conn L, et al. Disengaged: a qualitative study of communication and collaboration between physicians and other professions on general internal medicine wards. *BMC Health Serv Res.* 2013;13:494.

15. Interprofessional Education Collaborative. *Core Competencies for Interprofessional Collaborative Practice.* Washington, DC: Interprofessional Education Collaborative; 2016.

16. *Commission on Accreditation in Physical Therapy Education.* Standards and required elements for accreditation of physical therapy education programs. http://www.capteonline.org/AccreditationHandbook; 2018.

17. Accreditation Council for Pharmacy Education. *Accreditation Standards and Key Elements for the Professional Program in Pharmacy Leading to the Doctor of Pharmacy Degree.* Chicago, IL; 2015. Retrieved from: https://www.acpe-accredit.org/pdf/Standards2016FINAL.pdf.

18. Accreditation Council of Occupational Therapy Education. *Standards and Interpretive Guide, B.4.25.* North Bethesda, MD; 2020. Retrieved from: www.acoteonline.org.

19. Accreditation Council of Occupational Therapy Education. *Standards and Interpretive Guide, B.4.24.* North Bethesda, MD; 2020. Retrieved from: www.acoteonline.org.

20. Blechert TF, Christiansen MF, Kari N. Intraprofessional team building. *Am J Occup Ther.* 1987;41(9): 576–582.

21. Huynh T, Nadon M, Kershaw-Rousseau S. Voices that care: licensed practical nurses and the emotional labour underpinning their collaborative interactions with registered nurses. *Nurs Res Pract.* 2011;2011: 501790.

22. Wong R, Kitto S, Whitehead C. Other ways of knowing: using critical discourse analysis to reexamine intraprofessional collaboration. *Can Fam Phys.* 2016;62:701–703.

23. Robinson N. Training and other important needs for nursing assistants. *Narrative Inq Bioeth.* 2011;1(3): 147–151.

24. Maple G. Early intervention: some issues in co-operative teamwork. *Aust Occup Ther J.* 1987;34(4): 145–151.

25. Wackerhausen S. Collaboration, professional identity and reflection across boundaries. *J Interprof Care.* 2009;23(5):455–473.

26. Mickam S, Rogers S. Characteristics of effective teams. *Aust Health Rev.* 2000;23(3):201–208. quote p. 204.

27. Kester ES. Speech-language pathologists engaging in interprofessional practice: the whole is greater than the sum of its parts. *Perspect ASHA Spec Interest Group*. 2018;3(Part 1):20–26. SIG 16.

28. Gilbert JHV, Camp RD, Cole CD, et al. Preparing students for interprofessional teamwork in health care. *J Interprof Care*. 2016;14(3):223–235.

29. Meyer J, Leslie P, Ciccia A, Rodakowski J. Whose job is it? Addressing the overlap of speech-language pathologists and occupational therapists when caring for people with dementia. *Perspect ASHA Spec Interest Group*. 2021;6:163–166. p. 165. SIG 15.

30. Dombeck MT. Professional personhood: training, territoriality and tolerance. *J Interprof Care*. 1997;11: 9–21.

31. Merriman C, Chalmers L, Ewens A, Fulford B, Gray R, Handa A, Wescott L. Values-based interprofessional education: how interprofessional education and values-based practice interrelate and are vehicles for the benefit of patients and health and social care professionals. *J Interprof Care*. 2020;34(4):569–571. https://doi.org/10.1080/13561820.2020.1713065.

32. Haig KM, Sutton S, Wittington J. SBAR: a shared mental model for improving communication between clinicians. *J Qual Patient Saf*. 2006;32(3):167–175.

33. Croker A, Grotowski M, Croker J. Interprofessional communication for interprofessional collaboration. In: Levett-Jones T, ed. *Critical Conversations for Patient Safety: An Essential Guide for Health Professionals*. Sydney: Pearson; 2014:55–61.

34. Salvatori P, Mahoney P, Delottinville C. An interprofessional communication skills lab: a pilot project. *Educ Health*. 2006;19(3):380–384.

35. Spencer J. Virtual meetings: 10% technology, 90% psychology. *PTinMOTIONmag.org*. 2019:6–7.

36. Starmer AJ, Spector ND, West DC, et al. Integrating research, quality improvement, and medical education for better handoffs and safer care: disseminating, adapting, and implementing the I-PASS program. *J Comm J Qual Patient Saf*. 2017;43:319–329.

37. Leonard M, Graham S, Bonacum D. The human factor: the critical importance of effective teamwork and communication in providing safe care. *Qual Saf Health Care*. 2004;13(suppl 1):i85–i90.

38. Soskin P, Duong D. Social worker as SBIRT instructor to emergency medicine residents. *MedEdPORTAL Publ*. 2014;10:9840.

39. Corbally M, Timmins F. The 4S approach: a potential framework for supporting critical care nurses' patient assessment and interprofessional communication. *Critic Care Nurs*. 2016;21(2):64–67.

40. Betz C. Generations X, Y, and Z. *J Pediatr Nurs*. 2019;44:A7–A8.

41. Pulcini CD, Turner TL, First LR. Generational empathy: an approach for addressing generational differences. *Pediatrics*. 2021;147(3). https://doi.org/10.1542/peds.2020-0191.

42. Campoe K. Interprofessional collaboration during COVID-19. *MEDSURG Nurs*. 2020; 29(5):297–298.

43. Coppard BM, Lohman HL. *Introduction to Orthotics: A Clinical Reasoning and Problem-Solving Approach*. St. Louis, MO: Elsevier; 2015:394.

44. Navin MC, Wasserman JA, Opel DJ. Reasons to accept vaccine refusers in primary care. *Pediatrics*. 2020;146(6). https://doi.org/10.1542/peds.2020-1801.

45. Norsen L, Opladen J, Quinn J. Practice model: collaborative practice. *Crit Care Nurs Clin North Am*. 1995;7(1):43–52.

46. Leask J, Kinnersley P, Jackson C, et al. Communicating with parents about vaccination: a framework for health professionals. *BMC Pediatr*. 2012;12:154.

47. Rose L. Interprofessional collaboration in the ICU: how to define? *Nurs Crit Care*. 2011;16(1):5–10.

48. Opel DJ, Heritage J, Taylor JA, et al. The architecture of provider-patient vaccine discussions at health supervision visits. *Pediatrics*. 2013;132(6):1037–1046.

49. Sigmon LB. Interprofessional collaboration made easy. *Am Nurse J*. 2020;15(11):36–38. www.MyAmericanNurse.com.

50. Diekema DS and American Academy of Pediatrics Committee on Bioethics. Responding to parental refusals of immunization of children. *Pediatrics*. 2005;115:1428–1431.

51. Doherty RF, Peterson EW. Responsible participation in a profession: fostering professionalism and leading for moral action. In: Braveman BH, ed. *Leading and Managing Occupational Therapy Services*. 3rd ed. Philadelphia, PA: FA Davis; 2022.

CHAPTER 9

Respectful Communication in a Technology-Driven Age

The reader will be able to

- Compare and contrast modes and models of communication;
- Distinguish ways to convey respect in face-to-face, in-person, and virtual patient communication;
- Identify four important factors in achieving successful verbal communication;
- Discuss various factors that affect health literacy;
- Assess three problems that can arise from miscommunication in health care delivery;
- Discuss two voice qualities that influence the meaning of spoken words;
- Identify two types of nonverbal communication and describe the importance of each;
- Describe how attitudes and emotions such as fear, grief, or anger/frustration affect communication;
- Give some examples of ways in which time and space awareness differ among individuals and cultures;
- Recognize best practices for communicating through synchronous and asynchronous telehealth encounters; and
- Identify critical elements of effective listening.

Prelude

> ... *my left side is a little bit weak and almost paralyzed. Just getting to an appointment is a task for me... Going down my stairs to my computer, it's better.*
>
> R.E. POWELL ET AL.[1]

Patients rely on verbal and nonverbal communication to try to explain what is wrong or seek comfort or encouragement from health professionals. Health professionals also rely on verbal and nonverbal communication to ask questions, provide support and information, and assess patient status. Since communication is much more than words, patients may have difficulty with language or health literacy, finding the right terms, or they may literally be unable to speak and must resort to gestures. Patients also face collateral challenges with communication in today's digital world including access to technology such as computers, iPads, and cell phones.

In the aftermath of COVID-19 with stay-at-home orders and limited social contact, we have seen major changes in how we exchange information and all that involves. Different types of electronic/virtual communication are developing rapidly. Health professionals are not the only ones turning to communication technology to assist in the delivery of care, patients as well are increasingly citing advantages of a broad array of technologies that assist them in managing their health. As the patient in the prelude explained, some patients prefer virtual communication with health professionals in certain situations because it is less stressful for them. Thus advances in communication technology will surely continue as well as the need for fundamental skills in patient-centered communication (PCC) on the part of the health professional. This chapter contains an overview of key points in communication in health care—a critical element of the health professional and patient interaction. Additionally, as emphasized in Chapter 8, good interprofessional collaboration relies on effective communication between health professionals. All the tools described herein to avoid miscommunication and make the most of exchanges of accurate information to improve patient care also apply to interprofessional collaboration.

Talking Together

Understandably, a lot of health professional and patient interactions rely on verbal communication. The greater responsibility for respectful communication between you and a patient lies with you, although both must assume responsibility. By examining interdependent components of communication and the skills that are required such as using silence effectively, posing open-ended questions, listening mindfully, and responding empathetically to strong emotions, you will gain insight into this critical area of human interaction.[2]

In your work as a health professional, you will be required to communicate verbally with a patient to (1) establish rapport, (2) obtain information concerning their condition and progress, (3) confirm understanding (your own and that of the person with whom you are communicating), (4) relay pertinent information to other health professionals and support personnel, and (5) educate patients and their family/caregivers. Periodically, you are expected to offer encouragement and support, give rewards as incentives for further effort, convey bad news, report technical data to a patient or colleague, interpret information, and act as a consultant or advocate. Naturally, you will be more comfortable with some activities than with others, per your own specific abilities and experiences. Nevertheless, all health professionals should be prepared to perform the entire gamut of communication activities.

Verbal communication is instrumental in creating understanding between you and a patient. However, this is not always the result. You will often be able to trace the cause of a misunderstanding to something you said, perhaps it was the wrong thing to say, or it was said in the wrong way or at the wrong time. The way words travel back and forth between individuals has been the subject of considerable study in the communication field. Several models have been proposed to graphically describe what happens when two people exchange the simplest of words.

Models of Communication

Although the following quotation focuses on the exchange of information between a physician and patient, the same can be said of all health professionals as they communicate with patients. As you read the quote, recall the differences between how patients tell their stories that were elaborated in Chapter 6 and the traditional "interview" model described here in which the health professional questions the patient to arrive at a diagnosis.

> It is revealing to examine how this flow back and forth between physician and patient is shaped, what is revealed or requested, when, by whom, at whose request or command, and whether there is reciprocal revelation of reasons, doubts, and anxieties. When we look at the medical context, instead of a free exchange of speech acts we find a highly structured discourse situation in which the physician is very much in control. Some patients perceive this sharply. Others more vaguely sense time constraints and a sequence structured by physician questions and terminated by signals of closure, such as writing prescriptions.[3]

Communication understood in this way involves the transfer of information from the patient to the health professional so a diagnosis or plan for treatment can be made. The focus is on the "facts" and generally begins with a question about what problem or concern brought the patient to the health professional. Often, once the patient identifies a problem, little time or attention is devoted to eliciting other patient-centered concerns.

Think of some reasons this model is problematic. For example, the first complaint that a patient mentions may not be the most significant. More importantly, the patient may take a health professional's hurried rush through a series of questions as an overt sign of disinterest and disrespect. Most interactions with patients continue to take the form of interviews rather than a conversation or dialogue. Health professions students take great pains to learn interview techniques designed to reveal, by the process of data gathering and elimination, the patient's health problem. The interview becomes a means to an end, the end being a diagnosis, problem identification, and treatment plan. As was noted in Chapter 6, this end may not be the one the patient is seeking. Furthermore, by strictly following the interview model of communication, the health professional effectively controls the introduction and progression of topics. In emergent situations when time is of the essence, a predetermined line of questions to get at the cause of a health problem can be justified. In less dramatic situations, other approaches to communication could be used that rely less on the use of power and authority to give patients time to speak to topics that concern them.

There is more than one way to reconsider how communication with patients could be conceived. One method, *PCC*, "involves exchanging information, fostering healing relationships, managing uncertainty, responding to emotions, shared decision-making, and enabling self-management" which improves outcomes, satisfaction, and trust in the health professional.[4] The focus in PCC is on mutual understanding between health professional and patient about the patient's values and needs plus the sharing of responsibility.[5]

Another unique way to view the interaction between health professional and patient is to think of it as improvisation. For example, even though health professional and patient interactions are often structured, they are not scripted in that "neither knows exactly what the other will say or do."[6] *Improvisation skills* can be effective tools in health professional and patient communication by "improving active listening, clear information delivery, and collaborative narrative building."[6] An underlying principle of improvisation is the "yes-and" response, which helps affirm what the speaker is saying. Including questions and prompts such as "Tell me more about that" or "What have you tried that helps?" also offers greater opportunity for communication than mere "yes" and "no" types of questions. Also, keeping quiet and letting patients tell their stories are especially effective to build trust and gain a sense of what is most important to patients.

Communication, both verbal and nonverbal, can be conceptualized as the bridge between you and a patient or the building blocks of the scene you and the patient are constructing as in the earlier examples from improvisation (Fig. 9.1). The model also includes some of the primary and secondary cultural characteristics introduced in Chapter 4 that influence what each party brings to the dialogue. These factors (and others not listed in the figure) have an impact on the interaction.

The Context of Communication

Where, with whom, and under what circumstances the dialogue or conversation takes place also can have a profound influence on the process and outcomes of the interaction (Fig. 9.1). Clinical encounters between you and your patients are often time limited and stressful for both parties because the content is highly personal. Thus the internal context of a health care exchange between you and the patient sets it apart from everyday conversations. The environmental context also has an impact on the process and outcome of your dialogue and can include barriers to communication such as a noisy environmental setting, lack of privacy, or a cluttered or messy environment.

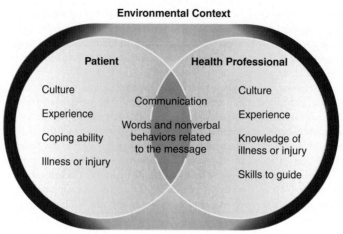

Fig. 9.1 Essential and influencing variables of the communication environment. From Keltner NL, Steele D. *Psychiatric Nursing*. 8th ed. St. Louis, MO: Elsevier; 2019.

Wherever communication occurs, make sure that you create a quiet, private place to talk that is well-lit and without distractions.

REFLECTIONS

- Reflect on barriers you have personally encountered to communication.
- What have you done to overcome them?
- Reflect on your own self-perceptions as a communicator such as what modes of communication are you most comfortable using. What modes are you most skilled in? What modes make you nervous?

In addition to the context of the interaction, other spatial factors impact communication. For example, if someone is literally right in front of you, the type of interaction is different from what occurs on the telephone or through an e-mail message, text, discussion board, blog, or virtual meeting room on the Internet. What varies most between in-person interactions and those that occur across distances is proximity, the quality of messages portrayed through nonverbal communication, the use of the senses of smell and touch, and the degree of relative anonymity. Direct personal contact with another person provides fewer places to hide fear, distaste, or discomfort for the person or about something in the interaction. In fact, knowing this, some health professionals specifically choose areas of practice in which they will have little direct contact with patients.

The value of direct contact is that when you can meet in person with a patient, all the possible ways of communicating can be engaged. Each sense can be a source of information about the other. This explains, in part, why the exchange is that much richer. During your career, there is a good chance you will use a variety of devices and modes to communicate with patients. In-person interactions with health professionals will continue but will be increasingly supplemented by ever-evolving forms of communication technology (Fig. 9.2). We begin by exploring face-to-face, in-person interactions with individuals and groups in different contexts.

ONE-TO-ONE INTERACTIONS

Before you begin any type of interaction with a patient, you should make sure the patient knows who you are and what you do. This sounds so basic that it hardly seems worth mentioning. However, some health professionals are so focused on getting on with the clinical task that they

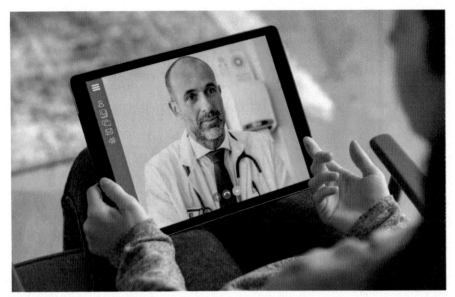

Fig. 9.2 Online communication with patients has both advantages and drawbacks. © Ridofranz/istock-photo.com.

forget the introductions. Many patients want to be greeted by a handshake or other means of personally "greeting" them in a culturally appropriate manner and verbal personalized contact with an explanation of your role.[7] If you have met before, but there has been some time between your interactions, it does not hurt to reintroduce yourself and explain your role. In addition, always wear your identification with your name and professional role clearly displayed.

If you are meeting a patient for the first time, be sure to use his or her full name. Do not presume to address a patient, unless the patient is a child, by his or her first name until the patient gives you explicit permission. Ask the patient how to pronounce his or her name if there is any doubt about the correct pronunciation and inquire regarding preferred pronouns. All these gestures convey respect for persons and set the stage for future communication.

After you introduce yourself, in a few sentences tell the patient what your role is regarding their care. It is helpful to practice this explanation with a sympathetic audience such as relatives or friends who will tell you if you are being too technical or confusing. Having established this initial rapport, you can now devote your attention to the patient before you and vice versa. We will address matters such as facial expression, gestures, and touch later in this chapter. All nonverbal forms of communication may override verbal messages, and this is especially obvious in face-to-face interactions.

GROUP INTERACTIONS

Working with an individual patient is different in some significant ways from working with a group of patients. Because you will have opportunities to interact with groups of patients or patients and their families or friends, knowledge about group functioning is important as the group has an impact on the roles individuals play within the group. For example, some people will take on a "gatekeeper" role that assures everyone in the group is on the same page before moving on to the next point of discussion. Others might take on roles that impede the work you want to accomplish within a group such as talking too much or undermining the role of the group leader. However, groups are helpful for much of what you communicate to individual patients regarding education about standard treatments, procedures, follow-up care, etc. The groups you interact with as a health professional may be spontaneously formed for a short period, such as family members at a care conference or a group of patients with a similar diagnosis being treated in an ambulatory clinic, such as a diabetes disease management group; or they may be groups that will interact for longer periods, such as a support group for patients who experienced a brain injury in a rehabilitation setting.

THE SETTING OF THE INTERACTION: INSTITUTION OR HOME

In Chapter 5, we discussed a variety of settings in which patients receive care today. Whatever the environment in which you encounter patients, for social, psychological, and financial reasons, there is a strong tendency to medicalize the setting. Even when in settings such as a rehabilitation setting or the patient's home, medical props and devices shape the atmosphere.

It is often evident to health professionals who work in patients' homes that they are viewed as guests at best or intrusive strangers at worst. Delivery of care in the home health setting places the health professional on the patient's turf and thus shifts control over the environment to the patient. Respect for the patient requires that health professionals in the home should be more deferential, more attuned to asking before doing. Other health care environments, such as intensive care units (ICUs) or emergency departments, do not even pretend to be "homelike" beyond the professional courtesies. The sights, sounds, smells, and urgency of these high-tech environments have a profound impact on patients, particularly because these environments are often foreign and perceived as threatening. Consider this excerpt from a poem involving a mother who gets her first glimpse of her child in the context of a critical care unit in a hospital.

Intensive Care

I am called.
   But nothing prepares me for what I see, my child

in her body of pain, hooked to machines. Grief
   comes up like floodwater. Her body floats on a sea

of air that is her bed, a force field of sorrow
   that pulls me to her side, I touch pain I know

I have never felt, move into a new land
   of nightmare. She is so still. Only one hand

moves, fingers oscillate like water plants risking
   the air. Machines line the desks,

the floor, the walls, confirm the deep pink
   of her skin in rapidly ascending numbers. One eye blinks. . .

L.C. GETSI[8]

REFLECTIONS

- How does the mother describe the "context" of the ICU setting? What impact might the setting have on further communication with the mother?
- Consider the opening lines of the poem. The mother is "called" to her child's bedside in the ICU. What words might have helped prepare her for what she was about to see and hear?
- If you were to enter this patient's room and come upon this mother, what would your first words to her be?

Sensitive communication depends on an appreciation of the effect of the environment on what transpires between you and the patient.

Choosing the Right Words

The success of verbal communication depends on two important factors: (1) the way material is presented (i.e., the vocabulary used, the clarity of voice, and organization) and (2) the tone and volume of the voice.

VOCABULARY AND JARGON

As we note in Chapter 8, the descriptive vocabulary of the health professional is a two-edged sword. Technical language is one of the bonds shared among health professionals themselves. In contrast, highly technical professional jargon is almost never appropriate in direct conversation with patients because it cuts off communication. It is imperative that you learn to translate technical jargon into common language when discussing a patient's condition or conversing with families and patient caregivers. Even when the patient happens to be a health professional, it is important to communicate in understandable language.

HEALTH LITERACY

Effective strategies for health care communication include health literacy. The Institute of Medicine (renamed the National Academy of Medicine) estimates that nearly half of all American adults (90 million people) have difficulty understanding and acting on health information.[9] *Health literacy* is "the degree to which individuals have the capacity to find, understand, and use information and services to inform health-related decisions and actions for themselves and others."[9] Think of all the items a patient might need to read to manage their health, such as wording on medication bottles, food labels, appointment slips, telehealth portal instructional emails, medical forms, insurance applications, medical bills, and health education materials. Another skill necessary to understand and manage certain aspects of health care is *numeracy* which is defined as "the ability to access, use, interpret, and communicate mathematical information and ideas, to engage in and manage mathematical demands of a range of situations in adult life."[9]

Not only do patients have to have a basic ability to read and comprehend what is written and use and interpret mathematical information, but they must also deal with "the increasing complexity of health care requires an understanding of digital communication, which may in turn require health, computer, numeric, computational and information literacy."[10] As mentioned in Chapter 8, generational differences in technological competency may result in older adults being less likely to be online than their younger counterparts and with the increasing use of digital health information, the divide will likely increase. Furthermore, vulnerable groups such as people who live in rural areas with poor Internet access and bandwidth and people who cannot afford the necessary technology to access digital communication will be less likely to use electronic patient portals or other types of digital communication not because of lack of ability but lack of access and support.[11,12]

Beyond the abilities of the patient, several other factors affect health literacy, including the quality of the information provided, the teaching method used, the context in which information is shared, the ability of the health professional to teach and communicate, and the patient's readiness to learn. Health professionals have a duty to teach patients effectively and evaluate their understanding and ability to use health information. Considerable attention has been dedicated to the research and development of various tools to screen patients for health literacy. Rather than spend time trying to determine each patient's health literacy abilities, organizations such as the American Medical Association and the Agency for Healthcare Research and Quality endorse adopting universal literacy precautions in much the same way as universal precautions for the protection of patients and health professionals from the spread of contagious disease.[13,14] In other words, health professionals should strive to communicate with all patients in simple, plain language, using lay language whenever possible to minimize the risk for any patient misunderstanding of the information provided. Additionally, there are communications tools like Ask3 that empower patients to ask three basic questions at the end of every clinical encounter The questions are: What is my main problem? What do I need to do? Why is it important for me to do it? These questions serve as a two-way street to better communication as such questions frame important points for both patients and health professionals. In particular, the last question, "Why is it important for me to do it?", is an opportunity to correct any misunderstandings about the reason for a treatment or therapy.[15]

LANGUAGE BARRIERS

Another common area for miscommunication is when the health professional and patient literally speak different languages. The health care environment is English-language dominant in the United States. As was mentioned in Chapter 4, an increasing number of patients will require the assistance of medical interpreters because of the influx of a variety of refugees and immigrants into the United States. It is rare that a health professional does not routinely encounter language barriers with patients because approximately 8.6% of the total US population is considered to have limited English proficiency.[16] More than 65 million (21.6%) of the nation's population aged five and older speak a language other than English at home.[16] Patients, or families in the case of pediatric patients, who do not speak English or have limited English proficiency are sometimes seen as a burden by health professionals. As one health professional noted, "Non–English speaking patients take at least twice the time of others. Everything one says should be understood, and some of it jotted down, by the interpreter before being relayed to the patient. It is not the patient's fault, but I can already picture the irritated waiting room."[17]

Numerous options exist for bridging these language barriers, including trained medical interpreters (in-person or through video conferencing/phone), bilingual health professionals, and trained volunteers. Implementing the use of professional medical interpreters has been shown to have the following positive benefits: a reduction in disparities, improved clinical outcomes, enhanced pain control, and improvement of patient satisfaction.[18] Furthermore, interpreters are uniquely equipped to assess how well information has been communicated with all parties involved. In-person interpreters have the added benefit of enabling a genuine dialogue by conveying patients' desires, questions, and fears.[19] It should be clear that the use of untrained volunteers or family members as medical interpreters should be avoided for the following additional reasons:

1. Untrained interpreters are more likely to make errors, violate confidentiality, increase the risk of patient dissatisfaction and poor outcomes.[20]
2. Family interpreters often speak as themselves rather than merely providing accurate information between parties.[21]
3. Untrained interpreters often lack knowledge of medical terms, which can lead to miscommunication and misdiagnosis.
4. Untrained interpreters may be emotionally harmed because of the stress of performing an essential activity for which they are not prepared.[22]

Patients may not initially trust formally trained interpreters, especially when they interact through the phone or video conferencing rather than in person, for a variety of social and cultural reasons including the intrusion of equipment into the interaction, but the risk for misunderstanding and errors without interpreter services is great enough to warrant their use. If possible, a combination of the languages involved, and nonverbal signs might be the best alternative when a patient refuses a trained interpreter. The main goal is to find a neutral and accurate means of communicating across language barriers in which both parties, patient and health professional, know what is being said.[23]

Of course, the way to respectful communication is to try as much as possible to talk to patients as equals (because that is what most patients want), seek assistance from medical interpreters when indicated, and remain flexible in your style to meet individual patients' needs.

Inefficiencies From Miscommunication

Several problems arise when miscommunication occurs because the health professional is unable to communicate with the patient in terms understandable to them. In situations in which language barriers and other impediments to communication have been remedied but the health professional is still having difficulty understanding the patient's attempts to explain their symptoms or problem because of a vague explanation or a reticent patient, it could be tempting to give up and turn to the objective criteria of laboratory and diagnostic findings or clinical experience to plan a treatment program. Yet, it is worth the effort to find other effective means of communicating as miscommunication can leave patients frustrated and anxious and so uncertain that it affects their ability to adhere with treatment.[24]

Another common area for miscommunication is when the health professional and patient are both using the same word but ascribing different meanings to it. One example noted earlier in this chapter is the professionals' use of the word *complaint*. This ordinary clinical jargon can convey a different meaning to the patient than to a health professional. In the attempt to understand a patient's situation, the professional is searching for the complaint or chief health problem the patient is experiencing. If the term "complaint" is used in the patient's presence, it may make the patient think they are a nuisance, when in fact the professional is simply searching for the relevant clinical signs, symptoms, or diagnosis.

Another problem that can result from using technical language is that the person to whom you are speaking will not be convinced you really want to know how they feel. When the health professional persists in using "big words" or technical language, the patient may interpret this as a sign that their problems are not important. Consequently, the very words meant to help can unintentionally hurt the patient. The complexity and impersonality of a health facility will undoubtedly be communicated to the patient if health professionals are unwilling to explain carefully to the patient, in understandable terms, their condition and its treatment. If the patient cannot understand what is being said, little will be accomplished, and poor health outcomes, including *adverse events*, which is "an event, preventable or unpreventable, that caused harm to a patient as a result of medical care" can result.[25]

The mastery of appropriate vocabulary includes being able to communicate with your interprofessional colleagues while at the same time being willing to converse with patients in words they can understand. When this is accomplished, patients will more likely comprehend what is requested, respond accurately to questions, and be convinced that you care about them.

LACK OF CLARITY

In addition to using words that are too technical for the patient to understand, a health professional may not speak with sufficient clarity to free the patient from uncertainty, doubt, or confusion about what is being said. What is the difference between the two? Lack of clarity can result if you launch into a lengthy, rambling description of treatment options (e.g., not realizing that the patient was lost at the outset). Lack of clarity also can result when patients become preoccupied with one facet of what you are saying and consequently interpret everything else considering that preoccupation.

It is surprising to some professionals that patients may be too embarrassed to ask them to repeat something, and so patients rely on what they think they heard. Patients are sometimes hesitant because they are a bit awed by you as the health professional and so try to act sophisticated instead of asking you to repeat what you said. Patients may be awed primarily because they realize that health professionals have skills that can determine their future welfare and that, regardless of their influence in the business or social worlds outside of health care, they are at your mercy in this situation. Some ways to help enhance the clarity of your communication follow.

Explanation of the Purpose and Process

Clarity begins with helping the patient understand who you are, why you are there, and what you plan to do. As mentioned earlier in this chapter, you first establish the purpose of your interaction when you introduce yourself and explain your role. This general introduction should be followed by a statement of the purpose of this encounter (i.e., what is going to take place now and why). Thus you and the patient know what the goal of the interaction is from the start. Because the patient may be tired or uncomfortable, it is also helpful to state at the outset how long the interaction will take and what the patient will likely experience (e.g., "The head of this instrument may be a little cold at first when it touches your skin," or "Push this call button if you want to get out of bed or need assistance of any kind. Someone will answer through the speaker in your room, and you can tell them what you need."). Questions the patient asks will then help you decide what more you need to say.

Organization of Ideas

Think ahead about how you are going to present your information. You can quickly confuse a patient by jumping from one topic to the next, inserting last-minute ideas, and then failing to summarize or to ask the patient to do so. Failure to systematically progress from one step to the next toward a logical conclusion is usually caused by (1) your own lack of understanding of the subject or of the steps in the procedure or (2), ironically, a too thorough knowledge of the subject or procedure. The former causes the patient to have to figure out the relevant facts, whereas the latter causes the speaker to leave out points that are obvious to him or her but not to the listener. In either case, it is advisable to organize the description of a procedure, test, or treatment into its component parts and then to practice describing it to a friend who is not familiar with the content. That person will be able to identify any obvious steps that have been omitted. Complicated information should be broken down into manageable chunks so that the patient is not overwhelmed by everything that follows. This is especially true when the information involves bad news.

Augment Verbal Communication

Verbal information and instructions alone are not always adequate to ensure clarity. When information is shared verbally there should also be written information for the patient. For example, it is hard to remember changes in medication dosing over a short period of time, like eye drops, that need to be given four times a day for a week, then three times for a week, then two times, etc. The same could be said regarding restrictions on activity post-op when the amount of movement could change daily in some cases. For situations like this, a calendar with instructions for each day or week is especially helpful.

Written notes or instructions, diagrams, videotapes, and nonverbal demonstrations are highly desirable adjuncts to the spoken word because they may help the person organize the ideas and information more fully and can be used for future reference. The augmented instructions or follow-up information for patients should be written in clear, direct language in the order required such as telling a patient at the outset not to eat or drink any fluids after midnight when providing instructions for an upcoming surgery. Beyond the specific words in written or spoken communication, there are factors that influence the meaning behind the words, which we examine next.

Tone and Volume

Paralinguistics "are the components of spoken communication that may or may not include words."[26] Although paralinguistics are considered part of the realm of nonverbal communication, we will discuss tone and volume here because they are so closely connected to the content of speech. Sometimes, a person's voice or volume belies their words. Any vocalized sound a person makes could be interpreted as verbal communication, so besides your words, you will communicate "volumes" with the tone, inflection, speed, and loudness of the words you use.

TONE

Tone is a voice quality that can support or reverse the meaning of the spoken word. Each of us tries to communicate more than the literal content of our messages by using different tones of voice of the same spoken message. A low tone of voice is often associated with authority. Also, the rise in pitch at the end of a sentence called high-rising terminal speech or "upspeak" indicates a question is being asked or approval is being sought.[27] However, upspeak is no longer reserved for questions. The rising intonation at the end of a sentence is more common among women than men and increasingly common among young people. Listen to your own voice as you interact with others to catch any unconscious rise in pitch when you are not asking a question to decrease the uncertainty in your tone. Changing intonation can thus change the meaning. An expression as short as "oh" can be used to express anger, pity, disappointment, teasing, pleasure, gratitude, exuberance, terror, superiority, disbelief, uncertainty, compassion, insult, awe, and many more. Try this exercise with "no," "yes," and other simple words or phrases to fully grasp the rich variety of meanings a word can convey simply by varying the tone and inflection.

Tone can be reassuring or off-putting. When the patient's response is puzzling to the health professional, the latter should be alert to the tone in which the patient communicated a message or reacted to a statement.

> **REFLECTIONS**
>
> Give several meanings to the simple question, "What are you doing?" by varying the tone in which it can be spoken. Try to mimic the tones of the following people: (1) a man telephoning his wife at midday; (2) the man's wife, who has just caught their 2-year-old son writing on the living room wall with a purple crayon; and (3) the 2-year-old son trying to make up to the mother after being scolded.

VOLUME

Tone and volume are closely related voice qualities. An angry person may not only spit out the words indignantly but also may alter the volume of the message. For instance, it is possible to communicate anger either by whispering words through gritted teeth or by shouting them.

Voice volume controls interaction in subtle ways. For instance, if one person stands close to another and speaks in an inordinately loud voice, the listener invariably backs away. On the other hand, a soft whisper automatically causes the listener to move closer. Thus literally and symbolically the volume of the voice does control distance between people.

Whatever you say, you must make certain the patient can hear you. An easy way to assess if you are speaking loudly enough is to ask the patient to repeat instructions rather than just solicit "yes" or "no" responses. Make sure the patient can see your face when you speak because some patients need the physical cues of your expression and the movement of your lips to understand what is being said. The requirement of wearing a facial mask during the COVID-19 pandemic made it particularly trying for people, patients, and health professionals alike, who rely on physical and visual cues to understand what is being said to them.

Choosing the Way to Say It

Your educational experience will provide you with the right words, but you will send many other messages to patients in addition to the spoken word. The most basic of nonverbal forms of communication is the way you think, feel, or act—your attitude. We will begin our discussion of attitudes by presuming inherent good intent in responding to one another. We presume an attitude of mutual trust and respect. Most health professionals maintain a caring attitude toward patients, and their way of speaking to them helps communicate this genuine concern and respect.

ATTITUDES AND EMOTIONS

One variable that is frequently overlooked and has considerable impact on the exchange of information is the patient's emotional and mental state and attitudes. Examples are fear or anger that complicate communication and the management of his or her condition. If you want to effectively communicate with patients, you must be knowledgeable about their mental state. You do not have to perform an exhaustive mental status examination to determine a patient's ability to comprehend, orientation to the task at hand, or ability to follow directions. You can obtain this information as you interact with the patient. If there is any doubt as to the patient's general cognitive ability, you can use one of the many screening tools available to assess general mental functions.

The emotional state of the health professional also has an impact on effective communication as well as the patient's. The attitude that a health professional has toward the patient will help to determine the effectiveness of spoken interaction, too. Attitudes and emotions that are commonly encountered on the part of the health professional are fear, grief, and anger/frustration.

Fear

Patients are often afraid for many reasons. Fear may manifest as stony silence, clenched fists, profuse sweating, anxiety, or an angry outburst. Patients may not recognize the emotion they are experiencing as fear, so you must be watchful for the signs of fear and do your best to help reassure the patient.

The specific situations in which health professionals' fears arise are just as numerous as those for patients. How will your fear manifest itself during spoken communication? Fear can arise when the health professional is inexperienced, or the patient is threatening in some way. Developing skills to de-escalate situations in which patients or family members are increasingly agitated is essential, especially if you work in high-stress areas such as emergency departments or psychiatric/mental health/behavioral facilities.

Grief

Patients deal with grief in a variety of ways. It is likely that you will see some people at the worst time of their lives and come to witness many different reactions to profound loss. It is important to prepare yourself to comfort patients and family members who are grieving and to try to effectively address your own feelings. Some of the topics outlined as benchmarks of professional respect in Chapter 1 are useful at such a time. For instance, reacting with deep sorrow or tears to a patient's plight may at times be deemed "unprofessional" because it suggests pity or overidentification with the patient's or family's unique situation. However, if you remain stoic, patients may conclude you do not care. Striking the right balance between maintaining one's role as a professional in this situation (you are not a friend or family member) and conveying authentic human care for their situation warrants reflection every time you are faced with the other's suffering. That there is no a specific formula for such a situation is evident in the following account of a struggle by a neurosurgical resident when she had to tell a patient he has a terminal brain tumor:

I sat down and delivered the news. I hinted at the ultimate implications of his diagnosis, but I didn't want to hit this too hard too soon. I wanted to give him some time to digest the shock of the unexpected. I looked at his wife, his infant daughter, and at him. He nodded his head, slowly, calmly. I wanted to provide them with some hope so I started, reflexively, to enumerate all the treatments he could receive that would give him the best possible chance. I reassured him that he was young and healthy, which would put him in a more favorable category.

I felt I had done enough talking at that point, so I stopped and sat in silence, a natural invitation for questions. I looked at the three of them. His wife was starting to cry, silently.

Then, without warning, I started to cry, too, then sob, interrupting the silence. My usual calm professional demeanor had broken down. I was struck by a harsh paradox: the vision of this young vibrant family sitting with me in the present, clashing with my knowledge of biology and how this tumor was about to change their lives. I could see the future too clearly.

The patient continued to look at me, stoically, nodding his head. He exhaled audibly and then thanked me. I didn't deserve much thanks, though. I worried that my unbridled outpouring of grief had wiped out any shred of hope.[28]

REFLECTIONS

- Because the prognosis was bleak, the message that the neurosurgeon related was accurate, but was it appropriate?
- Would the patient necessarily lose all hope as the neurosurgeon feared?
- What might be another outcome of the neurosurgeon's expression of grief?
- What else might the neurosurgeon have said or done after her expression of grief?

Anger or Frustration

Health professionals often struggle with patients who are rude, demanding, or seem to lack consideration for other patients whose needs could be greater than their own at a given time. Dealing with this type of patient interaction is explored more fully in Chapter 15. Changes in the communication style of the health professional with patients who are a challenge are often one of distancing. Health professionals may try to manage underlying negative emotions by pulling away from genuine warmth to a more aloof demeanor. Sometimes this is referred to as "putting on a professional face" to hide their feelings. However, the anger just below the surface has a way of making itself known to patients largely through nonverbal signs such as a curt tone of voice, lack of eye contact and limited, reassuring physical contact on the part of the health professional.

Of course, positive emotions and attitudes can also impact communication between the health professional and patient. For example, patients may use humor to communicate a range of emotions such as the need to protect themselves or a way to safely express frustration. One of the authors experienced this sort of exchange with a surgeon during a post-operative visit. The surgeon was examining the chest incision where he recently removed a venous access port from the author. Although the incision was healing well, the area surrounding it was one large, purple bruise. The surgeon commented, "Wow! It looks like you got kicked by a horse." The author replied, "I guess that makes you the horse." Both the author and the surgeon laughed, probably for different reasons. Additionally, the relationship between the two people involved was long-standing. They were not only fellow health professionals but also friends which would allow for this kind of humorous exchange to lighten the mood. Humor is highly subjective and must be carefully used as a means of communication between patients and health professionals.

Communicating Beyond Words

In this section, we turn our attention beyond vocal utterances designed to engage us in dialogue and conversation to consider all the additional (or substitute) ways we enter communication with patients and others. Collectively these means are often referred to as *nonverbal communication*. As important as effective verbal communication is, the majority of communication is nonverbal, with estimates of 7% of the message being verbal and the other 93% being nonverbal communication.[29] Supportive nonverbal behaviors such as leaning forward, making eye contact, nodding, smiling, gesturing, and using a warm tone of voice were positively associated with health outcomes and reducing the distance between health professionals and patients.[30] These nonverbal behaviors and others that follow are easy to adopt, so they become second nature when you interact with patients.

FACIAL EXPRESSION

Earlier in this chapter, you were asked to consider the variety of messages conveyed by altering the tone and volume of the spoken word "oh." It is possible to omit the word altogether and, with only a facial message, convey a variety of emotions.

Eye contact generally communicates a positive message. There is a powerful, immediate effect when we gaze directly at another person. If two people genuinely like each other, they will position themselves so that they look into each other's eyes. The distance between them as they face each other further communicates how they feel about each other. Distance as a form of nonverbal communication is discussed later in this chapter.

Even without eye contact, the rest of the face reveals many things. The presence or absence of a smile and the genuineness of a smile are all clues to a person's emotional state. Grimaces from pain, the vacant stare of a child with a fever, and the bland affect of a depressed patient provide important information that speaks volumes without the use of words. Your own facial expression can stimulate good feelings. For example, a genuine smile indicates that you are approachable, cooperative, and trustworthy. Certainly, face masks that were mandatory for health professionals who cared for patients during the COVID-19 pandemic changed the messages that are sent by the entire face and not just the eyes. As a result, gestures and body language discussed below were even more important.

GESTURES AND BODY LANGUAGE

Gestures involving the extremities, even one finger, can communicate the meanings of a message. Consider the mother who folds her arms when a child begins to sputter an excuse for coming home late, the man who clenches his fist, or the colleague who incessantly taps her fingers on the table at a dull department meeting. What unspoken messages are they sending? A common reaction to nonverbal gestures of patients that are misinterpreted as anxiety or irritability is the administration of sedatives or restraints when other communication strategies would be more appropriate and less upsetting and harmful to the patient.[31]

Many health professionals develop the skill of truly reading the meaning of the gestures and behaviors of patients. For example, staff members such as nursing assistants in nursing home settings have demonstrated the predictive value of certain changes in nonverbal behavior in patients and the development of acute illness. One study found that the nursing assistants' documentation of nonspecific signs and symptoms of illness such as "patient is not as usual," evidence of restlessness, or change in food intake was shown to be significantly correlated to the later development of an infection.[32] Another study noted that family members can also play a role in the timely detection of changes in health status in their loved ones in the following ways: noticing signs of changes in health, informing care staff about what they noticed, and educating care staff about their family members' changes in health.[33] Understanding subtle and obvious gestures is an important component of learning respectful communication. Patients can also read the health professional's body language. Your words might say one thing to the patient, but your body language says something else which sends mixed messages to the patient. When you are stressed, it is a good habit to take a moment to assume a relaxed posture, take a deep breath and shake off tension to ready oneself for effective communication.

PROFESSIONAL DRESS AND APPEARANCE

Stereotypes are commonly formed from outward appearances. In some instances, a person tries to adopt a stereotyped manner of dressing or speaking in the hope of being identified with a particular group.

Some health professionals adopt or are required to wear a stereotyped manner of dress (the uniform) to be identified easily within the world of health care. The "uniform" may include clothing such as scrubs, a patch, a pin, a lab coat, or a name tag or lanyard with a badge. Certain instruments also identify the person: the nurse's stethoscope dangling from the neck or the laboratory technologist's tray. Regardless of the symbols that can help patients identify health professionals, keep in mind that the first impression patients have of you will be how you look as you approach them. Thus clean, unwrinkled clothes and footwear, attention to personal hygiene and hair arranged in a manner that doesn't impede safe care are important to convey a professional appearance.

> **REFLECTIONS**
>
> - What are the implications of wearing a white coat, scrubs, stethoscope, and other readily identifiable professional attire while engaging a patient?
> - In today's highly complex health settings with an increasing number of people caring for patients, do uniforms help patients identify who is caring for them, or do uniforms create greater distance?

TOUCH

In all societies, individuals come into physical contact with each other all the time, but the context is crucial (e.g., they tend not to put their hands on each other except in well-defined social and cultural rituals). However, on entering a health facility, regardless of if they like or dislike physical contact, people may have to allow themselves to be palpated, punctured with needles, squeezed, rubbed, cut, examined, manipulated, and lifted.

These unusual touching privileges are granted to health professionals by society. Licensing of health professionals is primarily a protection against the charge of unconsented touching *(battery)*. In Chapter 2, we focused on boundaries, including physical ones, that must be maintained, even when legitimate touching is recognizable as part of the therapeutic encounter.

Fortunately, the comforting touch is usually regarded as legitimate, and you have in it a powerful tool for communicating caring (Fig. 9.3). Touching a patient on the arm, hand, or shoulder for less than a few seconds can create a critical human bond. The positive effects of a caring touch are sometimes observable in the patient. For example, you may observe one or more of the following: a lowering of the patient's voice, a slowing and deepening of the patient's breathing, or a spontaneous verbal response like a sigh or "I feel relaxed." A physician who was seriously ill commented on how much caring touch meant to him: "The nurse giving a back rub was so incredibly important to me. It was profoundly human—an act of caring. Even with painkillers, there's suffering and pain. Those back rubs were . . . somebody affirm[ing] that I mattered."[34]

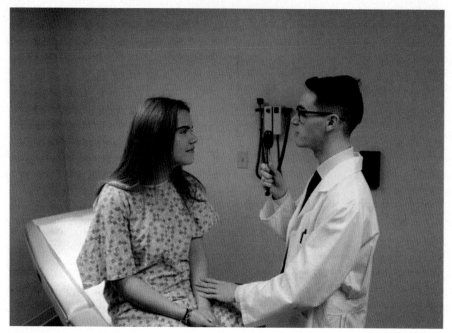

Fig. 9.3 A health professional who uses touch in an appropriate manner communicates caring to the patient. Courtesy Maren Haddad.

People pick up signals conveyed by your manner of touching. This is often related to the appearance of your gesture, the speed and ease with which you move, and the quality of your touch. Patients should be touched with respect for the person who lives inside the body being manipulated. Even if your touch is less than perfect, perhaps a bit clumsy, patients are generally deeply grateful for being handled with care by another.

Patients will be much more aware of this touching than the health professional, who has become used to touching, holding, facilitating, and moving patients. The experienced health professional probably has so firm a concept of his or her good intentions that the question of inappropriateness or improper familiarity never arises. However, touch, as one form of non-verbal communication, does involve risk. It may be seen as a threat because it invades an otherwise private space, or it may be misunderstood. So, an explanation before touching a patient is always in order. Speaking of space, we now turn our attention to the use of space in human interactions.

Proxemics

Proxemics is the study of how space is used in human interactions. For example, authority can be communicated by the height from which one person interacts with another. If one stands while the other sits or lies down, the person standing has placed himself or herself in a position of authority (Fig. 9.4).

Height is sometimes an unwitting message to a patient when the person is confined to a bed, a treatment table, or is a wheelchair user. In many instances, the patient interaction will be improved if the health professional moves down to the patient's level. An important rule for respectful interaction whenever you are talking to a patient is to sit down. This signals to the patient your willingness to listen and gives the impression, even if this is not true, that you are not going to

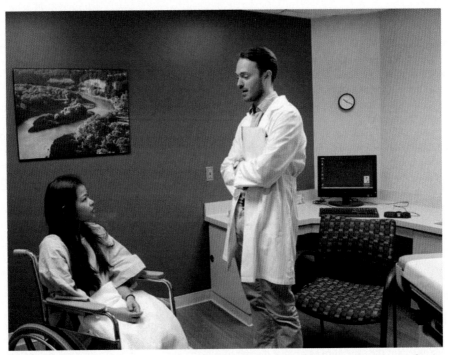

Fig. 9.4 Standing over a patient in a wheelchair is an example of inappropriate nonverbal behavior. Courtesy Maren Haddad.

rush through your time together. During stressful times, it is also a strategy for you as a provider to channel presence and be mindful of the patient encounter at hand.

Another aspect of proxemics is the distance maintained between people when they are communicating. In his now classic *The Hidden Dimension*, an intriguing book that explains the difference in distance awareness among many different cultural groups, anthropologist Edward T. Hall defines four distance zones maintained by healthy, adult, middle-class Americans.[35] In examining these zones, you may also be better able to understand how they differ from those of other cultural and socioeconomic groups. The four distance zones are as follows:

1. Intimate distance, involving direct contact.
2. Personal distance, ranging from 1 to 4 feet. At arm's length, subjects of personal interest can be discussed while physical contact, such as holding hands or hitting the other person, is still possible.
3. Social distance, ranging from 4 to 12 feet. At this distance, more formal business and social discourse take place.
4. Public distance, ranging from 12 to 25 feet or more. No physical contact and very little direct eye contact are possible.[36]

At least for the near future, the term "social distance" will have a different meaning since this is the term that was used to gauge how distant people should be from each other in public spaces, that is, 6 feet, to reduce the spread of COVID-19.

Health professionals perform many diagnostic or treatment procedures within the personal and intimate distance zones that evoke feelings of warmth and closeness supported by understanding, on the part of the patient, the reason for such closeness.[36] You may have to invade the patient's culturally derived boundaries of interaction, sometimes with little warning.

When you work with an ethnic or cultural subgroup outside of your own experience or travel to other parts of the world, culturally defined uses of space are clear. In addition, you may become aware of some things that you did not expect to be part of the interaction. For instance, body odors become more apparent when you are working at close range. In mainstream American society in which people are socialized to smell like a deodorant, a mouthwash, a hair spray, or a cologne, but not a body, it is not surprising that some health professionals find the patient's body odor offensive, sometimes nauseous; some admit that it so repulses them that they try to hurry through the test or treatment.

Patients will respond to the health professional's odors, too. An X-ray technologist confided to one of the authors that one of her biggest shocks while working in a mission hospital in India came when her assistant reluctantly admitted that patients were failing to keep their appointments because she "smelled funny," making them sick. The "funny" smell turned out to be that of the popular American soap she was using for her bath.

Adhering to a patient's need to maintain an appropriate distance that honors their cultural preferences, reinforces the patient's ability to feel secure in the strange new environment of health care institutions. By handling distance needs respectfully, you are helping patients to feel more secure in the sometimes-frightening health care setting into which they have been cast.

Differing Concepts of Time

A culturally derived difference that affects nonverbal communication is how people interpret time. The right time and the correct amount of time are relative, depending on one's cultural perspective. One aspect of the time dimension that directly affects the patient and health professional interaction is the scheduling and maintaining of appointments. Most health professionals are punctual and expect their patients to be the same. In fact, the health facility operates each day on a strict schedule. In mainstream Western societies, punctuality communicates respect. However, in some other cultures to arrive exactly on time is an insult in that it says, "You are such an unimportant person that you can arrange your affairs easily; you really have nothing else to do." Rather, an appropriate amount of tardiness is expected.

The amount of time spent in rendering professional service also may vary from one culture to another. How should a given amount of time be spent so that the patient benefits most? For example, in an ambulatory setting in the United States, a commonly accepted standard is to greet the patient briefly and begin a treatment or a test without delay. When the treatment is over, the patient usually leaves immediately and perhaps is accompanied to the exit by a member of the health care team.

However, in some cultures, if the treatment does not begin as soon as the patient arrives, it does not matter. Rather than rush into the procedure itself, you should first inquire about the weather, the family, and other things that may be important to the patient, sometimes spending several minutes in this way. During the actual treatment or test, you may hurry, but goodbyes must not be short and rushed.

Ways of operating within and indicating time, then, are highly relative. As mentioned in Chapter 4, you should always take individual values and differences into consideration when working with people whose cultural backgrounds are different from your own, recognizing that both distance and time awareness are deep seated and culturally derived. A person is usually not consciously aware of how they interpret time and distance, and so neither factor is easily identified as a cause of misunderstanding. This is another striking example of how culture influences the interpretation of verbal and nonverbal communication, warranting the professional's respect.

Communicating Virtually

Much of this chapter has focused on communication between the patient and health professional where the two parties are within physical proximity of each other. In many cases today, because of the mobility of society, scarcity of health professionals, technological developments, and infectious diseases health professionals and patients have turned to communication methods that support dialogue and even virtual physical assessment across great distances. In addition, you may work with colleagues on the same complex patient problem and yet geographically be in two different physical sites, providing an expanded idea of the interprofessional care team. All the techniques to enhance communication, in general, apply to communication across distances, but they must be adapted to the special demands created by the technology itself and the actual physical miles between a patient and health professional. Online communication with patients has many positive attributes such as the verbatim record of the transaction between patient and health professional. However, electronic communication is not well suited to urgent problems, and it does not contain all the nonverbal components of communication discussed previously in this chapter that are crucial to understanding.

WRITTEN TOOLS

Written communication includes information about diagnostic tests and evaluation observations, preauthorization and patient self-report questionnaires, treatment notes about patients, care instructions to patients and family caregivers, informed consent documents, and quality assurance surveys to obtain information from patients about services rendered. Whatever the reason for the written communication, there are distinct advantages to its use over verbal communication. Written communication has the advantage of visual cues, further enhanced when graphics are included. The reader has control over the pace of absorbing the information and can reread the information any number of times. However, written communication demands a high degree of accuracy and adequate health literacy as was mentioned earlier in this chapter. All written communication, whether it is a pamphlet explaining a diagnostic test, a formal letter indicating a change in office hours, an e-blast, or a secure message in a patient portal, should clearly state and define the purpose of the communication. The content should be well organized. Clarity and brevity are also hallmarks of good written communication. Clear, concise written messages will be more easily understood, and problems prevented if both spoken and written forms of communication can be used.

DIGITAL SOURCES OF HEALTH INFORMATION

Patients often seek information through Internet search engines about their medical conditions and treatment. However, concerns have been raised about a patient's ability to effectively search for accurate information. More than one study has confirmed that the percentage of sites that provided unreliable information was higher than those that offered accurate information.[37,38] Then there is the problem of patients comprehending what they find on reputable sites and coping with the overwhelming volume and variety of the quality of information presented.[39] Health professionals should also be vigilant regarding the reliability of the information they retrieve from the Internet for their own information.

Additionally, social media offers yet another way to connect with patients but in addition to the opportunities it provides, there are challenges for you in your role as a student and eventually a health professional. In 2021, most Americans, roughly seven-in-ten, say they used any kind of social media site with YouTube and Facebook dominating the online landscape.[40] Through social media sites, users can create, share, edit, and interact with online content which sets it apart from merely viewing content on a website. Patients use social media sites as reference sources, whether accurate or not, to access and share health information. Health professionals communicate with patients through social media because it can be used to share credible health information. Social media sites such as LinkedIn and Twitter can also be used by health professionals to interact specifically with each other to share technical, clinical, and research information. Although there are clear benefits of using social media, there are risks as well. The sheer reach of social media is enough to give one pause before using it in any situation that could be connected to one's professional role. Also, there is the problem of "content permanence" in that once something is posted or distributed, it is difficult, if not impossible, to remove entirely. Some of the consequences of misuse of social media include breached patient confidentiality, possible exposure to lawsuits by patients or others who are entitled to confidentiality, boundary issues in professional relationships and for students and faculty, and impairment of program integrity.[41]

There are professional guidelines and standards for the use of social media developed by the American Nurses Association, the American Society of Health Systems Pharmacy, the American Medical Association, and the American Physical Therapy Association that all encourage members of each profession to adhere to ethical and legal standards with an emphasis on patient confidentiality, privacy, and appropriate boundary setting.[42-45] These standards serve as resources to both health professionals and patients as this communication technology continues to evolve.

TELEHEALTH ENCOUNTERS

Telehealth (or telemedicine/telepractice) includes a variety of platforms and offers conveniences to patients such as increased accessibility, decreased transportation barriers and patient empowerment.[1] Table 9.1 summarizes the various platforms, opportunities, and limitations of telehealth currently in use in health care. Although electronic communication methods may assist in communication, their use depends on the availability of a personal computer or smart phone and a knowledgeable user on both ends. Not everyone has access to such technology, but access is steadily increasing worldwide. In some cases, advanced communication technology may be the best solution to providing health care to people who would otherwise not be able to travel to places with the latest innovations in health care. The World Health Organization (WHO) views *telemedicine* as one of the most promising methods of health delivery to areas where the need for high-quality health care vastly outstrips the ability to deliver it. The WHO defines telemedicine as, "The delivery of health care services, where distance is a critical factor, by all health care professionals using information and communication technologies for the exchange of valid information for diagnosis, treatment and prevention of disease and injuries, research and evaluation, and for the continuing education of health care providers, all in the interests of advancing the health of individuals and their communities."[46] Telehealth encompasses both provider-to-patient and provider-to-provider communications and can take place synchronously (telephone and video), asynchronously (patient secure portal messages, e-consults), and through virtual agents such as chatbots and wearable devices.[47]

Two electronic tools have become commonplace for patient use in the last two decades: patient portals and secure messaging (SM). *Patient portals* are "secure online websites that require username and password and are linked to a patient's personal health record providing 24-hour access from anywhere with an Internet connection."[4] Portals have proven helpful in returning lab results to patients and expediting prescription refills and adjustment. Health professional and patients can communicate bi-directionally on such portals via *SM*, where patients can send nonurgent health-related

TABLE 9.1 ■ **Classification of Telehealth Encounters**

Platform	Opportunities	Limitations
E-consult: Asynchronous clinician-to-clinician communication based on record review (inpatient and outpatient)	Time efficient for specialists. Patient-initiated second opinion requests are possible.	Lack of physical exam or direct communication with patients.
Remote patient monitoring: Gather patient outside traditional health care setting via connected device or patient-reported outcomes (synchronous or asynchronous)	Respond to clinical data outside of regular clinic visits. Recordings can be automatically sent to clinicians.	Data should be integrated into the electronic health record for consistency of care.
Asynchronous patient portal messaging	Autonomous text-based communication. Secure communication. Record of exchange between patient and health professional.	Time gap between message sent by patient and health professional reply.
Telephone visit: Synchronous patient–health professional communication by phone	Universally accessible even with the most ill/low socioeconomic status patients. Particularly helpful for management of chronic conditions.	Devalued by most payers. Inability to conduct physical exam.
Video visit: Synchronous patient–health professional communication with both audio and video, with possible ancillary and telemetry equipment	Replaces face-to-face visits during pandemics. Less taxing for patients who have mobility issues. Improvement in clinical care. Enables treatment of patient/family in their native context (home) if technology is available.	Technology requirements generally unavailable in the outpatient setting in both the clinic and home setting make this kind of visit difficult. Inpatient setting requires a mobile/zoomable camera with microphone and speaker and staff to work with technology. Need to develop infection prevention/sanitation protocols for devices.

Adapted from Wosik J, Fudim M, Cameron ZF, Cho A, Phinney D, Curtis S, et al. Telehealth transformation: COVID-19 and the rise of virtual care. *J Am Med Inf Assoc*. 2020;27(6):957–962. p. 958. doi:10.1093/jamia/ocaa067.

messages to providers, upload photos, ask follow-up questions about a treatment, view test results, and make appointments. Although these electronic forms of communication will not replace in-person visits, they augment the health professional and patient relationship by providing a way to seek advice and follow up on tests or changes in prescriptions or a plan of care. Another advantage is that there is a written record of the exchange that both parties can refer to in the future.

Although there are many platforms and methods of communicating with patients during a virtual visit, general guidelines for best practices for verbal and nonverbal communication in the

TABLE 9.2 ■ A Guide to Best Practices for a Telehealth Patient Visit

Previsit

When scheduling the appointment, inform the patient/family about what to expect and the goals of the virtual visit

Select and use the most appropriate telehealth technology based on patient need, preference, and available technology[a]

Familiarize yourself with the technology in advance of the visit[a]

Arrive early to test the technology and work through any problems[a]

Eliminate any predictable background noise (silence phones, close doors, etc.)

Visit

Establish rapport by centering your face in the screen, speaking with clarity at a normal pace and volume, and avoid covering your mouth so that facial expressions remain visible[b]

Reassure patient/family/caregivers of privacy and security of technology[a]

If you anticipate distressing or embarrassing information will be a part of the visit, ask the patient if they would like to arrange for privacy on their end

Ask the patient or family how they are doing to elicit their concerns and establish aims of the visit[c]

Make sure only one person speaks at a time during the visit to ensure that participants do not speak over one another[c]

Address background noise or other distractions on the patient's end of the conversation in a helpful and respectful manner

Use silence appropriately and include empathetic facial expressions and gestures such as head nods and good eye contact[b]

Review goals of the visit and follow-up such as next visit, whom to call and when[b]

Post visit

Ask for feedback about the virtual visit including ways to improve[c]

Address any technology issues[c]

Document updates to patient plan of care

[a]Adapted from Brown M. *Creating Meaningful Connections in the Virtual World*. Teleios Collaboration Network; 2020. www.teleioscn.org/blog/creating-meaningful-connections-in-the-virtual-world-is-here-to-stay# 8/19/2020.
[b]Adapted from Weinstein BE. Optimizing telehealth, communication amid COVID-19. *Hearing J*. 2020;73:47.
[c]Adapted from Webb M, Hurley SL, Gentry J, Ayoub C. Best practices for using telehealth in hospice and palliative care. *J Hosp Palliat Care* 2021;23(3):277–285. doi:10.1097/NJH.0000000000000753.

virtual, synchronous context are still in development. The information in Table 9.2 presents an overview of best practices for communicating virtually with patients, family, and caregivers before, during, and after a virtual visit.

As you will note, this use of information and communication technologies includes all members of the health care team and for broader purposes than health delivery to patients who are at a distance. This in turn supports interprofessional collaborative practice and aims to increase quality care outcomes for patients and families.

While telehealth's expansion has changed the delivery of health care even as the pandemic continued to evolve,[48] it is increasingly important to revisit other important issues such as the impact of technology on the quality of care, access to care and technology, consent, data protection, and privacy.[49]

Effective Listening

A considerable portion of a health professional's day is spent listening to patients and colleagues in person, on the phone or in a video/audio conference online.

Listening requires time that is free from interruptions. To listen well you need to set up the space for communicating in person. Make the setting as welcoming as possible given the context. Make sure that key attendees are there and be prepared by knowing the patient's story and clinical details. In situations of high stress, it is important not to communicate by yourself to patients or family members. More than one member of the interprofessional care team should be present to ensure all elements are clearly discussed.

Most people lack the skills to listen effectively. If you are one of them, two goals for your further development are (1) to improve listening acuity so you hear the patient accurately and (2) to ascertain how accurately a patient has heard you. The first step to achieving these goals is to examine the reasons messages get distorted by health professionals. Besides the often overlooked but important possibility of a hearing deficit, there are other reasons a health professional may unintentionally distort a verbal communication.

First, frame of mind may distort meaning. It is the result of experience. In this case, a person fails to listen to the spoken words or to note subtle individual differences because he or she is sure of what the other person will say.

The rate at which incoming information can be processed varies significantly. This is partially but not entirely due to differences in innate ability to understand the information being conveyed by the patient. Overconfidence or too little confidence in predicting what will be said also determines whether you will cease to process incoming information. If you are overconfident, boredom settles in. If you have too little confidence the tendency for many people is to become overly anxious and tune out the message. Active listening also requires undivided attention. If distracted by too much sensory input, you will not be able to listen.

The rate and level of understanding at which you absorb communication will alter the ability to process the information. A listener's mindset and the need to defend existing beliefs or ideas determine how accurately they will hear a message. Sometimes you will be the poor listener, and, as we discussed earlier, other times the patient will be.

Taking all these factors into account, you cannot control how effectively a patient listens, but you can become a more effective listener yourself. By simply restating what the patient has said, you can confirm part of a message before proceeding to the next portion of it. In addition, the following are some simple steps to more effective listening[50,51]:

1. Set the stage by assuring the patient that you will only share information with patient-approved sources such as insurers, family, or other members of the health care team.
2. Listen without interrupting, judging, or minimizing.
3. Show empathy and try to understand the patient's point of view.
4. Attend to cues in the patient's verbal and nonverbal communication.
5. Let the patient finish talking before asking a question.
6. Use reflection at regular intervals during conversation to acknowledge emotion, ensure clarity and understanding. When possible, reflect verbatim and confirm assumptions.
7. Stay focused.

The underlying theme in most discussions about listening is that it is a deliberate act. You must make a conscious decision to be fully present and engaged in the patient encounter to really understand what a patient is trying to tell you.

Summary

The purpose of this chapter is to give you an overview of numerous components of respectful communication. You will communicate in many ways with your patients. It may seem impossible to pay attention to the context of communication, the words you choose, your attitude, nonverbal signs, and manage the technology often used to convey your message all at the same time. However, communication designed for effective interaction in your professional relationships is a skill that can be learned and for that reason is included among the core competencies of professionals. Developing communication skills is a life-long learning process achieved through constant practice, reflection, and observation.[2] Effective communication includes the ability both to convey clearly what you want to impart and actively listen, acknowledge a patient's concerns have been heard, and ensure their agenda is elicited and addressed. The effort to meet these challenges yields the reward of maintaining a relationship that honors professional respect for all persons involved.

References

1. Powell RE, Henstenburg JM, Cooper G, Hollander JE, Rising KL. Patient perceptions of telehealth primary care video. *Ann Fam Med.* 2017;15(3):225–229. https://doi.org/10.1370/afm.2095.
2. Shaw AC, McQuade JL, Reilly MJ, Nixon B, Baile WF, Epner DE. Integrating storytelling into a communication skills teaching program for medical oncology fellows. *J Cancer Educ.* 2019;34:1198–1203. https://doi.org/10.1007/s13187-018-1428-3.
3. Smith JF. Communicative ethics in medicine: the physician-patient relationship. In: Wolf S, ed. *Feminism and Bioethics: Beyond Reproduction.* New York: Oxford University Press; 1996.
4. Alpert J, Markham MJ, Bjarnadottir RI, Bylund CL. Twenty-first century bedside manner: exploring patient-centered communication in secure messaging with cancer patients. *J Cancer Educ.* 2021;36:16–24, p. 16. https://doi.org/10.1007/s13187-019-01592-5.
5. Asan O, Yu Z, Crotty BH. How clinician-patient communication affects trust in health information sources: temporal trends from a national cross-sectional survey. *PLoS ONE.* 2021;16(2):e0247583.
6. Watson K. Serious play: teaching medical skills with improvisational theater techniques. *Acad Med.* 2011;86(10):1260–1265.
7. Wallace LS, Cassada DC, Ergen WF, et al. Setting the stage: surgery patients' expectations for greetings during routine office visits. *J Surg Res.* 2009;157:91–95.
8. Getsi LC. Intensive care. In: Getsi LC, ed. *Intensive Care—Poems by Lucia Cordell Getsi.* Minneapolis, MN: New Rivers Press; 1992.
9. Institute of Medicine. *Health Literacy: A Prescription to End Confusion.* Washington, DC: National Academies Press; 2004.
10. National Network of Libraries of Medicine. *Health Literacy [Internet].* Bethesda, MD: NNLM. Available from: https://nnlm.gov/initiatives/topics/health-literacy.
11. Tauben DJ, Langford DJ, Sturgeon JA, Rundell SD, Towle C, Bockman C, Nichols M. Optimizing telehealth pain care after COVID-19. *Pain J Online.* 2020;16(11):2437–2445. https://doi.org/10.1097/j.pain.0000000000002048.
12. Roberts ET, Mehrotra A. Assessment of disparities in digital access among Medicare beneficiaries and implications for telemedicine. *JAMA Intern Med.* 2020;180(10):1386–1389. https://doi.org/10.1001/jamainternmed.2020.2666.
13. Weiss BD. *American Medical Association: Health Literacy and Patient Safety: Help Patients Understand.* Chicago, IL: American Medical Association Foundation; 2007.
14. *Agency for Healthcare Research and Quality.* Health literacy universal precautions toolkit. http://www.ahrq.gov/professionals/quality-patient-safety/quality-resources/tools/literacy-toolkit/index.htm; 2010 Last reviewed September 2020.
15. *Agency for Healthcare Research and Quality.* Quick start guide. htpps://www.ahrq.gov/health-literary/improve/precautions/quick/html; 2015 Last reviewed September 2020.
16. *U.S. Census Bureau.* American community survey 1-year estimates. https://factfinder.census.gov/faces/tableservices/jsf/pages/productview.xhtml?src=bkmk; 2016 Accessed August 29, 2021.
17. Srivastava R. The interpreter. *N Engl J Med.* 2017;376(9):812–813.

18. Karliner LS, Jacobs EA, Chen AH, et al. Do professional interpreters improve clinical care for patients with limited English proficiency? A systematic review of the literature. *Health Serv Res*. 2007;42:272–754.
19. LeNeveu M, Berger Z, Gross M. Lost in translation: the role of interpreters on labor and delivery. *Health Equity*. 2020;4.1:406–409. https://doi.org/10.1089/heq.2020.0016.
20. Juckett G, Unger K. Appropriate use of medical interpreters. *Am Fam Phys*. 2014;90(7):476–480.
21. Schapira L, Vargas E, Hidalgo R, et al. Lost in translation: integrating medical interpreters into the multidisciplinary team. *Oncologist*. 2008;13:586–592.
22. Seidelman RD, Bachner YG. That I won't translate! experiences of a family medical interpreter in a multicultural environment *Mt Sinai J Med*. 2010;77:389–393.
23. Watermeyer J. She will hear me: how a flexible interpreting style enables patients to manage the inclusion of interpreters in mediated pharmacy interactions. *Health Commun*. 2011;26(1):71–81.
24. Butow PN, Brown RF, Cogar S, et al. Oncologists' reactions to cancer patients verbal cues. *Psychooncology*. 2002;11:47–58.
25. *Office of Inspector General and US Department of Health and Human Services*. Adverse Events. https://oig.hhs.gov/reports-and-publications/feature-topics/adverse-events. Last updated June 16, 2022.
26. Abirami K, Barathi S, Koperundevi E, Durgamani MK, Babu MI. Enhancing paralinguistic feature through Dubsmash: a case study. *Int J Pure Appl Math*. 2018;119(7):2325–2331.
27. Social Science Matrix. *Interview With Robin T. Lakoff: What's Up With Upspeak?* Berkeley, CA: Social Science Matrix; 2015. https://matrix.berkeley.edu/research-article/whats-upspeak/.
28. Firlik K. *Another Day in the Frontal Lobe: A Brain Surgeon Exposes Life on the Inside*. New York: Random House; 2006.
29. Argyle M. *Bodily Communication*. 2nd ed. London: Routledge; 1988.
30. Ruben MA, Blanch-Hartigan D, Hall JA. Nonverbal communication as a pain reliever: the impact of physician supportive nonverbal behavior on experimentally induced pain. *Health Commun*. 2017;32(8):970–976.
31. Grossbach I, Stranberg S, Chlan L. Promoting effective communication for patients receiving mechanical ventilation. *Crit Care Nurse*. 2011;31(2):46–61.
32. Tingström P, Milberg A, Rodhe J, Ernerud J, Grodzinsky E, Sund-Levander M. Nursing assistants: "He seems to be ill" – a reason for nurses to take action: validation of the Early Detection Scale of Infection (EDIS). *BMC Geriatrics*. 2015;15:122. https://doi.org/10.1186/s12877-015-0114-0.
33. Powell C, Blighe A, Froggatt K, McCormack B, Woodward-Carlton B, Young J, Robinson L, Downs M. Family involvement in timely detection of changes in health of nursing home residents: a qualitative exploratory study. *J Clin Nurs*. 2018;27:317–327.
34. Klitzman R. Improving education on doctor-patient relationships and communication: lessons from doctors who become patients. *Acad Med*. 2006;81(5):447–453.
35. Hall ET. *The Hidden Dimension*. New York: Doubleday; 1966.
36. Andersen PA, Guerrero LK, Jones SM. Nonverbal behavior in intimate interactions and intimate relationships. In: Mancuso V, Patterson M, eds. *The Sage Handbook of Nonverbal Communication*. Thousand Oaks, CA: Sage Publications; 2006:260.
37. Ogasawara R, Katsumata N, Toyooka T, Akaishi Y, Yokoyama T, Kadokura G. Reliability of cancer treatment information on the Internet: observational study. *JMIR Cancer*. 2018;4(2):e10031. https://doi.org/10.2196/10031.
38. Abola MV, Prasad V. The use of superlatives in cancer research. *JAMA Oncol*. 2016;2(1):139–141. https://doi.org/10.1001/jamaoncol.2015.3931.
39. O'Mathúna DP. How should clinicians engage with online health information? *AMA J Ethics*. 2018;20(11):E1059–E1066, p. E 1059.
40. *Pew Research Center*. Social media use in 2021. www.pewresearch.org; 2021.
41. Westrick S. Nursing students' use of electronic and social media: law, ethics, and E-professionalism. *Nurs Educ Perspect*. 2016;37:16–22.
42. American Nurses Association. *ANA's Principles for Social Networking for the Nurse*. Silver Springs, MD: American Nurses Association. https://nursingworld.org/anas-principles-for-social-networking-and-the-nurse; 2011 Accessed October 20, 2022.
43. American Society of Health-System Pharmacists. ASHP statement on use of social media by pharmacy professionals. *Am J Health Syst Pharm*. 2012;69:2095–2097.

44. *American Medical Association*. Professionalism in the use of social media. https://www/ama-assn.org/delivering-care/ethics/professionalism-use-social-media; 2010 Accessed August 13, 2021.

45. *American Physical Therapy Association*. Succeeding on social media. http://www.apta.org/social-media/succeeding-on-social-media; 2019.

46. World Health Organization. *Telemedicine: Opportunities and Developments in Members States, Report on the Second Global Survey on eHealth (Global Observatory for eHealth Series, 2)*. Geneva: WHO Press; 2009.

47. Wosik J, Fudim M, Cameron B, Gelland ZF, Cho A, Phinney D, Curtis S, et al. Telehealth transformation: COVID-19 and the rise of virtual care. *J Am Med Inf Assoc*. 2020;27(6):957–962, p. 957. https://doi.org/10.1093/jamia/oc067.

48. Brody, J.E. A pandemic benefit: expansion of telemedicine. *The New York Times*. 2020. https://www.nytimes.com/2020/05/11/well/live/coronavirus-telemedicine-telehealth.html; 2020 Accessed May 11, 2020.

49. Kaplan B. Revisiting health information technology ethical, legal, and social issues and evaluation: telehealth/telemedicine and COVID-19. *Int J Med Inf*. 2020;143:104239. https://doi.org/10.1016/j.ijmedinf.2020.104239.

50. Downes R, Foote E. HIV and communication skills for practice. *HIV Nurs*. 2019;19(4):86–93. 88.

51. Doherty RF. *Ethical dimensions in the health professions*. 7th ed. St. Louis, MO: Elsevier; 2021.

Respectful Interactions Across the Life Span

Introduction

Having studied the basic foundations of respectful interaction, you now have an opportunity to apply your learning to several types of patients you will see throughout the course of your professional career. We have chosen to address them by age group, over the life span, being mindful that individual differences often outweigh the similarities we are emphasizing in these different cohorts.

Life span development encompasses constancy and change in an individual's behavior throughout the life span. Development is not bound by a single criterion—it is multidimensional and multidirectional. Any process of development entails aspects of growth (gain) and decline (loss), and these relate to an individual's adaptive capacity. Each lifetime also presents different paths. Often illness or disability takes patients and families down an unfamiliar path. Your role as a health professional and member of the interprofessional care team is to help these individuals navigate that path, adjusting and adapting along life's journey.

Section 5 begins with Chapter 10, highlighting the joys and challenges of working with infants, toddlers, and preschoolers. The family is a key element of consideration, and the principles of patient- and family-centered care serve as guideposts for the interprofessional care team working with this age group. Chapter 11 moves the focus of your attention to school-age children and adolescents. The evolving needs of the child and family as they mature are discussed, particularly as they relate to supporting health through transitions and adversity during these important developmental stages.

In Chapter 12, we discuss your interaction with people who become patients during young and middle adulthood. Only in recent times have these life periods been given more than a cursory glance, and we share some of the insights that researchers and others are finding. Identity development across cultures, expansion of caregiving roles, onset of chronic conditions, and stressors related to adult responsibilities are discussed.

Chapter 13 examines key issues related to working with older adults. Of all age groups, this one is increasing more in diversity and size worldwide than any other population. Research and theories on healthy aging are presented, given their importance in supporting older patients for optimal physical, cognitive, and mental health.

Throughout the life span, the person who becomes a patient is faced with many of the challenges we have been discussing so far. Injury and/or illness can disrupt a person's life patterns and development, challenging the acquisition of "typical" life skills. You have a substantial role in respectfully helping your patient meet and overcome these challenges.

CHAPTER 10

Respectful Interaction: Working With Newborns, Infants, and Children in the Early Years

The reader will be able to

- Assess skills and activities that reflect respect toward newborns, infants, toddlers, and preschoolers;
- Distinguish some basic developmental differences that need to be considered in one's approach to newborns, infants, toddlers, and preschoolers;
- Discuss in general terms Erikson's sequential view of the psychological development of infants and toddlers;
- List some everyday needs of the infant that may help explain an infant's response to the health professional;
- Identify how a consistent approach builds trust in interactions with patients and families in early childhood;
- Describe six types of play and show how each can facilitate respectful interaction with a pediatric patient;
- Appraise how the young child's developing need for autonomy enters into the health professional and patient relationship;
- Appreciate the impact of the COVID-19 pandemic on early childhood education and development;
- Define early adversity and understand its impact on early childhood development; and
- Recognize the responsibility health professionals hold in reporting abuse and neglect.

Prelude

Lou and I walked back to Alex's isolette. We peered in at the uncomfortable little being who was still pulling at his feeding tube and now making a faint mewing sound. I put my hands through the portholes in the side of the box and stroked his arms down away from the tube. I couldn't get myself to talk to him. I stared at him but could not make sense of what I was seeing. Who was this new person? "Spastic diplegia." Would he even walk? I couldn't picture anything. I left the hospital that day with an empty feeling.

V. FORMAN[1]

This is the first of several chapters that examine respectful interaction with patients across the life span. It begins with our smallest patients—neonates and newborns—and transitions to working with infants, toddlers, and children in the preschool years. The section on growth and development includes information that applies across childhood, although working with each age group has its own opportunities and challenges. Provided here is a wide range of relevant topics concerning the interaction with young patients that provide a basis for more in-depth exploration in your other coursework and lifelong education.

Almost all health professionals interact at some point with newborns and children in the early years, including infants, toddlers, and preschoolers. Some health professionals work solely with these groups and others with their parents, grandparents, guardians, or siblings. These small patients must be treated with the respect they deserve as unique individuals like everyone else. Furthermore, the opportunity they are given to experience human dignity and support in their time of illness, injury, or other adversity can become a resource to help them and their families manage future difficulties. As the opening quote reminds us, we meet our youngest patients within the context of their families. It is through the loving care of family caregivers that infants bond, have their basic needs met, learn, and develop on their journey through early childhood.

Most of us take for granted that a newborn will live into his or her seventh or eighth decade of life. This has not always been so and is not the case in many countries. Today, the global average infant mortality rate is 29 infant deaths per 1000 live births.[2] In the United States, the infant mortality rate is 5.6 infant deaths per 1000 live births. Although the US infant mortality rate is declining, it currently is higher than in other economically developed countries, with the United States ranking 33rd among 36 countries in the Organization for Economic Co-operation and Development.[3,4] The top five causes of infant mortality in the United States are birth defects, preterm birth, maternal complications of pregnancy, sudden infant death syndrome, and injuries or accidents.[5,6]

Perhaps, the most significant to health professionals (and the public health sector) is that the overall infant mortality rate is not shared equally by all groups. Mortality is higher for infants and children living in poverty. The mortality rate for Black infants is more than twice that for White and Hispanic infants. The causes of these disparities are multidimensional, including social determinants of health, maternal health and behaviors, economic status, structural racism, insurance, and health care access.[7,8]

Better opportunities for health education and overall longevity in White and European Americans point to deep social inequities and health disparities, the consequences of which must be reckoned with. As a health professional, you will need to call on your skills and knowledge to reach solutions that help close the disparities gap. As discussed in Chapter 4, being aware of unconscious biases, advocating for social justice, and acting to decrease health disparities can enhance high-quality, culturally informed, and nondiscriminatory health care delivery.

Useful General Principles of Human Growth and Development

Growth and development occur in numerous ways—physical, emotional, intellectual (or cognitive), social, and moral—and all aspects of development affect one another. Some theories are hierarchical models of development, whereas others are dynamic. Although professionals often talk about growth and development simultaneously, *growth* can be thought of as quantitative (e.g., changes in height and weight) and *development* as qualitative (changes in performance influenced by the maturation process).

HUMAN GROWTH

Human growth proceeds in accordance with general principles of (1) orderliness, (2) discontinuity, (3) differentiation, (4) cephalocaudal, and (5) proximodistal and bilateral. Each is instrumental in helping you understand what occurs in the growth process, when, and why.

Orderliness

Growth and changes in behavior usually occur in an orderly fashion and in the same sequence. Thus infants can turn their heads before they can extend their hands. Almost every child sits before he or she stands, stands before walking, and draws a circle before drawing a square. Most babies babble before talking and pronounce certain sounds before others. Likewise, certain cognitive abilities precede the next. Preschoolers can categorize objects or put them into a series before they can think logically.

Discontinuity

Although growth is orderly, it is not always smooth and gradual. There are periods of rapid growth—growth spurts—and increases in psychological abilities. Parents sometimes speak of the summer that a child "shot up" 2 inches. Many adolescents experience a sudden growth spurt after years of being the ones with the smallest stature in their class.

Differentiation

Development proceeds from simple to complex and from general to specific. An example of differentiation in the infant is seen in an infant's ability to wave his or her arms first and later develop purposeful use of his or her fingers. Motor responses are diffuse and undifferentiated at birth and become more defined as the child grows. Beginning motor activity in the toddler involves haphazard and unsystematic actions, progressing to goal-directed, controlled actions and outcomes.[9]

Cephalocaudal

Cephalocaudal development means that the upper end of the organism develops earlier than the lower end. Increases in neuromuscular size and maturation of function begin in the head and proceed to the hands and feet. For example, after birth an infant will be able to hold his or her head erect before being able to sit or walk.

Proximodistal and Bilateral

Proximodistal development means that growth progresses from the central axis of the body (the trunk) toward the periphery or extremities. Thus the central nervous system develops before the peripheral nervous system. Bilateral development means that the capacity for growth and development of the child is symmetric—growth that occurs on one side of the body generally occurs on the other side of the body simultaneously. These principles apply throughout the life span, from infancy to old age.

HUMAN DEVELOPMENT

Development can be discussed in domains of human performance: cognitive, affective, and psychomotor or through standardized language/classification systems of human function and abilities such as the International Classification of Function, Disability and Health (ICF) developed by the World Health Organization.[10] The ICF dimensions of functioning and disability are body structure and function, activities and participation, and personal and environmental factors. We will focus primarily on cognitive development because it entails how a person perceives, thinks, and communicates thoughts and feelings. Time is also spent on psychosocial development because of the profound impact this has on the health professional's interactions with patients.

Cognitive Development

Cognitive development is the way a child learns to think, explore, and figure things out.[11] It is vital to the child's overall growth and development as it helps them understand and problem solve

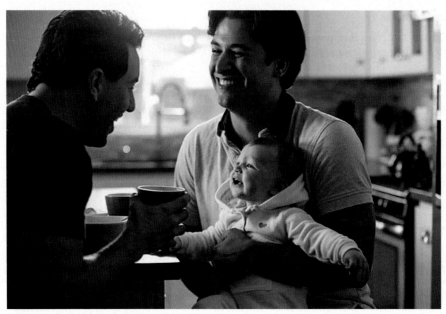

Fig. 10.1 Infants develop cognitive skills through verbal and nonverbal interactions with caring adults. © monkeybusinessimages/iStock/Thinkstock.com.

the world around them. Traditionally, health professionals have based their interventions with children on the stages of cognitive development described by Jean Piaget (1896–1980).[12] Piaget's theory is a logical, deductive explanation of how children think from infancy through adolescence. Piaget described the earliest stage of cognitive development as *sensorimotor*. At this stage, infants take in a great deal of information through their senses. Tactile and verbal stimulation and auditory and visual cues can have positive, long-range results. The early beginnings of cognitive development can be stimulated by talking to the infant and by face-to-face interactions (Fig. 10.1).

Piaget labeled the cognitive abilities of toddlers *preoperational*. Toddlers learn to think and understand by building each new experience upon previous experiences. Miller[13] summarized Piaget's depiction of the cognitive stage of toddlers in terms of egocentrism (seeing the world from a "me-only" viewpoint), rigidity of thought ("Mom is always right"), and semilogical reasoning ("My dog died because I was a bad boy"). Children in this stage are confused about cause and effect, even when it is explained to them, and think in terms of magic (e.g., wishing something makes it so). However, more current researchers refute Piaget's beliefs and claim that he may have underestimated the cognitive abilities of toddlers. These researchers suggest that children have far more potential to understand complex illness concepts than they have previously been given credit for.[14] Thus some toddlers can appreciate the perspective of another and adapt their behavior accordingly. Others propose that, rather than viewing the toddler as incapable of thinking a certain way, one should view him or her as a novice. Children have much less life experience than adults. Thus when children gain experience through chronic illness, for example, or perform tasks involving their own expertise, they can demonstrate adult-like performance and more sophisticated thinking and reasoning.[15] The debate on cognitive development is ongoing. For example, researchers in the field of evolutionary developmental psychology consider genetic and ecological mechanisms, as well as the effect of cultural contexts. They have recently added their voices to discussions regarding early childhood brain development.[16–18] The insights of various developmental theorists are important to explore because they have direct implications for how best to work with young children.

As with cognitive development, there are numerous stage/phase theories about *psychological and social development*. Development, seen this way, is a process or movement. The child matures and gains knowledge through a process of achieving intellectual mastery and more integrated ways of functioning over time. [19]

Almost all theories stress the importance of bonding or forming attachments as the primary developmental task. No one has done more to promote this idea than Erik Erikson, a psychologist who, in the 1950s and 1960s, proposed eight stages of psychosocial development.[20] According to his theory, the development of trust, introduced in Chapter 2 as fundamental to the effective patient and health professional relationships, is one of the tasks facing the child in all relationships they are engaged in. During infancy, the child is introduced to trust and begins to experience (or not experience) its power.

The psychosocial development of the toddler involves acquiring a clearer sense of himself or herself that is separate from that of the primary caregiver, becoming involved in wider social relationships, gaining self-control and mastery over motor and verbal skills, and developing independence and a self-concept. Later in this chapter, we consider specific examples of how you can effectively interact with infants, toddlers, and preschoolers by anticipating the developmental tasks specific to their age group. However, a caveat about relying on developmental stages is that it is difficult to place a child in a specific stage solely based on chronological age. Behaviors occur in context, and the environment or task-specific demands can alter function during that process.

Early Development: From Newborn to Preschooler

Between the first day of life and the first day of kindergarten, development proceeds at a lightning pace like no other. Consider just a few of the transformations that occur during this 5-year period:

1. The newborn's avid interest in staring at other babies turns into the capacity for cooperation, empathy, and friendship.
2. The 1-year-old's tentative first steps become the 4-year-old's pirouettes and soccer kicks.
3. The completely un-self-conscious baby becomes a preschooler who can describe themself in detail. Their behavior is partially motivated by how they want others to view and judge them.
4. The first adamant "no!" turns into the capacity for elaborate arguments about why the parent is wrong and the preschooler is right.
5. The infant, who has no conception that his blanket came off because he kicked his feet, becomes the 4-year-old who can explain the elaborate (if messy) causal sequence by which he can turn flour, water, salt, and food coloring into play dough.

It is no surprise that the early childhood years are portrayed as formative. The supporting structures of virtually every system of the human organism, from the tiniest cell to the capacity for intimate relationships, are constructed during this age period.[21]

NORMAL NEWBORN

The anticipation of the birth of a child is fraught with emotions ranging from joy to fear. In economically developed countries the birth process has largely moved from the home to the hospital. Many hospitals attempt to duplicate the comforts and familiarities of home by designing birthing suites complete with WiFi and comfy seating. With the move to shorter lengths of stay for a normal delivery, it is unlikely that you will have much opportunity to work directly with these tiniest of patients unless you choose to work in labor and delivery or neonatology. At the same time as noted earlier, many family members may be involved in one way or another with the birth event, and all health professionals should be prepared for a respectful response to the whole family.

Normal newborns experience relationships through their senses.[22] They are highly vulnerable but also amazingly adaptable to the new environment outside the womb. The newborn period ends at the first month of life. After that, newborns are called *infants*. Newborns have many needs, especially when health problems are present at birth. They are human beings worthy of full respect.

LIFE-THREATENING CIRCUMSTANCES

New technology is changing the possibility for survival in neonates and newborns. A full-term pregnancy lasts for 40 weeks. Some full-term newborns along with increasingly smaller neonates who have had gestations as short as 21 weeks in the womb are seen in neonatal intensive care units (NICUs). In the clinical setting, you may hear these patients referred to as *fragile neonates* or *preemies*. Many variables impact survival for these tiny patients.

Newborns in these settings range from those with high-intensity care needs (such as mechanical ventilation) to those with lower intensity care needs (such as monitoring of oxygen levels or postoperative support for corrective neonatal surgery). Sometimes a neonate who weighs more than the fragile neonate in the next isolette is the one who does not survive. Each year tens of thousands of babies end up in a NICU. In each case, parents and health professionals share a common goal—to make each baby healthy. New medical technologies are saving babies who until only recently would not have survived. For some of these families, however, the result may be a baby whose future involves lifelong chronic health conditions. With little or no preparation, parents often find themselves in times of great uncertainty and are asked to decide when the technology is doing more harm than good. Many parents do not feel prepared for such decisions and are burdened by this weighty responsibility.[23,24] Respectful interaction with parents of these fragile newborns requires that you take extra care to develop trust, communicate with clarity, and inform them in a timely manner about the status and progress of their children. More generally speaking, one essential key to respectful interaction with parents is your understanding and empathy for the complex stresses and, for some, losses they are experiencing as they cope with their new roles as parents.[25]

MOVING INTO INFANCY

When working with an infant, you, along with other members of the interprofessional care team, will be able to make key clinical judgments about the patient's best interests and observe the interaction between parents and their new baby. Happily, the parents almost always provide the primary supportive bridge between you and the infant patient, interpreting the baby's expressions, babbles, and postures and providing insight into how continuity of approach to the infant can be maximized. During this time, parents must learn cues from their infants, and sometimes you can teach the parents, as well as learn from the parents' comments and behavior. The needs of infants are sometimes difficult to determine because these small patients are vulnerable and lack sufficient verbal skills to express their wants and needs. Professionals who rely solely on a patient's ability to ask for what he or she needs take a narrow view of needs assessment. As with any nonverbal patient, the health professional must learn to read the infant's signals and collaborate with the family caregivers to determine the infant's needs.

INFANT NEEDS: RESPECT AND CONSISTENCY

There are two contexts by which to view the infant's needs. The first focuses on the stage of psychosocial development that we have already discussed and the second on immediate concrete needs such as the need for a drink of water, food, pain relief, or a diaper change. You have an opportunity to demonstrate respect for the infant by responding effectively to each type of need.

Remember that parents often have explicit ways of doing things for their infant that can help, too. For example, parents may hold the infant in a certain way or play a favorite game such as pretending to sneeze or rubbing the baby's back that will, at a minimum, help calm the infant while you look for other reasons for the infant's distress.

A primary approach is characterized by the three "Cs": consistency in approach, constancy of presence, and continuity of treatment. Consistency is especially important because it builds trust (infant self-confidence) through the following steps[26]:

1. An infant's need exists.
2. The infant exhibits generalized behavior.
3. The caregiver responds.
4. The need is satisfied.
5. The need recurs.
6. The infant predicts the caregiver's response.
7. The infant repeats the previous behavior.
8. The caregiver responds in a consistent manner.
9. The need is satisfied.
10. The infant's trust toward the caregiver develops.
11. The need recurs.
12. The infant is confident that the caregiver will respond appropriately.

Of course, all infants have different temperaments, which will create differences in responses to you, the health professional. These individual differences are welcomed by health professionals because they support the belief that humans are unique, each deserving of a distinct approach to care.

EVERYDAY NEEDS OF INFANTS

By now you have discovered in this book that the "solutions" to challenges during interaction with patients are sometimes concrete and dictated by common sense. Fussy, irritable, crying infants are in the vulnerable position of becoming the least liked (and potentially least cared for) patients in the pediatrics unit. Crying is one way infants try to communicate distress.

More likely than not, because of the infant's age and stage of development, this distress is related to a concrete, immediate need. Respectful interaction with infants in distress requires careful attention to several types of details.

Attention to the Comfort Details of Care

Small children most often become irritable when they experience physical discomfort. Careful attention to comfort is key to their sense of security and well-being. This becomes even more reason to check for factors that could lead to discomfort whenever possible. It is too easy to assume that a baby's crying or other belligerence is because they are a fussy or cranky baby.

REFLECTIONS

Which of these comfort detail questions should health professionals ask themselves?
- Is the onesie, diaper, or crib sheet wet from urine, sweat, or a spilled medication?
- Are they wrinkled and creating pressure spots?
- Does the baby have abrasions, punctures, or other bodily tenderness that causes contact pain? Is tape pinching the baby, or has an intravenous line infiltrated?
- Are the infant's throat and mouth dry?
- What did the baby eat and when? Is he or she taking fluids?
- Is a bowel movement creating skin irritation?

- Is the infant hungry or thirsty?
- Is the infant having some predictable side effects from a medication?
- What is the environment like? Is it too noisy? Too bright? Too dark?

What other comfort questions can you name?

HEALTH PROFESSIONAL DETAIL

Discomfort also can be caused by what you are wearing or doing. Think about the kind of clothing and adornments such as name tags that you wear in clinical practice.

1. Is your uniform scratching the baby? Is the color or design too complex?
2. Are you wearing jewelry that scratches, pokes, or pinches?
3. Are your hands clammy and/or cold?

Think about the number of providers evaluating or treating the infant.

1. Is the baby constantly being dressed and undressed?
2. Has the baby been assessed by several different members of the interprofessional health team without the opportunity to rest?
3. Is the baby overstimulated by machines and mechanical or procedural-based handling (vs. skin contact and loving touch to facilitate bonding with providers)?

Your conduct is like a mirror to the baby. If you are anxious or uncomfortable with caring for an infant, the infant will sense it. In addition to the immediate discomfort, you may cause an infant by inattention to these details, a more persistent negative response could be a sign of deeper discomfort. A good general rule is to remain consistent, approaching the infant similarly in each interaction in hope that the familiarity itself will be a comfort. Also, watch how the infant interacts with others, especially those who appear to be successful in calming them. Try altering your approach to match those that seem to calm the infant. Always orient the infant to your presence and provide comforting touch when procedural touch is also required.

Environmental Detail

Like all of us, infants have various comfort zones, which include temperature, space, noise, and other environmental factors.

REFLECTIONS

Look around the room that you are currently occupying, and imagine it is one that includes an ill infant.
- Is the room too warm or is there a source of cold air that is directed on you?
- Have you adjusted your clothing because you were sweaty or chilled?
- Are there distracting noises in the area from nearby construction, an open window, or a piece of electronic equipment?
- Are there different smells in the air such as the fumes from painting in the hallway, a disinfectant, or food preparation nearby?
- What else do you notice about the environment that could have an impact on an infant's well-being?

In short, this section is a reminder of ways you should be attentive to the behavior of the young patient and to the people who are associated with his or her care. One of the primary developmental goals of infancy is social attachment. Attention to comfort of the infant, the family care providers, and the environment is essential so that the infant can trustingly engage with others.[27]

CASE STUDY

Lucy Bahal is a 2-month-old infant referred to Bayside Early Intervention for an interprofessional developmental evaluation because of failure to thrive. Lucy was born at 37 weeks of gestation and transitioned home from the hospital with her family on her fifth day of life. Lucy was a little "slow to eat," so the care team recommended that she be bottle fed until the mother, Lydia, and Lucy could get into a routine. Lydia is a 29-year-old operating room nurse who breastfed her other two children without any difficulties. Lucy, however, is just "not taking to it," which is frustrating Lydia. You arrive at the Bahal home for the intake visit. Lucy is in a portable crib on her back. She is fussy and the two other children (aged 28 months and 4 years old) are arguing over which cartoon show they would like to watch. Lydia greets you by saying "just another day in paradise." You talk with Lydia about your role and start to take a developmental history of Lucy. Lydia reports that Lucy is her "hardest baby." She has not been able to breastfeed and reports that she is "very fussy." You ask Lydia what a typical day is like, and she reports that she is so overwhelmed by it all and there is no typical day. Lydia says all she really wants to do is sleep and that she does not feel like eating or playing with Lucy.

- What additional questions do you have for this postpartum mother? Besides the infant's failure to thrive, what other health issues might be going on in this family?
- How might you show respect and consistency for Lucy, while attending to the principles of patient- and family-centered care presented in Chapter 7 and cultural humility presented in Chapter 4?

Early Development: The Toddler and Preschool Child

Much of the material related to respectful interaction with the infant patient and his or her family can be applied to the child past the stage of infancy into other stages of early childhood. As a child grows, however, new challenges confront both parents and health professionals. This is especially true of the toddler and preschooler. These years are ones of rapid physical, social, emotional, and cognitive growth. Children begin to walk, run, and climb. They have increased control over feeding and toileting habits and start learning about limits. A review of Erikson's stages shows that the young patient's psychosocial tasks in moving from infancy to becoming a toddler and then an older child focus on becoming one's own "self," separate from others. Unique personalities develop, and at this early age respect for a toddler and preschool-age child can be enhanced when the child asks for what they want.

All children develop at their own pace, and some, like Lucy in the case study, may experience delays in reaching a milestone in a select area of growth and development. You often hear this reflected in the comments of parents who recall how one of their children did not talk until almost 2 but has not stopped talking since. Variations in the growth and development trajectory are not atypical but do require close monitoring. In recent years, educators, health professionals, and governmental agencies have worked interprofessionally to educate parents and caregivers regarding what normal child development typically looks like in efforts to improve childhood health outcomes. The Center for Disease Control and Prevention has developed an extensive resource for parents. It can be accessed at https://www.cdc.gov/ncbddd/actearly/milestones/index.html. This multimodal website includes information in English and Spanish and a milestone tracker app that is written in keeping with best practices in health literacy. The app includes a checklist, photos and videos, and an appointment tracker. It is a great example of an asynchronous technological tool that can serve to enhance provider communication as discussed in Chapter 9.

When children fail to reach multiple milestones over key developmental periods, and parents and health professionals have concerns about the child's day-to-day functioning, developmental testing is indicated. Early monitoring and developmental testing are vitally important because developmental disabilities are typically diagnosed in the early years.[28] Given their effect on early childhood functioning, developmental disabilities such as autism spectrum disorder (ASD) are being diagnosed much earlier than in years past. It is not uncommon for diagnosis to occur in the 18-month-old to 2-year-old child. The median age of ASD diagnosis is 4.2 years, yet most parents report seeing signs and symptoms of it as early as 6 months–1 year of age.[29]

PLAY

Play is an important vehicle through which a toddler patient's sense of worth can be fostered. According to developmental psychologists, play may be the child's richest opportunity for physical, cognitive, social, and emotional development. Play evolves over time and in addition to sensorimotor development, it is the primary tool through which the child learns social and cultural roles and norms. Play can be structured or unstructured. The literature describes several types of play, any of which can be encouraged as part of treatment or other aspects of interaction with the child and family. These include the following:

1. *unoccupied play* (0–3 months), which is when infants discover how their body moves through making a lot of movements with their arms, legs, hands, and feet;
2. *solitary play* (0–2 years), when a child plays alone, not quite interested in playing with others yet;
3. *onlooker play* (2 years), which involves intently watching others, such as when the health professional entertains the child or when the child observes others at play but does not actively participate;
4. *parallel play* (2+ years), which is side-by-side play characterized by activity that is interactive only by virtue of another's presence. (Participation by observation and side-by-side types of play may help decrease a young patient's loneliness, even though he or she cannot fully interact with others.) (Fig. 10.2);
5. *associative play* (3–4 years), which children start to interact; involves shared activity and communication but little organized activity; and
6. *cooperative play* (4+ years), which the child plays with others, having an interest in both the activity and the other children involved; requires following group rules and achieving agreed-on goals.[30]

Toddler and Preschooler Needs: Respect and Security

Attention to personal detail outlined in the section on infants applies to interaction with the toddler as well. Fortunately, in most cases, toddlers can verbalize their basic needs ("Me hungry," "Me go?" "More," or "No") and express their curiosity by pointing to something and asking, "Dis." Their illness, the intimidating surroundings, or their shyness, however, may make young children even more reticent than most patients to make their needs known in this direct manner. They often show their feelings of insecurity about what is happening to them by being cranky or acting overly fearful and demanding.

Children, like all patients, tend to regress when they become ill. Having so recently moved out of infancy, toddlers sometimes return to infant-like behavior. This is a normal tendency and should not be the cause to condemn young patients who do not "act their age."

One of the authors recalls hearing a health professional tell a pediatric patient that the patient was acting "like a baby," to which the patient confidently responded, "Well, I may not be a baby, but I am only 5!" Remember, even the smallest patients need care providers to validate their emotions. Tone and cadence of speech matter greatly in respectful interactions with children. In the

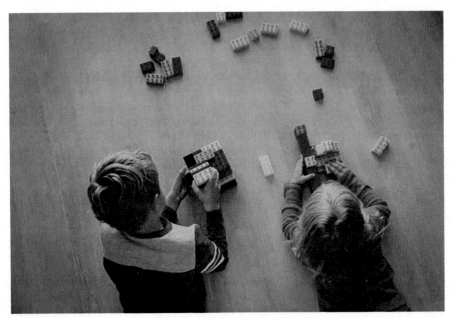

Fig. 10.2 Parallel play can be encouraged as part of treatment or other aspects of interaction with a young child. © Nadezhda1906/iStock/Thinkstock.com.

following story, a nurse tells of a toddler with Burkitt's lymphoma, a particularly fast-growing cancer, who was not doing well and was essentially silent:

> *I don't know how I knew this, but something said to me that he needed to be held right then. I asked him if he would like to rock in the rocking chair, and of course he didn't answer but he did not resist when I picked him up. We sat in that rocking chair for an hour and a half, and I could feel him settling in. I had on this knit sweater with a print, and when he finally sat up I laughed and said, "Jason, you've got waffles on your face!" He said, "I know, I've got them on my knees, too." That was the first time he spoke, and after that we couldn't shut him up.[31]*

A combination of gentle support for age-appropriate behaviors and tender care, such as holding and rocking, can encourage the young child to feel nurtured and secure. As they age, predictable routines, respectful responses, and consistent guidance allow young children to explore, learn, and develop a sense of who they are as individuals.

School Readiness

Because the early years are such a critical period in learning and development, it is during this stage that school preparedness begins. Children 3–5 years of age understand rules, share, begin to navigate conflict, initiate separation from their caregivers, explore social relationships, play, listen, and take turns. They begin to develop preliteracy skills (alphabet) and prenumeracy skills (counting) and are categorized as "preschoolers." Research shows that children who participate in high-quality preschool programs have better health, social-emotional, and cognitive outcomes than those who do not.[32] Despite this, participation in preschool activities varies greatly. Some children start preschool at 2.9 months of age, yet others may not enter until the start of kindergarten at age 5 or 6. In the United States, public funding for preschool varies from state to state. According to the US Department of Education, in 2019, 49% of 3–4-year-olds and 60% of 5-year-olds were enrolled in preprimary programs (preschool or kindergarten).[33] The COVID-19 pandemic has had an extended impact on preschool education and child development. As a result of the pandemic, children had less access to preschool, fewer attended state-funded preschool or Head Start programs, many of the children who did enroll "attended" virtual preschool, and preschool regulations were both tightened and relaxed to deal with the pandemic.[34] For health professionals who practice in the school and early childhood education settings, this means that the elementary school setting may be the first time a child meets a health professional or has a developmental need identified. Positive parenting and following principles of patient- and family-centered care, as described in Chapter 7, will help support respectful interaction with children and their families in the early years.

Early Adversity

Participation in typical childhood activities may be disrupted as a result of environmental factors such as deprivation, isolation, abuse, or exposure to violence.[35] *Early adversity*, or an *adverse childhood experience*, is the personal experience of abuse, neglect, or trauma associated with proximity to an unstable family member (i.e., a close family member who has a substance use disorder or mental illness, is incarcerated, and/or is a victim of domestic violence) or a suddenly departed family member (i.e., divorce, death, and abandonment).[36] Advances in biology are providing deeper insights into how early experiences are "built into the body" and the lasting effects of these stressful experiences on learning, behavior, and health.[37,38] Just as each personal or environmental situation is unique, so is each child's response to early adversity. Children who have experienced early adversity commonly develop insecure attachments, and research has shown that these experiences are biologically linked to an increased risk for cardiovascular disease, cancer, type 2 diabetes, substance use disorders, chronic inflammation, anxiety, and depression in adulthood.[39,40] For these reasons, it is essential that health professionals attend to the impact of early adversity and work to support at-risk children, families, and communities. Approaching children who have experienced adversity with consistency and reassurance helps garner their trust. Building resilience through the development of early coping skills and strengths based training models are key tools and interventions that can be carried through childhood into the adult years.

Abuse and Neglect

Legally, the parents or another formally appointed guardian are the voice of the young child, except in rare instances in which government agencies intervene to protect the child from caregivers whom the state deems are not acting in the child's best interest. The most grievous situation results when there is growing suspicion or knowledge that the patient is a victim of *child abuse* or *neglect*. In the case of a dysfunctional family in which abuse is suspected, you must turn your attention to the protection of the victimized child. The Child Abuse Prevention and Treatment Act (CAPTA), originally enacted in 1974, has been amended several times. It was most recently amended in 2019 and reauthorized under the Victims of Child Abuse Act Reauthorization Act of 2018 (P.L. 115-424). CAPTA is the key federal legislation addressing child abuse and neglect. It mandates reporting and provides support for community-based grants to prevent child abuse and neglect.[41] CAPTA defines child abuse and neglect as "any recent act of failure to act on the part of a parent or caretaker, which results in death, serious physical or emotional harm, sexual abuse, or exploitation, or an act or failure to act which presents an imminent risk of serious harm."[42] Younger children are more frequently maltreated than older children, with those younger than the age of 1 being at the greatest risk. A good general rule is to be suspicious of maltreatment when reports of the history of the child's injuries do not coincide with physical findings. Furthermore, you must become acquainted with appropriate reporting procedures for persons in your chosen profession. Most health professionals and educators are mandated reporters, although reporting procedures vary from state to state. Parents and other caregivers who maltreat children are deeply troubled. Your support of policies and practices that address maltreatment of children as a family affair is a valuable contribution to society.

In summary, despite the occasional problematic family situation, the family is usually a sound and reliable bridge to building a better understanding of the needs of infants, toddlers, and young children. Involving family systems in care is critical because families are the primary social context in which children live and receive care and nurturing.

Summary

This chapter beamed attention on the ways respectful interaction applies to the youngest patients and their families. To help highlight some unique and special characteristics of such relationships this chapter presented an overview of a variety of theories that seek to explain how human beings develop biologically, psychologically, and socially over the life span. The progression from birth to infancy to early childhood is shaped by the environment, the most important element of which is the family. As an infant develops into a toddler, then a preschooler, they start taking steps, literally and figuratively, toward a lifelong journey that is unique to each child. Recognizing the distinctness of the child as an individual, as well as being a product of a developmental phase, will help readers to better understand the many dimensions in which respect can be conveyed, and how the success of patient- and family-centered care will be maximized.

References

1. Forman V. *This Lovely Life: A Memoir of Premature Motherhood*. Boston, MA: Houghton Mifflin Harcourt; 2009:109.
2. *WHO*. WHO Global Health Observatory (GHO) data: infant mortality. https://www.who.int/data/gho/data/themes/topics/indicator-groups/indicator-group-details/GHO/infant-mortality. Accessed February 15, 2022.
3. United Health Foundation. *America's Health Rankings Annual Report*. Minnetonka, MN; 2019:40. https://www.americashealthrankings.org/learn/reports/2019-annual-report/international-comparison.
4. *Centers for Disease Control and Prevention. Division of Reproductive Health*. Infant mortality. June 22, 2022 https://www.cdc.gov/reproductivehealth/maternalinfanthealth/infantmortality.htm.
5. Jacoba J. US infant mortality rate declines but still exceeds other developed countries. *JAMA*. 2016;315(5):451–452.
6. Vilda D, Hardeman R, Dyer L, Theall KP, Wallace M. Structural racism, racial inequities and urban–rural differences in infant mortality in the US. *J Epidemiol Community Health*. 2021;75(8):788–793.
7. As S. Why the mortality rate for black infants is so high. *Hum Life Rev*. 2020;46(3):94–96.
8. Sedig MB, Pacquaio DF. Action on social determinants of black maternal and infant mortality in the United States. *J Nurs Pract Appl Rev Res*. 2021;11(2):67–75.
9. Chien C-H, Lee T-Y, Lin M-T. Factors affecting motor development of toddlers who received cardiac corrective procedures during infancy. *Early Hum Dev*. 2021;158. https://doi.org/10.1016/j.earlhumdev.2021.105392.
10. World Health Organization. *International Classification of Functioning, Disability and Health*. Geneva: ICF; 2002. http://www.who.int/classifications/icf/training/icfbeginnersguide.pdf.
11. *Help Me Grow Minnesota*. Cognitive development. n.d. https://helpmegrowmn.org/HMG/HelpfulRes/Articles/WhatCognitiveDev/index.html; Accessed November 10, 2021.
12. Piaget J. *Six Psychological Studies*. New York: Vintage; 1964.
13. Miller SA. *Developmental Research Methods*. Englewood Cliffs, NJ: Prentice Hall; 1987.
14. Myant K, Williams J. Children's concepts of health and illness: understanding of contagious illnesses, non-contagious illnesses and injuries. *J Health Psychol*. 2005;10(6):805–819.

15. Menendez D, Klapper RE, Golden MZ, et al. "When will it be over?" U.S. children's questions and parents' responses about the COVID-19 pandemic. *PLoS ONE*. 2021;16(8):e0256692. https://doi.org/10.1371/journal.pone.0256692.

16. Luby JL, Rogers C, McLaughlin KA. Environmental conditions to promote healthy childhood brain/behavioral development: informing early preventive interventions for delivery in routine care. *Biol Psychiatry Glob Open Sci*. 2022;2(3):233–241. https://doi.org/10.1016/j.bpsgos.2021.10.003.

17. Kenrick Douglas. Discovering the next big question in evolutionary psychology: a few guidelines. *Evol Behav Sci*. 2020;14(4):347–354.

18. Lally JR, Mangione P. Caring relationships: the heart of early brain development. *Young Child*. 2017;72(2):17–24.

19. Saracho ON. Theories of child development and their impact on early childhood education and care. *Early Child Educ J*. October 29, 2021 https://doi.org/10.1007/s10643-021-01271-5.

20. Erikson EH. *Identity and the Life Cycle*. New York: WW Norton; 1959.

21. *National Scientific Council on the Developing Child*. Connecting the brain to the rest of the body: early childhood development and lifelong health are deeply intertwined working paper no. 15. www.developingchild.harvard.edu; 2020.

22. Dosman C, Andrews D. Anticipatory guidance for cognitive and social-emotional development: birth to five years. *Paediatr Child Health (1205-7088)*. 2012;17(2):75–80.

23. Fairhurst N, Long T. Parental involvement in decision-making in the neonatal intensive care unit: a review of the international evidence. *Paediatr Child Health*. 2020;30(4):119–123.

24. Parish O, Williams D, Odd D, Joseph-Williams N. Barriers and facilitators to shared decision-making in neonatal medicine: a systematic review and thematic synthesis of parental perceptions. *Patient Educ Couns*. 2021;105(5):1101–1114.

25. Sweeney J, Heriza C, Blanchard Y, Dusing S. Neonatal physical therapy. Part II: practice frameworks and evidence-based practice guidelines…second article of a 2-part series [corrected] [published erratum appears in PEDIATR PHYS THER 2010 Winter;22(4):377]. *Pediatr Phys Ther*. 2010;22(1):2–16.

26. Schuster CS, Ashburn SS. *The Process of Human Development*. Boston, MA: Little, Brown; 1986.

27. Cronin A, Mandich MB. *Human Development and Performance Throughout the Lifespan*. 2nd ed. Clifton Park, NY: Thomson Delmar Learning; 2015.

28. O'Connor Leppert ML. Developmental evaluation. In: Voigt Robert G, Macias Michelle M, Myers Scott M, Tapia Carl D, eds. *AAP Developmental and Behavioral Pediatrics*. 2nd ed. Washington, DC: American Academy of Pediatrics; 2018:165–186.

29. *CDC*. Autism spectrum disorder. Data and statistics. https://www.cdc.gov/ncbddd/autism/data.html; 2021.

30. *Pathways.org*. How kids learn to play: 6 stages of play development. https://pathways.org/kids-learn-play-6-stages-play-development/; 2020 Accessed November 15, 2021.

31. Montgomery CL. *Healing Through Communication*. Newbury Park, CA: Sage; 1993.

32. *U.S. Department of Education*. A matter of equity: preschool in America. https://www2.ed.gov/documents/early-learning/matter-equity-preschool-america.pdf; 2015.

33. *U.S. Department of Education, National Center for Education Statistics*. Preprimary education enrollment. Fast facts. https://nces.ed.gov/fastfacts/display.asp?id=516; Accessed November 11, 2021.

34. *National Institute for Early Education Research (NIEER)*. The state of preschool 2020. National Institute for Early Education Research; 2021. https://nieer.org/wp-content/uploads/2021/04/YB2020_Full_Report.pdf.

35. Whitcomb DA, Carrasco RC, Neuman A, et al. Correlational research to examine the relation between attachment and sensory modulation in young children. *Am J Occup Ther*. 2015;69: 6904220020.

36. Lynch A, Ashcraft R, Tekell LM. Understanding children who have experienced early adversity: implications for practitioners practicing sensory integration. *SIS Q OT Pract Connect*. 2017;2(3):5–7.

37. Snow PC. Psychosocial adversity in early childhood and language and literacy skills in adolescence: the role of speech-language pathology in prevention, policy, and practice. *Perspect ASHA Spec Interest Groups*. 2021;6(2):253–261.

38. Morris AS, Wakschlag L, Krogh-Jespersen S, et al. Principles for guiding the selection of early childhood neurodevelopmental risk and resilience measures: HEALthy Brain and Child Development Study as an Exemplar. *Advers Resil Sci*. 2020;1(4):1–21. https://doi.org/10.1007/s42844-020-00025-3.

39. Shonkoff JP, Boyce WT, McEwen BS. Neuroscience, molecular biology, and the childhood roots of health disparities: building a new framework for health promotion and disease prevention. *JAMA.* 2009;301(21):2252–2259.

40. McFarland DC, Nelson C, Miller AH. Early childhood adversity in adult patients with metastatic lung cancer: cross-sectional analysis of symptom burden and inflammation. *Brain Behav Immun.* 2020;90:167–173.

41. Child Welfare Information Gateway. *About CAPTA: A Legislative History.* Washington, DC: U.S. Department of Health and Human Services, Children's Bureau; 2019.

42. Child Welfare Information Gateway. *Definition of Child Abuse and Neglect.* Washington, DC: U.S. Department of Health and Human Services: Children's Bureau; 2019.

CHAPTER 11

Respectful Interaction: Working With School-Age Children and Adolescents

The reader will be able to

- Discuss the key developmental tasks of children and adolescents;
- Identify developmental challenges that require consideration in the health professional's approach to school-age children and adolescents;
- Describe how the concepts of play introduced in Chapter 10 are relevant—or not relevant—to respectful interaction with children;
- Describe how a child's developing need for connection enters into the health professional and patient relationship;
- Identify strategies to help minimize the disequilibrium of the family during a child's illness;
- Understand the impact of social media on identity development in school-age children and adolescents;
- Describe high-risk behaviors in adolescence that can lead to long-term health problems; and
- Describe reasons for giving respectful attention to an adolescent's desire to exercise authority regarding health care decisions, and describe legitimate limits on that authority.

Prelude

The important thing about you is that you are you. It is true that you were a baby, and you grew, and now you are a child, and you will grow, into a man, or into a woman. But the important thing about you is that you are you.

M.W. BROWN[1]

Much of the material related to respectful interaction with the infant or toddler and their family can be applied to older children. As a child grows, however, some new challenges and opportunities confront the child, parents, families, and interprofessional care team. In this chapter, we add to the groundwork we laid in Chapter 10 to highlight some of the most important differences and focus on the distinct needs of adolescent patients.

The Child Becomes a Self

A young child's psychosocial tasks of moving from early to middle childhood focus on the need to recognize that one has a "self," separate from others, but also that ultimately, many aspects of that self must survive and thrive in relationships with others. Therefore much activity and energy are focused on being different from others. At the same time, much is invested in learning how to be accepted by others and having some say in relationships. As we address later in this chapter, these tasks become paramount during the adolescent years, but the fundamental building blocks begin much earlier.

NEEDS: RESPECT AND RELATING

A significant part of the child's developmental task is becoming a "self" different from others. In general, children want to make it alone and have learned not to accept the full dependence of infancy. The toddler and preschool years are not yet independent either. As highlighted in earlier stages of development discussed in Chapter 10, when children become patients, the dependence side of the scale tips. The independence that the child was gaining suddenly escapes. In this confusing never-never land of being neither fully child nor fully adult, children must try to reestablish some sense of equanimity and self-identity during their time as patients. Additionally, when their child enters the health care system, caregivers also face fear and loss of control as they must hand over some of their parental control to the health care team.[2] This situation increases the health professional's challenge of finding means to convey respect for the young patient and their caregivers.

Most children beyond the preschool years have learned to communicate verbally and have many more experiences to rely on compared to an infant or a toddler. Thus, their resources for relating to other children and adults are greater than in earlier years. The school-age years expand the child's world to interactions with many new and different people. These are mainly authority figures, such as teachers, coaches, and other role models, as well as peers, playmates, and older children.

Health professionals often present types of authority that are unfamiliar to the child. Interacting with family and school authority figures usually does little to prepare children for the health care setting and its unique challenges and choices. Additionally, relating to figures of authority differs for children from different backgrounds and socioeconomic strata. Children raised in middle-class households tend to have a more robust sense of entitlement, are familiar with negotiation, and may see adults as equals. In contrast, there are typically clearer boundaries between children from working-class backgrounds and the adults in their lives.[3]

THE IMPORTANCE OF PLAY

Regardless of background and socioeconomic status, play is a child's primary occupation and universal right.[4] In 1989, world leaders adopted an international legal framework protecting the rights of children called the United Nations Convention on the Rights of the Child. Included in one of the articles is the child's right to "engage in play and recreational activities appropriate to the age of the child."[5] In the health care setting, play, appropriate to the child's age and social development, serves as a means of easing the tension a child is feeling about relating to people. In Chapter 10 we introduced six types of play and noted that play changes as children develop new motor, cognitive, and social–emotional skills. Age, peer group, and play opportunities are important contributors to play. Regardless of the environment (hospital, school, or home), children *need* to play. In fact, pediatric patients who are anxious and scared may benefit even more from the distraction of play and laughter. Art, music, and pet therapy are all valuable options.[6] However, with limited funds or access to these resources or environments, the health care provider must be creative to distract young patients with fun activities and humor.

Some older children who become patients may regress to an earlier stage of play, but many will assume roles at the higher levels of play, which will allow them to act out their predicament of being in a new situation. For example, associative play can involve playing "hospital" with a health professional or family member. Observing the child role-playing the nurse or someone else in charge may reveal anxieties and illustrate how the child perceives their situation. Their perception of the health care provider and clues to how their tension could be eased may be deduced from how they interact with their play patient. Cooperative play involving modified sporting activities, such as catch with a balloon, or video games, for example, can serve as an effective way of relating to children.

Young patients often play with toys too, so building blocks, puzzles, or other objects may be an effective means of helping to establish a relationship. At the same time, children can be sensitive about being "too old" for certain types of toys, so health professionals and others must think carefully about which toys to offer and how to integrate family and siblings into their sessions. You will recall the discussion of the danger of stereotyping from Chapter 4. Stereotypes are beliefs about traits in a specific group or social category. The same risks hold for making assumptions about preferred play based on a child's age or gender. Rather than stereotyping masculine or feminine toys, the health professional should use open-ended questions to learn from the young patient about their preferences. They will likely enjoy sharing about their favorite game or toy.

Health professionals must also be sensitive to the fact that some children may not have access to toys and books. The poverty threshold for a family of four in the United States is $26,172.[7] In 2019, 14% of those under the age of 18 were living in poverty.[8] Children living in poverty are often vulnerable to environmental, health, educational, and safety risks. They are also at particular risk for developmental challenges. Thoughtful considerations on how to help families modify environments and maximize access can bring about meaningful change in the number of opportunities for children to engage in play (e.g., repurposing everyday items as toys and accessing library services).

REFLECTIONS

The COVID-19 pandemic saw a resurgence in the sale of puzzles and coloring books for adults.[9] This resurgence was related to stay-at-home orders but also attributed to the calming effects of play.
- When was the last time you engaged in "play"?
- How did you feel during the activity? After the activity?
- How did it contribute to your mood?

TRANSITIONS IN SCHOOLING

Starting school is a rite of passage and a significant transition for children and families. As discussed in Chapter 10, some children start the transition to school as early as age of 2 years, when they begin preschool. Others transition at the start of kindergarten. Regardless of the age at which they transition, every child goes through both the challenge and the excitement of new roles, routines, and learning experiences. Each school-based transition brings a period of adjustment to new rules, teachers, friends, and environments. Emotions related to school transitions include excitement, happiness, sadness, and worry.[10] When school-age children become patients, health professionals are faced with additional challenges. Even a short illness or injury may disrupt school attendance, put the child behind in schoolwork, and have social consequences. During the school years, children organize most of their relational activity around family and school and risk missing out on valuable social interactions when removed from the educational environment.

Consider the impact of school closure during the COVID-19 pandemic on children and adolescents. To limit the spread of the virus, schools around the world closed and transitioned to virtual learning formats affecting more than 55 million children from kindergarten through 12th grade in the United States.[11] While there were certainly concerns about the lack of academic gains made during the "lost year," it is important to remember that schools provide children with many other services beyond academics. Schools can be the main source of food for children.[12] Many children, especially those from minoritized backgrounds or with lower socioeconomic status, rely on school for health care and mental health services.[11] Additionally, as described above, schools are an important source of social interaction and development. The pandemic provided an acute awareness of the multiple benefits of school and psychological consequences of being out of school. At the very least, patient-centered respect for the child requires you to be aware of this loss and show interest in any school-related activity being carried on at the moment. The COVID-19 pandemic and stay-at-home orders limited teachers and school counselor's ability to monitor for signs of abuse toward children and adolescents and report to the proper authorities. In instances where children may be out of school for a prolonged period, the role of the health care provider in screening patients and being vigilant for signs of child and adolescent abuse is vital.[13]

Most children with chronic illnesses or long-term disabilities will receive special attention regarding education through the school system itself. Over the past 30 years, the definition of disability has changed. In the 1970s and 1980s the concept of a disability referred to an underlying physical or mental condition that reduced one's abilities. Disability was thought to begin where health ended. Today, disability is seen as a complex interaction between a person and their environment, and there is a focus on functioning in society regardless of the reasons for limitations. The development of the international classification of functioning, disability, and health by the World Health Organization (discussed in Chapter 4) reflects this new perspective. In this classification, *disability* is an umbrella term for impairments, activity limitations, and participation restrictions. This perspective acknowledges that any individual can experience a decline in health at various points in their life span, hence experiencing disability. It is a biological, individual, and social perspective of health rather than a diagnosis or label.[14] There is also a shift in thinking about disability to focus on participation and well-being.

In the United States, the number of children with developmental disabilities and mental health conditions is on the rise. A study from the Centers for Disease Control and Prevention (CDC) and the Health Resources and Services Administration found that 17% of school-age children had a developmental disability. Notably, this percentage increased over the two time periods compared, 2009–11 and 2015–17. In this study, some groups of children were more likely to have been diagnosed with a developmental disability than others, such as

- boys compared to girls;
- non-Hispanic White and Black children compared to Hispanic children or children of other races;
- children living in rural areas compared to children living in urban areas; and
- children with public health insurance compared to uninsured children and children with private insurance.[15]

Children living in poverty consistently experience the highest overall rates of disability; with a documented 28.4% rise in disability rates among children living in households at greater than 400% of the poverty level.[15] Regardless of sociodemographic trends, these statistics highlight the need for health, educational, and social services for school-age children and their families.

The Individuals with Disabilities Education Act (IDEA) is the federal law that governs the provision of special education services. It requires public schools to make available to all eligible children with disabilities a free, appropriate public education in the least restrictive environment appropriate to their individual needs.[16] However, the law does little to address the accompanying problems that sometimes arise, such as peer cruelty toward differently abled children, and parents disagreeing with the individualized education program (IEP) and feeling as if they have little recourse. Additionally, teachers may feel as if they have insufficient time to devote to the needs of all the children in their classrooms, and children with serious but not permanent conditions may not qualify for services.[17] When you encounter families trying to work through some of these issues, you can direct them to the appropriate resources when problems arise. For example, the IEP team's job is to work together to meet the needs of the child. However, if parents disagree with the IEP, IDEA allows for three different ways to solve the problem: (1) mediation, (2) complaint, and (3) a due process hearing.[18]

In short, during the school-age years, a child's feelings of self-worth and experiences of relatedness are usually tied to school. Any means by which you can convey empathy for the child's predicament and respect for their interests will enhance the child's self-esteem and help ensure success in the relationship.

Family: A Bridge to Respectful Interaction

All of the family dynamics described in Chapter 7 apply as the child grows older. However, the growing child does present some additional challenges to the family and health professional working with the family. The needs of the school-age child revolve around tasks, hobbies, and activities. During this stage, 7- to 12-year-olds develop a sense of values to guide decision-making and interests.

A child's desire to become more independent is one of the major developmental tasks of this growth period, while at the same time, they may feel incredibly lonely and insecure when illness strikes. The family is often torn between wanting to support the child as increasingly independent and being attentive to their needs. They may also be dismayed by the child's obvious regression or respond to their own feelings of guilt with overprotectiveness.

Not surprisingly, parents of children in a pediatric intensive care unit described that it is vital that providers keep them informed. Parents perceived that they were good parents when they focused on their child's quality of life, advocated for the child during discussions with the health care team, and put their child's needs above their own.[19] Wei et al. found that parents of pediatric patients valued when health care providers cared about the child and the whole family. They appreciated it when health care providers tried to understand what they were going through emotionally and physically. Encouragement and facilitation to maintain the parental role are critical. Notably, when parents observed the interprofessional care team working together, they described their burden being lowered.[2]

Your caring professional attention to family and caregiver struggles and needs are essential ingredients for success. Family members warrant your due respect. They are the people who are most knowledgeable about the child and are key collaborators in clinical decision-making. Lawlor and Mattingly put this best when they stated: "Collaboration is much more than being nice. It involves complex interpretive acts in which the practitioner must understand the meanings of illness or disability in a person and family's life and the feelings that accompany these experiences."[20]

CHILDREN AS ACTIVE PARTICIPANTS IN CARE

Children are sometimes described as silent consumers of health care[21] and yet they should not be. Respect for the child's input, especially when their opinions seem to differ from their parents', is essential. Although developmental psychology has often used age as an indicator of reliable decision-making capacity (i.e., in clinical terms, patient *competency*, with decisions based on the patient's informed consent), this view is being challenged and replaced by the principle that maturity and experience are more reliable markers of the ability to participate in decisions related to the child's health care.[22,23] Although the legal age of consent is 16–18 in a majority of the United States; many policies now acknowledge the importance of listening to children and having them *assent* to care decisions. Assent in children honors respect for persons and should be sought from the age of 7 upward. It ensures that children have the opportunity to understand

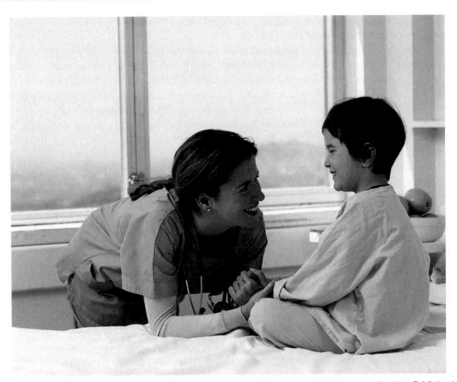

Fig. 11.1   The health professional must listen to what the child has to say during an examination. © Michael Blann/Digital Vision/Thinkstock.com.

their condition, share their views, and participate in decisions regarding their care.[23] Assenting to decisions allows children to communicate a choice and have a say in what happens.[24] Children often express their preferences through body language and actions. However difficult the discussion may be, many children should be invited to participate in the care planning process. It is through this participation that they learn the life skills necessary for decision-making and illness management. Remember that not all children are familiar with negotiation, and some may require more encouragement and facilitation than others. Children are also often aware of their parent's anxiety, opposition, or denial and may try to act as referees among family members or between health professionals and family.

Children can and should have the opportunity to participate in a meaningful way in discussions about their health care (Fig. 11.1). When children aged 7–11 years were asked what the best thing about their hospital experience was, children responded that interacting with people (including health professionals and educators) especially those associated with sympathy and competence was a positive experience. They also saw hospitalization as the opportunity to have their parents constantly present and have family and friends visit. Going back to the concept of the importance of play, children interviewed also emphasized enjoying access to books, games, and watching television. They also valued the opportunity to get better and be cured from their illness and finally, the opportunity to eat their favorite foods. When asked about their worst experience, children described feelings such as being sick and not being able to leave the hospital, as well as pain and isolation. Procedures and examinations such as getting tests and injections stood out as the worst experiences. Highlighting the importance of school to young children, hospitalized children noted the time spent waiting for procedures and the absence from school and the daily routine as the worst experiences.[21,25]

Siblings are also affected by the stress that illness creates in the family. Siblings are the pediatric patients' first peers, often supporting them through various life situations such as illness, thus making them a significant part of family dynamics. In a study of sibling's perspectives on the perceived changes to family dynamics and daily functioning following a child's chronic pain diagnosis, Gorodzinsky et al. found conflicting themes. Patients reported minimal changes to family relationships as a result of their illness while siblings reported significant changes. Some siblings reported increased conflict while others reported a strengthened sibling relationship. Increased conflict is not surprising given that the pediatric patient with chronic pain may not have the additional cognitive or social resources to dedicate to their sibling relationship.[26] You can help siblings cope by providing support and information. Through the application of the principles of patient and family-centered care, supportive participation, information sharing, and collaboration, siblings feel engaged and supported. You can also help by keeping family disequilibrium at a minimum while acting primarily as an advocate for the child.

This balancing act is sometimes easier said than accomplished. For example, consider the case study below regarding Jai, his family, and the interprofessional care team.

CASE STUDY

When Jai was 9, he fell from a swing, had some joint pain in the lower left extremity, and could not fully extend his knee. Numerous radiographic studies were completed, and the results were largely normal. However, Jai could still not play soccer and continued to complain of tenderness. Finally, a magnetic resonance image revealed a lesion that turned out to be non-Hodgkin's lymphoma (NHL). Jai received combination chemotherapy and has been in remission for two and a half years. His mother has been his primary in-home caregiver. When the physician asked about Jai's father, Jai replied, "He can't deal with having a wimp for a kid." His mother said that she "had everything under control" and that Jai's dad was "a very busy man who spends a lot of time on out-of-town business." As Jai has gotten older, the team which has followed Jai and his family has grown somewhat concerned about his mother's overprotectiveness. Although it was less noticeable when he was first diagnosed, it has been the topic of conversation among the interprofessional care team when Jai and his mother have come to the clinic. For instance, she mentioned that she still will not let Jai go on a sleepover and accompanies him almost everywhere. She is also very aware of symptoms that she notes in him even though Jai tries to protest that they either did not occur or were just passing. You believe he is becoming more withdrawn on visits and that she increasingly overrides questions the team members try to pose to him directly.

REFLECTIONS

- If you were a member of the interprofessional care team following Jai and his family, what would you do at this point?
- How might you respect both the mother and Jai in their attempt to be heard?
- What are some key considerations given Jai's developmental stage and age?

When the health professional is faced with dilemmas concerning how much information to share with pediatric patients, the following suggestions may be beneficial:

1. *Make your position clear* to yourself and the patient's parents. Do you think the child can handle information about their condition? Why or why not? What is in the best interests of the child? Of the family as a unit? Under what conditions would you feel morally bound to disclose relevant health information to this child? Under what conditions would you withhold such information, even if you believed that doing so could increase the child's distrust in you?

2. *Explore the resources available in your health care setting* to support families as they work out their anxieties and difficulties. As one author notes, "The purpose is... to support, not supplant, the family. An atmosphere of acceptance and assurance allows each family to manage their own lives and to arrive at a solution most adequate for them."[27] Social workers and ethics committees are two examples of the many supports available to families and teams of care providers in these situations.

3. *Present information so the child can understand* with ample opportunity for questions and explanations from the child in their own words about what has been discussed. Present opportunities for alternative questions by asking, "Is there a reason that you were curious about x?" Assent in children should help the pediatric patient achieve a developmentally appropriate awareness of the nature of their condition while informing them about what to expect in the future.[28]

4. *Implement strategies to lower family stress.* Two major tasks can help lower family stress and ensure that they are involved. The first is providing information. As collaborators in the care process, families need ongoing information. Structured communication such as regular phone calls, frequent family meetings, and involvement in team rounds can help the family understand and cope with their child's prognosis.[29] The second is involving families in the care of their family member. Family involvement in various patient care tasks may help reduce the sense of powerlessness.

In summary, a child brings to the health care interaction hopes, fears, and dreams that reflect their need to establish autonomy while maintaining the security of relationships with family, friends, and others. The delicate balance between being an individual and being part of relationships that are difficult under the best of circumstances is further challenged by illness or other incapacities. The efforts of health professionals and family working together are required for successful adaptation or recovery. The benefit is that within a context of respect for the child as a unique individual, the health professional and family will work together to meet the patient's best interests.

Adolescent Self

Adolescents have significantly different health care needs than children and adults. The word *adolescent* means literally "to grow into maturity or adulthood." During the later stages of child development, all children are thrust into the difficult position of demonstrating individuality in the larger world, asserting who they are, commanding authority in some areas, and exploring the mysteries of developing sexuality. "Adolescence typically is defined as beginning at puberty, a physiological transformation that gives boys and girls adult bodies and alters how they are perceived and treated by others, as well as how they view themselves."[30] It is a time of rapid biological, cognitive, and social–emotional growth and development and lays the foundation for adult health.

EARLY AND LATE ADOLESCENCE

Most psychologists and others writing about adolescence divide it into two stages: early and late, each with developmental tasks. Early adolescence lasts for about 2 years and is characterized by growth spurts, maturing of reproductive functions and sex organs, increased weight, and changes in body proportions. These profound changes understandably may have profound psychological results and are heightened for transgender and gender nonconforming youth. Transgender youth are three times more likely to experience depression, anxiety, and suicidal ideation as a result of stigma and family and peer rejection.[31]

Teenagers are often described as irrational, impulsive, oversensitive, and, at times, oppositional. Anyone who is around early teens knows that their self-images govern much of what they do. The teen years are a time of intensely seeking one's "self." In its extreme form, the self is the way the body looks and nothing more. However, for many teens, the absorption with the self goes beyond bodily appearance alone. Adolescents are generally highly concerned with fitting in with their peers. They will try various roles to integrate their developing social skills with goals and dreams.

This early period of adolescence is so unsettling that psychologists and others have described it as a period of adolescent turmoil. However, other researchers indicate that adolescents may not be as fraught with emotional issues as previously thought. In an ethnographic study of early adolescent girls, both popular and not so popular, the findings revealed a close relationship with parents and indeed not the trauma and stress suggested by common discourses (or myths) about adolescence. Teachers, parents, and health care professionals may expect trouble from adolescents because of, or attributed to, "raging hormones," but in this study, the trauma did not materialize.[32] However, at a minimum, there is clearly a disconnect between physical development and psychosocial maturation, leading to many of the challenges of adolescence.

After this period of rapid and profound change, young people move into late adolescence. Here, self-identity fully emerges as they practice the various roles and responsibilities they will assume as adults. It should also be noted that some adolescents do not move on to this stage of development because of adolescent mortality rates. Teens 12–17 years old were, on average, more likely to be victims of violent crimes compared with young adults (ages 18–30). Additionally, adolescents aged 12–17 were more likely to be victimized by someone they knew (54%). While the presence of physical and dating violence reported by students declined between 2013 and 2017, high school females were more likely than males to report physical or sexual dating violence. Additionally, the prevalence of physical dating violence was greater for Black students than White or Hispanic students, and gay, lesbian, or bisexual students and those not sure of their sexual identity were more likely than heterosexual students to report physical or sexual violence in 2017.[33]

The World Health Organization reports that suicide is the third leading cause of death in people aged 15–19 years and depression is one of the leading causes of adolescent illness.[34] The differences in victimization between adults and teens, and teens by racial or ethnic group, and gender and sexual identity indicate the profound impact disparities and health behaviors can have on adolescent mortality. Adolescents in developing countries have to contend with poverty, starvation, and infectious diseases. Those in developed countries contend with obesity, gun violence, and eating disorders.[35] Attending to these statistics guides health professionals in effective care interventions and health policy for the teenage population.

FRIENDS AND PEER GROUPS

Adolescents tend to spend less time with family and more time in new environments such as work settings, peer relationships, and romantic relationships. They move toward a more mature sense of themselves and start to question old values without losing their identity. Friendships are an essential part of adolescent development. The impact of a peer's behavior on an adolescent is significant (Fig. 11.2). Research supports the biological science behind the influence of peers on teenage behavior and decision-making. Substance use (tobacco, marijuana, and alcohol use), violence (weapons and physical fighting), and suicidal behavior (suicidal ideation and attempts) have been shown to relate to a teen's friends' substance use, deviance, and suicidal behaviors, respectively.

Although the stereotypical adverse effects are often highlighted, there are also positive effects. Peers help teens learn social norms and provide the support needed during the challenging time of adolescence. Prosocial behavior in friends has been shown to negatively correlate with violence and positively influence academic performance, skill, and personality development.[36,37] Other factors, such as family function, depression, and social acceptance, influence adolescents' health-risk behavior as well, but parents continue to be the most influential people in teen's lives. Supporting parents to keep communication open with teens during this rapid time of change (and sometimes conflict) is of prime importance in the context of supporting family health.

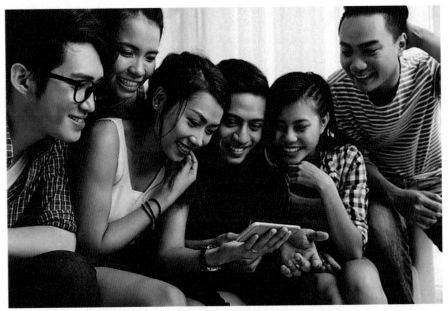

Fig. 11.2   An adolescent's behavior is influenced by that of their peers. © DragonImages/iStock/Thinkstock.com.

To highlight some challenges of showing respect for and working with adolescents and their families we return to the story of Jai and his mother introduced earlier.

CASE STUDY

Jai is now 15, and during a follow-up visit to the oncologist, it is discovered that he has a recurrence of NHL. Everyone is concerned; however, the prognosis for children with NHL has improved significantly over the last 35 years with a 5-year survival rate of between 79% and 97%.[38]

Jai is readmitted to the hospital for treatment. His mother visits for a minimum of 6 hours every day and remains steadfast at the bedside. In a recent conversation with the interprofessional care team during early morning rounds and before his mother arrives, Jai says, "Hey, since you guys are going to knock me out with all those killer chemo drugs again, what do you say we talk about saving my sperm? I talked with my buddies about sperm banking after reading about it in a survivor's blog, and we think it's a good idea. I mean, I want to have kids someday, too."

The physician approached Jai's mother about the team's desire to follow up with Jai regarding his recent question. She was shocked and enraged, stating: "Jai is just being provocative. He is too young to talk about such things. I bet he got this crazy idea from the girl he met at the cancer support group. And hard as I try, he is hanging out with boys I don't like. They are having a bad influence on him. This is not to be discussed with him under any circumstances." Although the team knows she is the legal decision-maker for Jai, many think she is limiting his participation in care planning and not making decisions in his best interests. The interprofessional care team's opinions on whether he should be allowed to sperm bank are divided.

REFLECTIONS

- What should you and the interprofessional care team do differently from your interactions with Jai and his family when Jai was younger?
- What questions do you want to raise with Jai and the care team about the most caring way to express respect toward Jai and his mother?

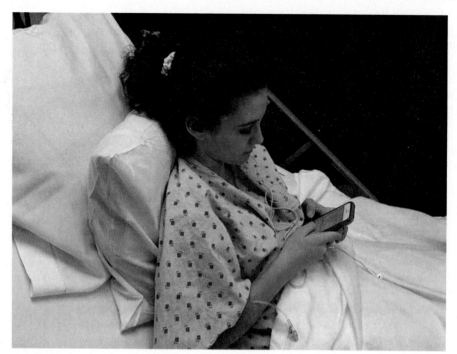

Fig. 11.3 Digital lives and social media influences in adolescent and school-age children. Photo courtesy R.F. Doherty.

Whether you follow a patient from childhood through to adolescence, the opportunity to express respect continues to be a major factor in respectful interaction. The rule of thumb is to always consider that the child's evolution of self-identity, independence of expression, and authority to speak on their behalf is somewhere on the continuum toward full adulthood. At the same time, family and other authority figures continue to exert a major influence on the pediatric patient's decision.

DIGITAL MEDIA

In today's digital world, a teenager's peer group extends beyond the individuals they interact with in school, sporting activities, and neighborhoods to include those in their digital life. A Nielsen report found that the typical age when children got a cell phone service plan was at the age of 10.[39] Parents' reasons for getting their children a cell phone was to reach them easily and keep track of them. According to the Pew Research Center, 95% of teens have a smartphone or access to one. The Internet and social media have become a place of social connection for many teenagers (Fig. 11.3) and 45% of teens report being online on a near constant basis.[40]

Teens are digitally connected behaviorally and biochemically. When asked about the influence of social media on their lives, many teens surveyed (45%) report that social media has neither a positive nor a negative effect on their lives.[40] However, research shows that electronic media have both positive and negative effects on adolescents.[41–44] Social media and gaming can influence the brain's reward circuitry, leading to a rush of the chemical dopamine being released, influencing adolescent brain development.[42] Among the positives are access to health information, social connections, and expanded learning opportunities. For example, Jai mentions that his request for sperm banking was initiated with his researching the topic online. The negatives include high-risk behaviors, sexting, cyber aggression, social isolation, Internet addiction, and digital invasions of privacy. The speed and pervasiveness of social media limits teens' abilities to control their digital footprint, and, in some ways, they lose the ability to make mistakes without consequences.[45] Health professionals and parents alike must educate teens on the impact of digital media on health and development. Health professionals must be aware of the influence of social media on their teenage patients and discuss appropriate digital health. Many health professionals who practice in the school system, such as school psychologists, school nurses, and physical and occupational therapists, have turned their attention to helping school-age children and adolescents critically evaluate which apps to choose, what information to share, and how to safely participate in social media platforms.

Needs: Respect, Autonomy, and Relating

Autonomous decision-making raises some delicate questions for health professionals who work with adolescent patients because adolescents often want to aggressively assert their authority in decisions. Only in recent years has there been an attempt to address the legal rights of adolescents. The most prominent view, referred to as the *Mature Minors Doctrine*, allows for parents or the state to speak on behalf of a minor's interests only if the minor is unable to represent themselves. Thus, the level of the young person's development emerges as a decisive factor. In keeping with the legality of the Mature Minors Doctrine, you can try to assess the maturity of an adolescent patient regarding their ability to cope effectively with illness or injury. The question of whether an adolescent is a "mature minor" must be decided by health care professionals independent of parental judgment.[46]

There are some compelling reasons to give decision-making authority to mature adolescents. Some adolescents would never consult a health care provider with a problem if they knew it would require parental consent before treatment. Also, in their developing autonomy, they would never share delicate information with the provider if they thought confidentiality would be violated. Coupled with the reluctance of adolescents to speak about risky behavior or other health issues, they often do not receive recommended and preventive counseling or screening services appropriate to their age group.[47]

Adolescence is often viewed as a relatively healthy time in a person's life. However, behavior patterns can change rapidly in adolescence and can include irregular dietary habits, lack of sleep, inactivity, experimentation with drugs, alcohol and tobacco use, sexual activity, and reckless driving. The connection between these behaviors and long-term consequences for health is being increasingly recognized

> [A] degree of experimentation and risk taking seem[s] to be an integral part of the transition from childhood to adulthood, and most young people come through this phase of life relatively unscathed. So the challenge to researchers and clinicians alike is to be able to identify those at most risk of adverse consequences, without interfering with normal development, and to evaluate possible interventions that will result in improved long-term outcomes.[48]

Programs to promote healthy lifestyles for adolescents should include information on nutrition, activity, stress management, family planning, prevention of smoking, alcohol and substance abuse, safety (particularly digital and motor vehicle safety), and sexual and mental health. Adolescents should be involved in the design of such health promotion programs so that they are both age appropriate and culturally relevant.

FAMILY AND PEERS: BRIDGES TO RESPECTFUL INTERACTION

The emphasis on the importance of the adolescent's autonomy and authority should in no way be seen as undermining the importance of treating the patient as a part of a family unit and a peer group. Most adolescents like to argue about adult rules, even those they accept. Listening to family exchanges about rules that the adolescent disagrees with often will provide insight into the conduct of the adolescent toward you too. In addition, the health professional should not assume that the adolescent's attitude toward parents means there is not a deep dependence on them or heartfelt caring from the family. Although adolescents frequently challenge authority figures, they need and sometimes want limits. Limits provide a safe boundary for teens to grow and function.[49]

REFLECTIONS

- What does it mean to "set limits"?
- How do you envision setting limits with patients and families in your professional practice?
- Do you anticipate that limit-setting will be an easy or hard task for you?

It is important to note that families, like individuals, also develop over time. The family dynamic changes as children and parents age. Normal life events such as job changes, relocations, changes in schools, changes in the family structure (e.g., loss of a grandparent, parent, or sibling), and changes in support systems all impact family function. Changes to family systems, such as divorce and remarriage, may also require additional developmental tasks to reestablish family cohesion. Families undergoing changes to their structure and dynamics may exhibit higher levels of conflict during a child's illness because individuals who typically do not interact with each other may need to come together around care.[30] Illness and disability are in no one's life plan or aspiration for their children. Many adolescents who experience injury, illness, or disability find themselves halted in their progression to adulthood. The quote below by a parent sums this up nicely.

> *Jeffery's accident struck him like a bomb as he was crossing the bridge to manhood. He was approaching independence .... Quadriplegic paralysis steals legs, arms, hands, fingers—and the future. Jeffery's paralysis stole our future ... because no dream included paralysis. Not one.*[50]

Health professionals often benefit from including an adolescent patient's close friends and peers in interactions. Peer group activity is essential for identity formation, and all illnesses or injuries are jolts to the adolescent's identity. Getting to know an adolescent patient's friends by name, seeking their support, and trying to understand their feelings about the patient's condition can be helpful to all. We did not discuss the function Jai's friends played in his decision, but you can reflect on it yourself as to whether the opportunity to bring them into your discussion with Jai should be considered.

Principles of patient- and family-centered care serve as continuing guides for family and health professionals during adolescence. The interprofessional care team will find the following suggestions helpful when caring for teenage patients and families.[42,51]

1. *Stay involved.* When communication begins to break down, make extra efforts to let the teen know that you care and are a dependable resource.
2. *Stay calm.* Argumentative or distant teens can fluster even the best of us. Try not to lose your temper or express anger. Talking to teens calmly regarding their positions and decision-making can help their brains process the information and learn.
3. *Set limits.* Teens need limits and enforcement of boundaries. Limits help teens maintain safety and learn practical life skills and health habits.

4. *Encourage self-awareness.* Teens are always asking adults why. Flip the question and help the teen reason through decisions and actions. Doing so helps encourage new ways of thinking and mindfulness.

5. *Emphasize the positive.* The adolescent years come with many ups and downs, for which the teenage patient may not have any perspective given their stage of development. Help teens see the positives of life events, reinforcing effective health coping strategies and positive adaptation.

Summary

In this brief overview of school-age children and adolescents, the theme of respect revolves around at least two ideas—patient autonomy and effective relatedness. There are numerous ways in which the young patient will try to exert autonomy and relate with you effectively. By leveraging compassion and, at times, patience—you will have an opportunity to build a close and rewarding relationship.

One of the greatest challenges for you as a health professional is to think of the development from birth to adulthood as a continuum, with some patients moving along it faster than others. We have provided some guidelines that will help you think about people as they pause—then continue to pass through—older childhood and adolescence. The patient will present themself as a unique individual still in the process of forming and refining an identity. You have a responsibility to be sure that, amid activities such patients may engage you in, their health care needs are met. Next, we move ahead to the unique challenges associated with treating people in their adult years.

References

1. Brown MW. *The Important Book*. New York: Harper Collins Publishers; 1949.
2. Wei H, Roscigno CI, Swanson KM. Healthcare providers' caring: nothing is too small for parents and children hospitalized for heart surgery. *Heart Lung*. 2017;46(3):166–171. https://doi.org/10.1016/j.hrtlng.2017.01.007.
3. Lareau A. *Unequal Childhoods: Class, Race, and Family Life*. 2nd ed. Berkeley, CA: University of California Press; 2011.
4. Williams NA, Ben Birk A, Petkus JM, Clark H. Importance of play for young children facing illness and hospitalization: rationale, opportunities, and a case study illustration. *Early Child Dev Care*. 2019;191:1–10. https://doi.org/10.1080/03004430.2019.1601088.
5. UN General Assembly. *Convention on the Rights of the Child*. United Nations Treaty Series; 1989. Available from: http://www.refworld.org/docid/3ae6b38f0.html.
6. Majzun R. Coloring outside the lines: what pediatric hospitals can teach adult hospitals. *Pediatr Nurs*. 2011;37(4):210–211.
7. Poverty Thresholds. US Census Bureau. https://www.census.gov/data/tables/time-series/demo/income-poverty/historical-poverty-thresholds.html; 2020 Accessed August 21, 2020.
8. Current Population Survey Annual Social and Economic Supplement (CPS ASEC). US Census Bureau. https://www.census.gov/programs-surveys/saipe/guidance/model-input-data/cpsasec.html; 2020 Accessed August 21, 2020.
9. Bodenheimer R. What's behind the pandemic puzzle craze? *JSTOR Daily*. Updated December 16, 2020. https://daily.jstor.org/whats-behind-the-pandemic-puzzle-craze/.
10. Caspe M, Elena Lopez M, Chattrabhuti C. Four important things to know about the transition to school. *FINE Newsl*. 2015;7(1). Harvard Family Research Project. https://archive.globalfrp.org/family-involvement/publications-resources/four-important-things-research-tells-us-about-the-transition-to-school.
11. Golberstein E, Wen H, Miller BF. Coronavirus disease 2019 (COVID-19) and mental health for children and adolescents. *JAMA Pediatr*. 2020;174(9):819–820. https://doi.org/10.1001/jamapediatrics.2020.1456.
12. Petretto DR, Masala I, Masala C. School closure and children in the outbreak of COVID-19. *Clin Pract Epidemiol Ment Health*. 2020;16:189–191. https://doi.org/10.2174/1745017902016010189.

13. Intimate partner violence and child abuse considerations during COVID-19. Substance Abuse and Mental Health Services Administration. https://www.samhsa.gov/sites/default/files/social-distancing-domestic-violence.pdf; n.d. Accessed August 21, 2020.

14. World Health Organization. *International Classification of Functioning, Disability and Health (ICF)*. Geneva: WHO; 2002. https://www.who.int/docs/default-source/classification/icf/icfbeginnersguide.pdf?sfvrsn=eead63d3_4.

15. Increase in developmental disabilities among children in the United States. Centers for Disease Control and Prevention: Developmental disability. https://www.cdc.gov/ncbddd/developmentaldisabilities/features/increase-in-developmental-disabilities.html; 2019 Accessed August 21, 2020.

16. U.S. Department of Education: Office of Special Education Programs: IDEA 04. Building the Legacy. https://sites.ed.gov/idea/.

17. Sullivan PM, Knutson JF. Maltreatment and disabilities: a population-based epidemiological study. *Child Abuse Negl.* 2000;24(10):1257–1273.

18. Insider tips for navigating IEP meetings. Center for Parent Information and Resources. https://www.parentcenterhub.org/video-8-tips-on-iep-meetings/; 2019 Accessed August 21, 2020.

19. October TW, Fisher KR, Feudtner C, Hinds PS. The parent perspective: "Being a good parent" when making critical decisions in the PICU. *Pediatr Crit Care Med.* 2014;15(4):291–298. https://doi.org/10.1097/PCC.0000000000000076.

20. Lawlor MC, Mattingly C. Family perspectives on occupation, health and disability. In: Schell BA, Gillen G, eds. *Willard and Spackman's Occupational Therapy.* 13th ed. Philadelphia, PA: Wolters Kluwer; 2019:196–211.

21. Loureiro FM, dos Reis Ameixa Antunes AV, Pelander T, Charepe ZB. The experience of school-aged children with hospitalisation. *J Clin Nurs.* 2020;30(3–4):1–9. https://doi.org/10.1111/jocn.15574.

22. Ruhe KM, Wangmo T, Badarau DO, Elger BS, Niggli F. Decision-making capacity of children and adolescents – suggestions for advancing the concept's implementation in pediatric healthcare. *Eur J Pediatr.* 2015;174(6):775–782.

23. Koller D. 'Kids need to talk too': inclusive practices for children's healthcare education and participation. *J Clin Nurs.* 2017;26(17/18):2657–2668.

24. Doherty RF. *Ethical Dimensions in the Health Professions.* 7th ed. St. Louis, MO: Elsevier; 2021.

25. Boztepe H, Çınar S, Ay A. School-age children's perception of the hospital experience. *J Child Health Care.* 2017;21(2):162–170.

26. Gorodzinsky AY, Davies WH, Tran ST, et al. Adolescents' perceptions of family dynamics when a sibling has chronic pain. *Child Health Care.* 2013;42(4):333–352. https://doi.org/10.1080/02739615.2013.842460.

27. Fleming SJ. Children's grief: individual and family dynamics. In: Corr CA, Corr DM, eds. *Hospice Approaches to Pediatric Care.* New York: Springer; 1985.

28. AAP Committee on Bioethics. Informed consent in decision-making in pediatric practice. *Pediatrics.* 2016;138(2):e20161484.

29. Leon AM, Knapp S. Involving family systems in critical care nursing: challenges and opportunities. *Dimens Crit Care Nurs.* 2008;27(6):255–262.

30. Call KT, Riedel AA, Hein K, McLoyd V, Petersen A, Kipke M. Adolescent health and well-being in the twenty-first century: a global perspective. *J Res Adolesc.* 2002;12(1):69–98.

31. Selkie E, Adkins V, Masters E, Bajpai A, Shumer D. Transgender adolescents' uses of social media for social support. *J Adolesc Health.* 2020;66(3):275–280. https://doi.org/10.1016/j.jadohealth.2019.08.011.

32. Finders MJ. *Just Girls: The Hidden Literacies and Life in Junior High.* New York: Teachers College Press; 1997.

33. Hullenaar K, Ruback RB. *Juvenile Violent Victimization.* U.S. Department of Justice; 2020. https://ojjdp.ojp.gov/juvenile-violent-victimization.pdf.

34. *World Health Organization.* Adolescent and young adult health. https://www.who.int/news-room/fact-sheets/detail/adolescents-health-risks-and-solutions; 2021.

35. Kassebaum N, Kyu H, Vos T, et al. Child and adolescent health from 1990 to 2015: findings from the global burden of diseases, injuries, and risk factors 2015 study. *JAMA Pediatr [Serial Online].* 2017;171(6):573–592.

36. Prinstein MJ, Boergers J, Spirito A. Adolescents' and their friends' health-risk behavior: factors that alter or add to peer influence. *J Pediatr Psychol.* 2001;26(5):287–298.

37. Khan A, Jain M, Budhwani C. An analytical cross-sectional study of peer pressure on adolescents. *Int J Reprod Contracept Obstet Gynecol [serial online]*. 2015;3:606–610.
38. Cairo MS, Pinkerton R. Childhood, adolescent and young adult non-Hodgkin lymphoma: state of the science. *Br J Haematol*. 2016;173(4):507–530.
39. Mobile kids: The parent, the child and the smartphone. https://www.nielsen.com/us/en/insights/article/2017/mobile-kids-the-parent-the-child-and-the-smartphone/; 2017 Accessed August 21, 2020.
40. *Pew Research Center*. Teens, social media, and technology. https://www.pewresearch.org/internet/2018/05/31/teens-social-media-technology-2018/; 2018.
41. Argo T, Lowery L. The effects of social media on adolescent health and well-being. *J Adolesc Health [Serial Online]*. 2017;2:75–76.
42. Jensen FE, Nutt AE. *The Teenage Brain: A Neuroscientist's Survival Guide to Raising Adolescents and Young Adults*. New York: Harper Collins Publishers; 2015.
43. American College of Obstetricians and Gynecologists' Committee on Adolescent Health Care. Concerns regarding social media and health issues in adolescents and young adults. *Obstet Gynecol [serial online]*. 2016;127(2):e62–e65.
44. Primack BA, Shensa A, Sidani JE, et al. Social media use and perceived social isolation among young adults in the U.S. *Am J Prev Med*. 2017;53(1):1–8.
45. Couros A. *Identity in a Digital World*. Presented at TEDxLangleyED; March 15, 2015. https://www.youtube.com/watch?v=pAllBTgYfDo.
46. Reynolds S., Grant-Kels JM, Bercovitch L. How issues of autonomy and consent differ between children and adults: kids are not just little people. *Clin Dermatol*. 2017;35(6):601–605. https://doi.org/10.1016/j.clindermatol.2017.08.010.
47. Alderman E. Original study: confidentiality in pediatric and adolescent gynecology: when we can, when we can't, and when we're challenged. *J Pediatr Adolesc Gynecol*. 2017;30:176–183.
48. Churchill D. The growing pains of adolescent health research in general practice. *Prim Health Care Res Dev*. 2003;4:277–278.
49. U.S. National Library of Medicine, National Institutes of Health. Adolescent development: MedlinePlus medical encyclopedia. https://medlineplus.gov/ency/article/002003.htm.
50. Galli R. *Rescuing Jeffery: A Memoir*. New York: St. Martin's Griffin; 2000.
51. Damour L. *Untangled: Guiding Teenage Girls Through the Seven Transitions into Adulthood*. New York: Ballantine Books; 2017.

Respectful Interaction: Working With Adults

The reader will be able to

- Compare the development tasks in young and middle adulthood;
- Describe the opportunities for growth and enrichment that arise through continued development during the adult years;
- Discuss "responsibility" as it applies to the middle years of life and how it may affect the patient's trust that health professionals are showing due respect to them;
- Discuss the meaning of work for adults;
- Describe at least three social roles that characterize life for most middle-aged persons and ways in which showing respect for a patient requires attention to those roles;
- Discuss how stress factors into attempts to carry out the responsibilities of each of the social roles and some health-related consequences of negative responses to stress; and
- List fundamental challenges facing health professionals who are working with an adult going through a midlife transition.

Prelude

Once you become an adult, you are not instantly thrust into stability with a manual on how to be mature. Adulthood is anything but stable; you are continuously learning about what it takes to function in the "real world," and even then, no one will ever become a model adult.

RAMIREZ[1]

Who Is the Adult?

Adulthood is often referred to as the least understood and least studied of all the developmental life stages. A common stereotype about adult life is that it is only a waiting period or holding place made up of work, establishing a family, or dealing with menopause or other physical changes, on the way to retirement and old age. In recent years, even the noun "adult" has been turned into the verb "to adult" or "adulting" which implies engaging in mundane adult-like behaviors and tasks (like doing taxes).[2] While adulthood is seen as the end of an epitomized youth, there is a wide variation in the types and timing of transitions and activities in adult life that is far richer than this stereotype suggests. For these reasons, it is important to examine some vital issues concerning life as an adult today.

Adulthood can be legally defined by chronological age or when a person begins to assume responsibility for themselves and others.[3] In the majority of the United States, the legal adult age of capacity is 18.[4] Adulthood can also be defined by the achievement of certain developmental tasks such as being independent, establishing long-term relationships, and reflectively establishing personal identity. Adults also strive to find a meaningful occupation, contribute to the welfare of others, make a contribution to family, faith community, or society at large, and gain recognition for accomplishments. Finally, adulthood can be defined in psychological terms—that is, by the level of maturity exhibited by a person. Mature persons can take responsibility, make logical decisions, appreciate the position of others, control emotional outbursts, and accept social roles. What it means to be an "adult" refers to far more than doing taxes or laundry but is instead a combination of many factors, the most important of which you will be introduced to in these pages. First, we will address biological development.

BIOLOGICAL DEVELOPMENT DURING THE ADULT YEARS

Aging can be defined as "the sum of all the changes that normally occur in an organism with time."[5] Biological development is sometimes treated as complete when a person shows the result of changes that occur during adolescence, but human beings continue to grow and mature throughout their life span. There is often a focus on the negative aspects of aging and the losses that accompany aging as well as negative stereotypes of decline and dependency. However, research has switched to focusing on the potential of development as humans age.[6]

Adult development is not marked by definitive physical and psychomotor changes such as those seen in early childhood (e.g., learning how to walk) or adolescence. Still, it is full of challenging and largely unpredictable opportunities and experiences. Interpersonal relationships that are established in childhood and adolescence evolve during adulthood. For example, relationships with parents evolve. The adult who is now a parent gains increased appreciation for what their parents went through. The adult may also become a caregiver to the parent. Understanding the complexity of the experience of adulthood is essential as an orienting position for entering a professional relationship that conveys genuine respect for the adult patient.

Adult life is marked by concepts such as independent life choices, midlife physical and emotional challenges and changes, and generativity. The concept of *generativity* came out of Erikson's theory of development across the life span, with each stage characterized by a specific challenge. Generativity (the focus of the seventh stage) coincides with middle adulthood and is concerned with nurturing and ensuring the success of future generations. In this stage, the individual is focused on leaving a legacy behind.[6,7] It is unsurprising that this stage often includes raising a family, facing the empty nest, the return of adult children, and the addition of grandchildren. Raising children and grandchildren is the most common means of leaving a legacy.

There may be differences in the way adulthood is experienced depending on one's gender identity. Additionally, the specific point in history when a person enters adulthood may have profound implications for adult life. For example, many women in Western societies who entered adulthood during the women's movement of the 1960s and 1970s faced more opportunities regarding work and sexual freedom than the previous generation of women. Finally, development also may differ because of sexual orientation, race, ethnicity, socioeconomic status, culture, and education, to name a few.

Demographers, social scientists, and developmental psychologists consider young adulthood to be roughly between the ages of 21 and 40 and middle adulthood to be between the ages of 40 and 65.[8] Aging, like adulthood itself, is complex and varies from one person to another. The rate at which individuals age is highly variable, but so is how they adapt to age-related changes and illness. Aging also gives rise to feelings of anxiety in a way no other area of human development does. Failing intellectual or biological functions in the middle years can become a preoccupation for patients in your care. For example, during this period, the pure joy of physical activity experienced in younger years may acquire a sober edge. One of us overheard a man who for years has enjoyed running tell his friend, "*Yeah, my running will probably guarantee that I live 5 years longer, but I will have spent that 5 years running!"* highlighting the perspective that often accompanies the aging process.

Adults may also worry about the age-related changes that begin to take place in their mental functions and body structure and function. Suddenly, forgetfulness is no longer taken lightly but could portend more serious problems generally associated with aging. Perhaps, the anxiety that aging provokes is due to the close relationship most of us think exists between biological development and illness, decline, and death.[9] Rather than view aging in this way, gerontologists have proposed the concept of *compressed morbidity*, which suggests that people may live longer, healthier lives and have shorter periods of disability at the end of their lives. The focus of health care then becomes one of prevention, maintenance of quality of life, health promotion, and postponement of chronic conditions and disability or death rather than cure.[10,11] In Chapter 13, we explore different views of aging and their impact on your interactions with older patients.

The human life span is thought to be about 110–120 years. In the first half of 2020, the life expectancy for the United States population was 77.8 years, although this varies by gender, race and ethnicity, and other variables. For instance, the life expectancy of males in 2020 was 75.1 years compared with 80.5 years for females. In this same period, the life expectancy was 79.9 years for Hispanics, 78.0 years for non-Hispanic Whites, and, by stark contrast, 72 years for non-Hispanic Blacks.[12]

The 10 leading causes of death for all age groups in the United States are listed in Table 12.1.[13] The cause of death varies according to race and gender, but this table provides a general idea of the types of illnesses you will encounter most often with adult patients. This, of course, does not consider that some entire populations within the United States and Western societies are refugees or immigrants from countries with a variety of stresses that affect their health and life course. Table 12.2 highlights the 10 leading causes of death globally.[14] As you compare these two tables, you will likely note some similarities and differences. As the World Health Organization emphasizes, "It is important to know why people die to improve how people live. Measuring how many people die each year helps to assess the effectiveness of our health systems and direct resources to

TABLE 12.1 ■ Leading Causes of Death in the United States

Causes of Death	Total Number of Deaths in the US Population
1. Heart disease	696,962
2. Cancer	602,350
3. COVID-19	350,831
4. Accidents (unintentional injuries)	200,955
5. Stroke (cerebrovascular diseases)	160,264
6. Chronic lower respiratory diseases	152,657
7. Alzheimer's disease	134,242
8. Diabetes mellitus	102,188
9. Influenza and pneumonia	53,544
10. Nephritis, nephrotic syndrome, and nephrosis	52,547

From *U.S. Department of Health and Human Services, Centers for Disease Control and Prevention, National Center for Health Statistics*. Leading causes of death. https://www.cdc.gov/nchs/fastats/leading-causes-of-death.htm; 2021.

TABLE 12.2 ■ **Leading Causes of Death Globally**

Causes of Death	Total Number of Deaths Globally (In Millions)
1. Ischemic heart disease	8.9
2. Stroke	6.19
3. Chronic obstructive pulmonary disease	3.22
4. Lower respiratory tract infections	2.6
5. Neonatal conditions	2.0
6. Trachea, bronchus, lung cancers	1.8
7. Alzheimer's disease and other dementias	1.6
8. Diarrheal diseases	1.5
9. Diabetes	1.5
10. Kidney diseases	1.3

From *World Health Organization*. The top 10 causes of death. https://www.who.int/news-room/fact-sheets/detail/the-top-10-causes-of-death; 2021.

where they are needed most."[14] With increasing awareness, the health professional can demonstrate increased sensitivity to each patient's situation to express due respect to them.

Many causes of death among all adult populations are the result of chronic diseases. While 6 in 10 Americans live with at least one chronic disease,[15] the burden of chronic disease among race and socioeconomic status is disproportionate.[16] Fortunately, conditions such as diabetes, depression, and cardiovascular disease are being diagnosed and treated earlier in adulthood than ever before; however, chronic disease management remains a critical health concern in the United States. The consequences of chronic disease were made evident to the lay public during the COVID-19 pandemic, where those most at risk of suffering from COVID-19 had underlying cardiovascular and pulmonary chronic conditions, which often included an increased prevalence amongst Black and Brown communities.[17] Complex social problems, such as health disparities, which disproportionately impact patients from minoritized backgrounds, often resist solutions by a single organization.[18] These problems may instead benefit from an interprofessional and collaborative approach. Given these observations, you can see why the interprofessional care team has become the norm for diagnosis and treatment interventions.

As science progresses, we learn more about how individual genes, biology, and behaviors interact with the social, cultural, and physical environment to influence health outcomes. Targeting prevention, illness management, and lifestyle modification in young and middle adulthood can increase the quality of life and prevent the development and severity of chronic disease in older adulthood. Young adulthood is often referred to as the healthy years and the hidden hazards. Individuals in early and middle adulthood tend to underestimate the impact over time that poor lifestyle choices or unpreventable environmental situations may have on their overall health quality and life span.

Emerging and Early Adulthood

As discussed in Chapter 11, it is during late adolescence that self-identity begins to form. These identity exploration and consolidation processes continue at the beginning of emerging or early adulthood (generally between the ages of 18 and 25). Adulthood is not defined by a single factor, rather by an integration of cognitive development, physical development, reflective judgment, and societal experience. The way an individual transitions through adulthood is heavily influenced by experiences in previous stages of life.

REFLECTIONS

The transition from adolescence to adulthood is a process.
- Can you identify two or three factors that influenced your transition to adulthood?
- How did your family or peers influence your transition?
- What were you looking forward to in adulthood? Looking back, was this a realistic view?

In the span of a few generations, the path to adulthood has changed dramatically. Through extensive research with young adults aged 18–29 in the United States, Arnett[19] identified several distinguishing features of emerging adulthood. These five main features are (1) identity exploration, (2) instability, (3) self-focus, (4) feeling in-between, and (5) possibilities. In general, today in the United States and other wealthy nations, young people are taking longer to leave home,[20] attain economic independence, marry, and form families than did their peers half a century ago.

In a 2019 survey of 3054 US adults and teenagers aged 15 and older, young millennials (aged 22–28) revealed that they delayed milestones such as moving out of their parent's home and buying a home of their own because of their student loan debt.[21] In March of 2020, nearly half the 18- to 29-year olds in the United States were living with one or both of their parents.[22] The rise in the number of young millennials who plan to move back home with their parents after college has resulted in this generation being called "The Boomerang Generation."[21,23]

There are numerous benefits to multigenerational households who share resources such as food, childcare, eldercare, transportation, and utility costs. Multigenerational homes can result in improved financial reserves, emotional support, decreased stress and loneliness, and improved social capital. Those who were foreign born may be especially accustomed to this sort of living arrangement and the growing number of immigrant populations may be one of the contributors to the increase in multigenerational homes in wealthy nations such as the United States.[20] However, there may be intergenerational cultural differences which can cause tension. While 82% of the parents surveyed said that they would welcome their children moving back from home,[21] these longer transitions can strain families and institutions (such as health care systems) that work with young adults. For example, adults who have children might think that they have moved through an adult developmental task of parenting, only to find their children returning home after a divorce or unemployment. Parents who might have been rejoicing in an empty nest may find their adult children under their roof once again, with grandchildren in tow. While the stigma around living at home in the early 20s is decreasing, in mainstream Western societies delayed acquisition of independence, earlier physical maturation characteristic of modern cultures, pressures on young people to take on appearances of being grown up, return of adult children to their parents' home, and delayed childbearing all complicate traditional views held about progression through adulthood.

Needs: Respect, Identity, and Intimacy

Along the life span, illness and injury invariably result in changes in the patient's *identity*. Identity is an understanding of the basic self that provides continuity over time and across problems and changes in life. Thus, there is a sense of maintenance of one's self through identity and yet room for change to accommodate the vicissitudes of life. Adult patients are generally more capable of entering a patient-centered professional relationship as an equal partner than younger people. Even though most adult patients can better protect their interests and make their wishes known, they are still worthy of the respect that we afford to younger, generally more vulnerable patients. Given the varying degrees of health literacy in the US population,[24] adults should not be assumed to have better self-advocacy skills purely based on their age. Respect, in its basic expressions of appreciation of the other, attention to specific characteristics, and individualized care, introduced in Chapter 1, continue to be helpful benchmarks of effective interaction in this period and all the others through the life span.

Intimacy is another developmental task of the adult. According to Erikson, adult development is marked by the ability to experience open, supportive, and loving relationships with others without the fear of losing one's own identity in the process of growing close to another.[3] You were introduced to the difference between personal and intimate relationships in Chapter 7, illustrating that the type of intimacy a patient will experience with family members, lovers, and friends is deeper and more complex than the professional, care-based relationships in which you and the patient will engage. It is that deeper intimacy that Erikson is talking about.

Adulthood sometimes involves people going back to previous developmental tasks such as establishing a basic identity if they did not resolve these issues previously in late adolescence or early adulthood. Researchers have begun to move away from the linear perspective of identity development, recognizing the importance these milestones hold over the life span. For example, some LGBTQ (lesbian, gay, bisexual, transgender, queer/questioning) adults may experience difficulties with self-identity and sexual identity development given the high levels of stigma and low levels of social support they experience.[25] As health professionals, being aware of the isolation that sexual gender minorities or other minoritized groups often encounter provides one avenue of professional respect that must be expressed. Attentiveness to this difference also is essential given that LGBTQ adults experience health challenges at higher rates, including mental illness, substance use, heart disease, HIV, and physical violence, than their heterosexual and cisgender peers.[26] Positive outcomes of reaching sexual identity milestones and adopting an identity include improved self-esteem, sense of community, sense of living authentically, and improved relationships with romantic partners and parents.[27] The major developmental facets of adult life are referred to repeatedly as we explore the social roles, meaning of work, and challenges of midlife.

Psychosocial Development and Needs

Part of being an adult often requires the acceptance of responsibility and empathy for others. The concept of achievement central to adult life can be defined in many ways. Some midlife challenges discussed later in this chapter stem from a person having assumed responsibility and realizing their achievement potential. In contrast, others arise when the individual has failed to do so. A profile of a person in the adult years of life will necessarily involve a consideration of their sense of "responsibility." Underlying the idea of responsibility is an assumption that the individual is a free agent (i.e., one who is willing and able to act autonomously). Thus, a person coerced into performing an act is not considered to have accepted responsibility for it. Given these conditions of ability and agreement, we want to know whether the person can be trusted to carry out the acts, regardless of whether the agreement was explicit (i.e., a promise to abide by the terms of a contract) or implicit (i.e., a promise to provide for one's own children or parents).

REFLECTIONS

Describe an activity you currently participate in and enjoy or feel a sense of responsibility for the outcome.
- What are the environmental, personal, and family or societal factors that facilitate your participation?
- How has this activity helped you find purpose/meaning in your life?
- How does this activity relate to those you were exposed to as a child or young adult?
- Do you project that you will still be doing this activity in the later stages of your adulthood? Why or why not?

During adulthood, another aspect of acting responsibly involves having a high regard for the welfare of others. The adult must find a way to support the next generation by redirecting attention from themselves to others. In other words, the adult learns to care.[28] This involves empathy for the predicaments that befall others in life. The acts may flow from free will, but the will must operate in accordance with reasonable claims and justifiable expectations of other people, traditions, and cultural expectations. The claims of society on a person peak during the middle years, so "acting responsibly" must be interpreted in terms of how completely the person fulfills the conditions of those claims. Another way to view the matter of responsibility in our culture is to review the concept of self-respect. During the adult years, most people perceive their self-respect as being vulnerable to the judgments of others. One's self-respect at least partially depends on the extent to which they command the respect of employer, family, and friends. This idea is related to our concept of "reputation." One commands respect by giving due consideration to society's claims. Hiltner[29] notes, correctly we think, that to a large extent, even the personal values of the middle years must include regard for others.

This period of middle adulthood is sometimes characterized by failure, loss, or tragedy which serves as a wake-up call. Brooks[30] refers to this journey, of moving away from the focus on the self to focus on others through service, as the "two-mountain life." Negotiating the first mountain likely involved finishing school, starting a career, and perhaps a family. The individual falls prey to societal pressure and pursues what they think they are supposed to. They may focus on their reputation and what others think of them. However, there are many whose life was interrupted, often by failure or tragedy, and they begin a larger journey that is less about self and more about others. For example, in 2020 many experienced devastating losses as a result of the COVID-19 pandemic. Brooks[30] highlights, "If the first mountain is about building up the ego and defining the self, the second is about shedding the ego and dissolving the self. If the first mountain is about acquisition, the second mountain is about contribution."

The second mountain is often characterized by relationships. For most, middle adulthood is a highly social period when interdependencies are complex and pervasive. Let us explore the social roles in adulthood further.

Social Roles in Adulthood

Several social roles most fully characterize this period involving primary relationships, parenting, care of older family members, mentoring the next generation, and involvement in the community in the form of political, religious, or other social or service organizations and groups.

PRIMARY RELATIONSHIPS

It is frequently during adulthood that a person decides with whom lasting relationships will be developed. Fortunately, an increasing number of older people are also developing new relationships, but they are usually people who could sustain deep and lasting relationships in the middle years.

The primary relationship takes priority over all others, the most common type being the relationship with a significant other. Choosing a life partner and becoming better acquainted (i.e., learning to know the person, discovering potentials and limits, similarities and differences, and compatibilities and incompatibilities) are processes interwoven with the more basic activities of eating, sleeping, acquiring possessions, working, worshipping, relaxing, and playing together.

Of course, one does not have to marry to develop a deep and lasting involvement with another. One of your first tasks of respectful interaction with an adult patient is to find out if there is a key person in their life and, if so, who that person is. This can be accomplished without unnecessary probing into the person's private life. Particularly in times of crisis, the patient looks to that key person for comfort, sustenance, and guidance. However, sometimes the person you assume would be the most supportive is not. Consider the case of Mary Ogden and Pam Carlisle.

CASE STUDY

Mary Ogden, age 52, is a single teacher who is hospitalized for treatment related to severe diabetes. The entire small community where she has resided and taught for 25 years adores her. Through the years, she has received numerous awards for community service. She is a cheerful person, who, despite her illness, continues to be an inspiration to everyone. She is especially fond of Pam Carlisle, the head nurse on the unit where Mary is being treated.

On the afternoon before Mary's planned hospital discharge, an unscheduled visitor comes to the nursing desk, insisting on speaking to Pam about a highly personal matter. The visitor is Agnes Ogden, an older adult, who informs Pam that she is the older sister (and only living relative) of Mary. The visitor seems sincere and asks that Pam provide details of her sister's condition so that Agnes might be better prepared to aid Mary with both her physical illness and personal affairs. Pam complies with her request, feeling relieved that there is someone to share this burden with her. The following morning Pam visits Mary's room and finds her furious for the first time. She informs Pam that she has not been on speaking terms with her sister for many years, considers her sister to be untrustworthy, and thoroughly resents her sister knowing her personal affairs and illness. Mary feels betrayed and expresses her distrust of Pam as her health care provider. She becomes withdrawn, agitated, and uncooperative.

REFLECTIONS

Besides violating the federal Health Information Portability and Accountability Act regulations, discussed in Chapter 5, and designed to protect Mary's privacy and confidentiality legally, Pam has also broken the trust that is fundamental to a respectful health professional and patient relationship.

We can assume that Pam shared the information with Agnes Ogden, believing that she was doing so with Mary's well-being in mind. Still, what could Pam have done differently to foster Mary's trust rather than destroy it? What would you have done when Agnes came to you requesting information?

How might you rebuild the trust that once existed between you and a patient should such a breakdown occur?

PARENTING OF CHILDREN

Another important social role of adult life often includes caring for children. Gender role stereotypes traditionally assigned to mothering, fathering, and coparenting are breaking down in many families so that both parents share the whole range of parenting skills. The concept of parenting is being expanded, too. As discussed in Chapter 7, families come in many forms, and parenting can be shared by several persons, including grandparents, especially in multigenerational homes. However, it should be noted that despite gains made, women generally spend twice as much time on household and child-care tasks compared to men[31,32] and this has implications for other life roles, which will be discussed later in this chapter.

REFLECTIONS

Parenting is often a part of adult life.
- Is it one of your life goals to be a parent? Why or why not?
- If you are already a parent, how did you transition into this role?
- What are some of the advantages and disadvantages of parenting children today?

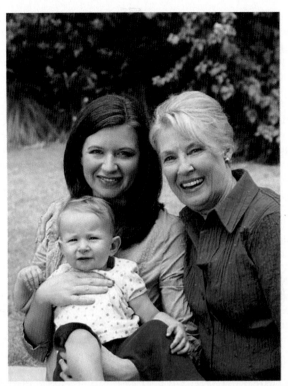

Fig. 12.1 Parenting relationships are among the most enduring and complex of human interactions. © David Woolley/Digital Vision/Thinkstock.com.

Whatever the challenges of each model, all share the assumption that the child's welfare depends on the quality of parenting. The age-old recognition that a child's physical and emotional well-being depends on adult care is now buttressed by more recent assertions that the child's potential for fulfillment and satisfaction in later years is also determined in the earliest years of life that the parent strongly influences. The least that can be said of parenting relationships is that they are among the most enduring and complex human interactions (Fig. 12.1). We saw in earlier chapters that parents play a crucial role in the delivery of patient- and family-centered care. The health professional who fails to consider parents respectfully neglects an integral part of the patient's identity.

CARE OF OLDER FAMILY MEMBERS

Not only do many adults care for children as a part of their daily responsibilities, but they also care for their parents, parents-in-law, and other older friends and relatives. Middle-age adults are often referred to as the "sandwich" generation because they are responsible for care of both young (children) and old (aging parents/family members). They are "sandwiched" between these two generations. The move toward supporting the older adult to age in place often increases the demands placed on adult children. In 2015 there were 43.5 million caregivers in the United States. That number has since risen to an estimated 53 million adult caregivers in the United States. Additionally,

61% of family caregivers are also working. While caregivers report that this role gives them a sense of purpose, caregivers often put the needs of their care recipients ahead of their own, and 23% report that caregiving has made their health worse.[33] As noted in Chapter 7, caregiving has both positive and negative outcomes. Caregiving responsibilities can disrupt employment, health maintenance, leisure, and social participation during adulthood.[34]

Just as family structure and functions differ from culture to culture, so do caregiving roles and expectations. A recent systematic review of the multicultural experiences of caregiving highlights some general themes that emerge in caregiving roles and expectations. Latino caregivers who were interviewed valued family decision-making regarding care. Asian-American caregivers experienced strained interpersonal relationships and shame in asking for help. Black or African American caregivers reported reliance on community and striving to maintain the cohesion of their family and Native American caregivers reported feeling pressure to provide care despite limited resources and a lack of formal resources.[35] This and other research highlight that the cultural lens is essential for accurately viewing this role of adult life.

MENTORING THE NEXT GENERATION

Earlier in this chapter, we referenced that adults are often focused on imparting knowledge and leaving a legacy behind. Some choose to make their mark by raising children and grandchildren. However, there are many opportunities for leaving a legacy behind such as professional achievements and contributions to society. Many choose to mentor the next generation. Mentoring as a social role in adulthood is explored next.

Mentoring

The International Mentoring Association defines mentoring as a complex process used to guide a protégé through career transitions and as a necessary part of training effective, reflective practitioners.[36] There are three consistent agreements about mentoring. The first is that mentoring is focused on the growth and development of another. The second is that several forms of support are used, including role modeling and psychological support, and finally, researchers agree that there is a degree of reciprocity associated with mentoring and that adult mentor gains as much from the relationship as the mentee.[37] Mentors are described as "socializing or influence agents, encouraging protégés to internalize the norms, behaviors, and values of the scientific community."[38]

As discussed in Chapter 4, diversifying the health professions is a vital step toward minimizing health disparities. The adult who chooses to engage in a mentoring relationship is a vital part of this process. Traditional mentoring programs are commonly used to foster the retention of historically disadvantaged students in health sciences programs.[39] Outcomes of mentoring programs include improved academic performance, increased sense of belonging, and support systems that build confidence.[40] Adulthood is a journey of discovery and becoming, evolving, trying different things, being ready to fail, and trying again; mentors serve as key guides along the many paths in this journey. Whether one serves as a mentor through a community agency such as Big Brother Big Sister or through professional organizations such as the American Nurses Association, these adult relationships provide the opportunity to build capacity and support the development of all those involved, mentor and mentee.

POLITICAL AND OTHER SERVICE ACTIVITIES

Involvement in political and social organizations has traditionally been at a peak during the adult years. Large-scale protests for racial equality characterized the summer of 2020. Pew Research data from June 2020 revealed that 41% of those who said they recently attended a protest focused on race were between 18 and 30 years old.[41] Responsibilities stemming from membership in political and social organizations are often second only to those of work if measured in terms of energy consumption and personal commitments beyond those toward family. A sense of identity in adulthood depends heavily on belonging to such groups, whether political, religious, service, or arts organizations. These service activities are a source of identity and a vehicle for contributing to one's profession, community, or nation.

In summary, there are many sources of claims on adults, but attending to primary relationships such as spouses or significant others, children, parents, and mentees while contributing to public initiatives constitute highly significant ones.

Work as Meaningful Activity

Work, like family and adulthood, is a concept that can be variably defined, and work as meaningful activity can occur in a variety of settings and assumes many patterns. Therefore, the meaning of work and the responsibilities it requires will depend on the person's value system, expectations, aspirations, and the specific environment, job title, and position within a hierarchy. For some, work is performed primarily in the home (especially during the pandemic when social distancing guidelines were in place). However, ordinarily, it entails a significant amount of time away from home for a great many. Adults are judged to spend about half of their waking hours engaged in work, and it is during middle adulthood that career consolidation typically occurs. The average US employee works 7.62 hours a day.[42] Women have a greater likelihood of working part-time compared with men.[31] The kind of work one does traditionally determines their income, lifestyle, social status, and place of residence. Because of the amount of time and energy expended, the type of information one acquires over a lifetime is often influenced by the working situation. Studies of professional socialization suggest that the kind of work one does also contributes to one's worldview.

Despite advances in gender equality, work-related responsibilities still differ for men and women. You have undoubtedly observed what most women experience in their work roles: expectations on them include not only doing a job in the labor force but also maintaining the quality and amount of work performed in the home. Women respond to these various needs or demands by trying to balance their impulse to care and the level of personal support available. When the limits of caregiving are reached, something else must give. Expectations of caregiving responsibilities for women often result in women working fewer hours and getting paid less in comparison to men.[43,44]

Two types of responsibilities are associated with the work role: (1) to do one's job well and (2) to fulfill the reasonable expectations of others (e.g., employer, peers, and family members). The professional relationship has the added dimension of caregiving that one is expected to help those who seek professional services.

Your task as a health professional is to assess how the patient views their work situation, what work means, and particularly the responsibilities and relationships in it. Whether a patient's work involves providing quality childcare, laboring on the section crew to replace railroad ties, or presiding over a meeting in the executive suite, the work entails responsibility toward both a job to be done and other human beings. Treatment goals must be tailored to help the patient carry out these responsibilities, modify them, or accept that work may no longer be possible or accomplished in the same ways.

Those who work with adult patients in the areas of occupational health are keenly aware of the relationship among health, injury, or illness and the worker's role. Consider the following case:

CASE STUDY

Jenny Chan has worked as a certified nursing assistant in a skilled nursing facility for the past 15 years. She is the sole provider for her three children, one of whom has just started college. Although Jenny attended the mandatory in-service sessions on proper body mechanics and lifting of patients, she did not always follow the appropriate procedure. Jenny stated to her fellow workers more than once, "I'm big and strong. I don't like waiting for help or lugging out the lift to get patients up. I can get them up and out of bed without help." Unfortunately, while getting a patient out of bed, Jenny injured her lower back and neck. She has been on workers' compensation leave for the past month and is now involved in a "work-hardening" program to determine if she can return to work in the nursing home. The health professionals working with Jenny observe that she is highly motivated to return to work but fearful of reinjury. Her confidence in her strength and sense of invulnerability have been badly shaken. During a particularly trying day in the work-hardening program, she tells her therapist, "If I can't work in the nursing home, I don't know what I'll do. It's the only kind of work I've ever done. All my friends are there."

REFLECTIONS

- What "meanings" do you think Jenny gives to her work?
- How does her identity tie to her work roles?
- How does your work tie into your own identity?

We have emphasized responsibility in terms of relationships and work roles in the adult years and that self-respect during this period is determined largely by meeting the justifiable expectations of others. However, self-respect unquestionably also depends on believing in and being true to oneself. Thus adults who meet all of society's expectations can still be unfulfilled. That is precisely what Brooks[30] is referring to in the two-mountain analogy. Conquering the first mountain focused on societal expectations can contribute to the challenges of midlife discussed in this chapter. The sense of "being somebody," such an integral part of adolescent development, must become more fully defined in the young and middle adult years. By middle adulthood, individuals are expected to show more clearly who they are and what they can contribute to the welfare of loved ones and society, that is, climb the second mountain.

Stresses and Challenges of Adulthood

In terms of social roles, adulthood is described generally as "a time when the individual is a responsible member of society under pressure to coordinate multiple roles (e.g., partner, worker, parent, and caregiver)."[45] The more responsibilities a person assumes, the more vulnerable they become to the symptoms associated with stress. Stress is recognized as a potential threat to well-being, and its adverse effects will increase if steps are not taken to respond positively. Major problems associated with negative responses to stress in adult life are finally gaining the attention of researchers, health professionals, workplace counselors, and religious groups. Given the associated negative health behaviors and outcomes of work and life stress, the identification of protective factors such as physical activity, mindfulness, and sleep for adult patients is essential.[46]

Chapter 3 addresses some sources of stress in professionals as they move through their student years and into becoming a professional. The specific sources of stress may differ, but how a young person has learned to cope and deal with stress will be carried into adulthood.

Some stresses result from personal life choices. The responsibilities assumed in marriage and other primary relationships (e.g., child-rearing, parent care, and work) all create stress, as do unemployment and some factors in the social structure itself. Each is discussed separately.

PRIMARY RELATIONSHIP STRESSES

Marriage relationships during the middle years have been studied more extensively than other types of primary relationships revealing that all such intimate relationships produce stressful situations. Common sources of stress in committed relationships include nonfulfillment of role obligations by a significant other, lack of reciprocity between partners, a feeling of not being accepted by a significant other, and unequal household and child-rearing responsibilities. Even with shared responsibility, there is the stress related to child-rearing. Research supports that sources of stress that are damaging to long-term relationships are those of an ongoing nature instead of those of a discrete event.[47–49]

Couples with children often experience stress around the departure of their children, leaving both (and not only the woman, as is often thought) with the "empty nest syndrome." In addition to the empty nest, women's middle age is often discussed in terms of menopause and new opportunities for activity and self-expression. Although a positive relationship has been established between successful aging and positive self-esteem in postmenopausal women, menopause can be perceived negatively among cultures that value fertility.[50,51]

A more violent expression of stress, the primary source of which may not arise from the relationship itself but is acted out within it, is domestic violence or intimate partner abuse. Domestic violence is defined as "willful intimidation, physical assault, battery, sexual assault, and/or other abusive behavior as part of a systematic pattern of power and control perpetrated by one intimate partner against another. It includes physical violence, sexual violence, threats, and emotional/psychological abuse."[52] According to the National Intimate Partner and Sexual Violence Survey, 1 in 4 women and 1 in 10 men have reported abuse by an intimate partner during their lifetime.[53]

Some persons involved in domestic violence situations receive attention from self-help groups and other organizations, but not all do. They will be present among your patients, exhibiting both overt and covert symptoms that deserve attention. It is important to note that domestic violence occurs across the socioeconomic spectrum and among all ethnic and other demographic groups. For many generations, abuse survivors have mainly remained hidden and silent, victimized by the fear of stigmatization, shame, and having no place to go for safety and support. For many, financial dependence is a common reason to return to an abusive partner. Increasingly, the inhumane situation abuse victims are left in has prompted health professionals, lawmakers, volunteers, and others to help provide an antidote to this devastating state of affairs. Currently, more educational and legal mechanisms are being put in place to provide professional caregivers with the tools to recognize, assess, and report certain or suspected domestic violence in a patient.

The professional who treats adult patients must be aware of clinical guidelines that express deep respect by discovering symptoms or behaviors, institutional policies regarding suspected or obvious abuse, local sources of support available to patients, and legal requirements to report intimate partner abuse. For example, any health professional can become familiar with the location of refuges or safe houses in many cities and sometimes in rural areas. In addition, an increasing number of health professionals are becoming involved more directly in the treatment and rehabilitation of those who have suffered abuse.

PARENTING STRESSES

The tremendous responsibility associated with parenting also leads to stress situations in young and middle adulthood. Parenting is socially constructed, and there are both burdens and benefits to parenting. Because there is no "instructor's manual" on how to manage the twists and turns of parenthood, patients in your care may turn to you for advice. As a health professional, you may be the first to recognize the signs of parental stress. Providing a listening ear and care for the caregivers are key first steps in helping parents cope with stress. This supports the health of the family as a unit. Child abuse and neglect (discussed in Chapter 11), which are increasing (or, perhaps, are being reported more systematically), are tragic examples of what can happen when stress is not controlled. Most stress related to child-rearing leads to less deplorable results, but nonetheless, it does take an immense toll on both parent and child.

STRESS IN CARE OF ELDERLY FAMILY MEMBERS

Family caregiving crosses generations; however, as previously mentioned, most of the burden for parent care falls on adult women. Many quit their jobs to fulfill the responsibility of caring for one or more elderly family members. The stress is often borne with considerable grace as adult children express the desire to care for their parents and the satisfaction and joy it brings them in concert with the burdens. This burden was particularly high during the pandemic when those with caregiving roles in their families were providing both financial and emotional support. It is hypothesized that this is one reason women were more vulnerable to various forms of mental health conditions (including depression, anxiety, and stress) during the pandemic.[54]

WORK STRESS

For many individuals in their middle years, stress related to work is their primary stress, manifesting itself in a wide range of disorders. Chronically elevated work-related stress is a risk factor for numerous physical and mental health outcomes, including depression and cardiovascular disease. Interestingly, work-related stress such as limited job control, low social support at work, and high job strain is associated with an increased risk for cognitive decline and dementia later in life.[55] Some jobs are in themselves highly stressful. One of the highest stress jobs is military personnel. Others are firefighters and airline pilots.[56] Studies have demonstrated that a job with high responsibility in which the consequences for a mistake are dire creates the highest stress. At the other end of the spectrum, boredom and repetition also create stress. Work-related stress can be a key factor in the development of serious health problems such as cardiovascular disease and alcoholism, or other substance abuse.

A form of stress related to the work role is caused by the inability to find or hold a job. In a society that rewards its members for paid work and in which adult responsibility is tied to societal contribution, the stress of working can be less threatening to health and well-being than the stress of being unemployed.

Thus, it becomes evident that the middle years, in which a person is in many ways at their prime, are also years of responsibility and stress. Although each taken alone may be a small constraint, the burdens sometimes have the overall effect of making the middle-aged person feel exhausted and overwhelmed. Authors Amelia and Emily and Nagoski highlight that to break the stress cycle, one needs to complete the stress response cycle. If we don't, we go into (and remain) in fight or flight mode which can lead to health problems. The authors recommend three ways to complete the stress response cycle: (1) engage in cardiovascular exercise, (2) seek safety in the means of a 20-second hug from a trusted friend or loved one, and (3) get a good night's rest (a particularly potent, although sometimes elusive restorative activity).[46]

REFLECTIONS

Think about all your current major life roles.
- Did you choose these roles or were they assigned to you?
- What are the behaviors expected by you in these individual roles?
- How do your roles influence your use of time? Do they conflict?
- How have you shaped this role? How has the culture in which you live shaped the role?
- What are the stressors associated with this role?
- What strategies have you developed to combat the stressors in your life and allow you to remain resilient?

Doubt at the Crossroads and Midlife Challenges

The task of assuming responsibility and its attendant stresses, the great desire to achieve, or transitions in career, family life, and health condition may at some critical moment trigger an opportunity to take stock. The feeling accompanying the experience is most clearly expressed as doubt. It differs from the vacuous zero point of boredom and lacks the volcanic fervor of other types of stress. Doubt allows no rest; indeed, it is a relentless churning that nakedly reveals almost all the dimensions of one's life. The masks that have allowed the masquerade to go on, the clatter that has accompanied the parade, and the walls that have kept fearful monsters from view all suddenly evaporate and leave a pregnant silence. The self stands alone. Middle-age adults may wonder, "Is this all there is?" and feel that "something is missing." Also, the focus on worldly aspirations may shift to more spiritual aspects of life and their place in the bigger scheme of things. Middle-age adults make more informed decisions about their futures.

The various transitions that are a part of adult life allow people to come to terms with new situations. Bridges[57] conceptualizes a transition as a three-phase psychological process people go through ending, neutral zone, and new beginning. A transition begins with an ending. Something must be left behind to move to the next phase. A transition may be sought or thrust upon a person.

CASE STUDY

Consider the case of Tanya Zorski, a claims processor at an insurance company for the past 10 years. Recently, Tanya's employer merged with another company, resulting in "downsizing," or firing of many people in the claims department, including Tanya. Tanya's transition begins with the ending of her job. The next phase of transition is the neutral zone. After letting go, willingly or unwillingly, she must examine old habits that are no longer adaptive.[51] As Tanya begins to look for another position, she will discover that the computer skills that had been adequate at her old job are not marketable. Employers want people with experience in leading-edge computer programs, and Tanya does not possess these skills. During the neutral zone phase, people start to look for new, better adapted skills or habits. People may take this opportunity to pursue a long-held dream. The final phase is the new beginning. Tanya decides to move into a new beginning in her life by pursuing a degree in nursing. She reasons that if she is going to invest the energy, time, and financial resources in learning new skills, she might as well do it in a profession that she has wanted to join since she was young.

REFLECTIONS

- Do you anticipate working in the same role for your entire career?
- What would lead you to "shift gears" in your work, living arrangements, or location?

Although changes in midlife have often been labeled as a "crisis," perhaps the language is too strong for most people. "Instead, perhaps, many individuals make modest 'corrections' in their life trajectories—literally, 'midcourse' corrections."[58] These corrections to one's life course are often the opportunity for growth and learning along the life span. As is the case with Tanya Zorski, the more life-changing an event, the more likely it is to be associated with learning opportunities. In the face of stress, adults with a strong learning goal orientation develop more effective, problem-focused coping styles.[59]

As we have previously acknowledged, the COVID-19 pandemic was a time of profound loss and suffering across the globe. However, for many, social distancing guidelines and the collective forced "time-out" provided the opportunity for introspection. Regardless of whether they were at midlife or not, many reflected on whether they wanted to emerge from this acutely stressful experience the same or have some sort of a transformation. Newport[60] calls this the "deep reset." Regardless of whether the pandemic triggered a positive change or not, the adult's task is to prepare for the adjustments and challenges still to come.

Working With the Adult Patient

This chapter deals primarily with the physical and psychosocial processes people face in their young and middle adult years. Some suggestions for maintaining respectful interaction have been offered, and we turn more fully to the health professional–patient relationship in this last section.

The patient you encounter in the adult years who arrives at the health facility may be working to maintain health or may be experiencing an illness-related symptom. Because these years are not "supposed to be" characterized by painful or other troubling physical symptoms, patients may feel especially angered or confused by this physical intrusion into their work of being a responsible person and pursuing goals. A woman of middle years who was being interviewed recently in a seminar reported that "being an adult was overrated!" Her father was in hospice for end-of-life cancer care, and two of her three sons required special education services for attention-deficit/hyperactivity disorder and learning disorders. Additionally, she was just told by her primary care physician that she needed to follow up with an oncologist for a positive mammogram. The ideas of being struck down in one's prime and that of the "untimely" accident or death are often applied to this age group. The denial, hostility, and depression that patients feel about being so attacked are factors to which you should give your attention, whether your interaction occurs only once or extends over a long period.

Because psychological and social well-being are preeminent for adults, treatment must be attuned to both. Of all the challenges presented by illness, injury, or disability, the loss of independence most epitomizes the overall loss experienced by the great majority of adult patients. Of course, the person's former self-image is threatened, too, but this is almost a direct outgrowth of the loss of independence. Patients who can no longer go about meeting the responsibilities expected of them and pursuing the numerous life roles and established goals may feel trapped, vulnerable, and frustrated. The primacy of these concerns in middle life should help you understand why a patient seems overly concerned about having to get a babysitter for an hour or having to return home at a given time, or why they are willing to forego treatment rather than take time from work for an appointment at a health care facility.

Furthermore, an adult patient experiencing acute stress poses special problems and challenges. Each one must be treated according to the manifestations of the stress. Part of the respect you must express is to assess physical or psychological symptoms that may be arising from stress. This, of course, is often done with a psychiatrist or psychologist, but not always. As you learned in Chapter 7, the skills of listening to the patient's narrative are tools to help you discern what is on a patient's mind. Listening may not only help decrease their anxiety at the moment but also may enable you to make adjustments in schedule, routine, or approach that will further diminish it.

Many of the suggestions given throughout this book apply to all age groups. However, if you are alert to some of the central concerns and roles of young and middle adulthood, you may well find that your success in achieving respectful interaction with the adult patient is heightened. In the next chapter, you have an opportunity to examine some changes that are faced by the person who has successfully lived through the middle years. As you will see, these changes involve some of life's greatest challenges, both positive and negative.

Summary

Biological capacities peak and begin to diminish in adulthood. It is during this time that adults have sufficient capacity for personally satisfying and socially valuable participation in life with all that it offers. The major life tasks for adults are establishing personal identity, developing intimate relationships, and feeling and acting on the desire to make a lasting contribution to the next generation. A key claim on adults is to accept responsibility through parenting, work, and public service activities. Although some individuals never resolve the issues that are brought into focus during the transitions of midlife, fortunately, most do allowing them to thrive while adulting. The COVID-19 pandemic heightened the adult period of introspection and "taking stock." Some emerged from the process with a new job, a new partner, or a new life view. The various aspects of adult development presented in this chapter are a sampling of how you can look at the complex process of how people grow, learn and develop as adults. Prioritizing these observations can help you be respectful in your relationships with adult patients and their families.

References

1. Ramirez K. *Why Adults Can Love Young Adult Literature Too.* Arizona State University; 2020. Retrieved from: https://www.studybreaks.com/culture/reads/adults-young-adults-literature.
2. Steinmetz K. *This Is What Adulting Means.* https://time.com/4361866/adulting-definition-meaning/; 2016.
3. Erikson EH. *Childhood and Society.* 2nd ed. New York: WW Norton; 1963.
4. *Black's Online Law Dictionary.* http://thelawdictionary.org/adulthood/; 2017.
5. Matteson ES, McConnell ES, Linton AD, eds. *Biological Theories of Aging in Gerontological Nursing: Concepts and Practice.* 2nd ed. Philadelphia, PA: WB Saunders; 1996.
6. Villar F. Successful ageing and development: the contribution of generativity in older age. *Ageing Society.* 2012;32(7):1087–1105.
7. Erikson EH. *The Life Cycle Completed.* New York: Norton; 1982.
8. Cronin A, Mandich MB. *Human Development and Performance Throughout the Lifespan.* 2nd ed. Boston, MA: Delmar Cengage Learning; 2015.
9. Cannon M. What is aging? *Dis-A-Mon [Serial Online].* 2015;61:454–459. Issues on Aging.
10. *U.S. Department of Health and Human Services Healthy People (Website).* https://www.healthypeople.gov; 2017.
11. World Health Organization. *International Classification of Functioning, Disability and Health (ICF).* Geneva: WHO; 2002. https://www.who.int/docs/default-source/classification/icf/icfbeginnersguide.pdf?sfvrsn=eead63d3_4.
12. *U.S. Department of Health and Human Services, Centers for Disease Control and Prevention, National Center for Health Statistics, National Vital Statistics System.* https://www.cdc.gov/nchs/data/vsrr/VSRR10-508.pdf; 2017.
13. *U.S. Department of Health and Human Services, Centers for Disease Control and Prevention, National Center for Health Statistics.* Leading causes of death. https://www.cdc.gov/nchs/fastats/leading-causes-of-death.htm; 2017.
14. *World Health Organization.* The top 10 causes of death. https://www.who.int/news-room/fact-sheets/detail/the-top-10-causes-of-death; 2021.
15. *Centers for Disease Control and Prevention, National Center for Chronic Disease Prevention and Health Promotion (NCCDPHP).* https://www.cdc.gov/chronicdisease/index.htm; 2021.
16. National Center for Health Statistics (US). *Health, United States, 2015: With Special Feature on Racial and Ethnic Health Disparities.* Hyattsville, MD: National Center for Health Statistics (US); 2016. Report no. 2016-1232. PMID: 27308685.
17. Duque RB. Black health matters too … especially in the era of Covid-19: how poverty and race converge to reduce access to quality housing, safe neighborhoods, and health and wellness services and increase the risk of co-morbidities associated with global pandemics. *J Racial Ethnic Health Disparities.* 2020;8:1–14. https://doi.org/10.1007/s40615-020-00857-w.
18. Siegel DJ. Why universities join cross-sector social partnerships: theory and evidence. *J Higher Educ Outreach Engagement.* 2010;14(1):33–62.
19. Arnett JJ. *Emerging Adulthood: The Winding Road from Late Teens Through Early Twenties.* 2nd ed. New York: Oxford University Press; 2015.
20. Muennig P, Jiao B, Singer E. Living with parents or grandparents increases social capital and survival: 2014 General Social Survey-National Death Index. *SSM-Popul Health.* 2018;4:71–75.
21. *TD Ameritrade.* Boomerang generation, returning to the nest. https://s2.q4cdn.com/437609071/files/doc_news/research/2019/Boomerang-Generation-Returning-to-the-Nest.pdf; 2019.

22. *US Census Bureau.* Estimated 17.8% of adults ages 25 to 34 lived in their parents' household last year. https://www.census.gov/library/stories/2020/09/more-young-adults-lived-with-their-parents-in-2019. html; 2020.

23. Friedman Z. 50% of millennials are moving back home with their parents after college. *Forbes.* 2019. Retrieved from: https://www.forbes.com/sites/zackfriedman/2019/06/06/millennials-move-back-home-college/?sh=4d3f432e638a.

24. Rikard RV, Thompson MS, McKinney J, et al. Examining health literacy disparities in the United States: a third look at the National Assessment of Adult Literacy (NAAL). *BMC Public Health.* 2016;16:975. https://doi.org/10.1186/s12889-016-3621-9.

25. Dirkes J, Hughes T, Ramirez-Valles J, et al. Sexual identity development: relationship with lifetime suicidal ideation in sexual minority women. *J Clin Nurs.* 2016;25(23/24):3545–3556.

26. The LGBT resident in long-term care, *CNA Training Advisor.* 2017;25(5):1–8. Retrieved from https://www.advanced-healthcare.com/wp-content/uploads/2011/07/May-2017-Inservice-2.pdf.

27. Riggle ED, Whitman JS, Olson A, et al. The positive aspects of being a lesbian or gay man. *Prof Psychol Res Pract.* 2008;39:210–217.

28. Malone J, Liu S, Vaillant G, et al. Midlife Eriksonian psychosocial development: setting the stage for late-life cognitive and emotional health. *Dev Psychol.* 2016;52(3):496–508.

29. Hiltner S. Personal values in the middle years. In: Ellis EO, ed. *The Middle Years.* Acton, MA: Publishing Sciences Group; 1974.

30. Brooks D. The moral peril of meritocracy. *The New York Times.* 2019. Retrieved from: https://www.nytimes.com/2019/04/06/opinion/sunday/moral-revolution-david-brooks.html.

31. U.S. Department of Labor Bureau of Labor Statistics. American time use survey summary. In: *Average Hours per Day Spent in Selected Activities by Sex and Day;* 2019. Retrieved from: https://www.bls.gov/charts/american-time-use/activity-by-sex.htm.

32. Bianchi SM, Sayer LC, Milkie MA, Robinson JP. Housework: who did, does or will do it, and how much does it matter? *Soc Forces.* 2012;91:55–63.

33. AARP and National Alliance for Caregiving. *Caregiving in the United States 2020.* Washington, DC: AARP; 2020. https://doi.org/10.26419/ppi.00103.001.

34. Piersol CV, Earland VT, Herge EA. *Meeting the Needs of Caregivers of Persons With Dementia: An Important Role for Occupational Therapy, OT Practice.* Bethesda, MD: AOTA Press; 2012:8–12.

35. Apesoa-Varano EC, Tang-Feldman Y, Reinhard SC, et al. Multi-cultural caregiving and caregiver interventions: a look back and a call for future action. *J Am Soc Aging.* 2015;39(4):39–48.

36. *International Mentoring Association.* What is mentoring? http://www.mentoringassociation.org/; 2003.

37. Crisp G, Cruz I. Mentoring college students: a critical review of the literature between 1990 and 2007. *Res Higher Educ.* 2009;50(6):525. https://doi.org/10.1007/s11162-009-9130-2.

38. Hernandez PR, Estrada M, Woodcock A, Schultz PW. Protégé perceptions of high mentorship quality depend on shared values more than on demographic match. *J Exp Educ.* 2017;85(3):450. https://doi.org/10.1080/00220973.2016.1246405.

39. Lewis V, Martina CA, McDermott MP, Trief PM, Goodman SR, Morse GD, Ryan RM. A randomized controlled trial of mentoring interventions for underrepresented minorities. *Acad Med: J Assoc Am Med Coll.* 2016;91(7):994–1001. https://doi.org/10.1097/ACM.0000000000001056.

40. Wilson AH, Sanner S, McAllister LE. An evaluation study of a mentoring program to increase the diversity of the nursing workforce. *J Cult Divers.* 2010;17(4):144–150. Retrieved from: http://tuckerpub.com/jcd.htm.

41. Barroso A., Minkin R. *Recent Protest Attendees Are More Racially and Ethnically Diverse, Younger Than Americans Overall;* https://www.pewresearch.org/fact-tank/2020/06/24/recent-protest-attendees-are-more-racially-and-ethnically-diverse-younger-than-americans-overall/; 2020.

42. *U.S. Department of Labor Bureau of Labor Statistics.* American time use survey summary. https://www.bls.gov/tus/; 2019.

43. Lee Y, Tang F. More caregiving, less working: caregiving roles and gender difference. *J Appl Gerontol.* 2015;34(4):465–483. https://doi.org/10.1177/0733464813508649.

44. World Bank. Gender differences in employment and why they matter. In: *World Development Report 2012: Gender Equality and Development.* Washington, DC: World Bank; 2011:198–253. Retrieved from: https://siteresources.worldbank.org/INTWDR2012/Resources/7778105-1299699968583/7786210-1315936222006/Complete-Report.pdf.

45. Helson R, Sato CJ. Up and down in middle-age: monotonic and nonmonotonic changes in role, status and personality. *J Pers Soc Psychol.* 2005;89(2):194–204.
46. Nagoski E, Nagoski A. *Burnout: The Secret to Unlocking the Stress Cycle.* New York: Ballantine Books; 2020.
47. Elam K, Chassin L, Eisenberg N, Spinrad T. Marital stress and children's externalizing behavior as predictors of mothers' and fathers' parenting. *Dev Psychopathol [serial online].* 2017:29.
48. Sampasa-Kanyinga H, Chaput J. Associations among self-perceived work and life stress, trouble sleeping, physical activity, and body weight among Canadian adults. *Prev Med.* 2017;96:16–20.
49. Timmons A, Arbel R, Margolin G. Daily patterns of stress and conflict in couples: associations with marital aggression and family-of-origin aggression. *J Fam Psychol.* 2017;31(1):93–104.
50. White AJ, Taliaferro D. Relationship between postmenopausal women's successful aging, global self-esteem, and sexual quality of life. *Int J Hum Caring.* 2016;20(2):102–106.
51. Sievert LL. Menopause across cultures: clinical considerations. *Menopause.* 2014;21(4):241–423.
52. *National Coalition Against Domestic Violence.* What is domestic violence? n.d. https://ncadv.org/learn-more.
53. Smith SG, Zhang X, Basile KC, et al. *The National Intimate Partner and Sexual Violence Survey (NISVS): 2015 Data Brief – Updated Release.* Atlanta, GA: National Center for Injury Prevention and Control, Centers for Disease Control and Prevention and Control, Centers for Disease Control and Prevention; 2018. Retrieved from: https://www.cdc.gov/violenceprevention/pdf/2015data-brief508.pdf.
54. Xiong J, Lipsitz O, Nasri F, et al. Impact of COVID-19 pandemic on mental health in the general population: a systematic review. *J Affect Disord.* 2020;277:55–64. https://doi.org/10.1016/j.jad.2020.08.001.
55. Sindi S, Kareholt I, Solomon A, et al. Midlife work-related stress is associated with late-life cognition. *J Neurol.* 2017;9:1996–2002.
56. Min S. The 10 most and least stressful jobs in America. *CBS News.* 2019. Retrieved from: https://www.cbsnews.com/news/10-most-and-least-stressful-jobs-in-america/.
57. Bridges W. *Managing Transitions: Making the Most of Change.* Reading, MA: Addison-Wesley; 1991.
58. Stewart AJ, Ostrove JM. Women's personality in middle age: gender, history, and midcourse corrections. *Am Psychol.* 1998;53(11):1185–1194.
59. Delahaij R, van Dam K. Coping style development: the role of learning goal orientation and metacognitive awareness. *Personal Individ Differ.* 2016;92:57–62.
60. *Cal Newport.* The deep reset. https://www.calnewport.com/blog/2020/05/14/the-deep-reset; 2020.

CHAPTER 13

Respectful Interaction: Working With Older Adults

Prelude

John Quincy Adams is well. But the house in which he lives at present is becoming dilapidated. It is tottering upon its foundation. Time and the seasons have nearly destroyed it. Its roof is pretty well worn out. Its walls are much shattered and it trembles with every wind. I think John Quincy Adams will have to move out of it soon. But he himself is quite well, quite well.

JOHN QUINCY ADAMS IN A RESPONSE TO A QUERY REGARDING HIS
WELL-BEING ON HIS 80TH BIRTHDAY[1]

One of the challenges confronting anyone who attempts to speak of the older adult is to earmark exactly when "old age" begins, even though it is a phase of life everyone enters if they are fortunate enough to live past middle age. According to many social policies, eligibility for financial and other support benefits for the older adult begins at the age of 65, but the usefulness of this age as a distinguishing line largely ends there. In fact, many people's feelings that they are "old" are determined by the presence (or absence) of illness, disability, or other limiting factors rather than simply by their chronological age. For the purposes of this chapter, the term "older adult" will refer to individuals in later adulthood—age 65 or older. Late adulthood can be divided into the young old, age 65–75; the middle old, age 75–85; and the old old, age 85 and older.

The older population in the United States currently represents 16.5% of the US population.[2] By 2060, nearly one in four Americans is projected to be an older adult.[3] The *baby boomer* genera- tion is largely responsible for this increase in the older adult population. (This term "baby boomer" and other generational distinctions is introduced in Chapter 6). Boomers comprise one of the largest generational cohorts in US history. The boomers began crossing into the older adult (65+) category in 2011, and they will continue to do so until 2030, shifting the US age structure and the face of health care and society. Though not all in this population are sick, the average patient in a US inpatient health care facility is likely to be older than 75 years of age. Additionally, the older population—the heaviest users of the health care system—will be far more racially and ethnically diverse and will be women, especially among those older than 85 years.[4]

In Chapter 4, you learned about implicit bias and the pervasiveness of stereotypes. Most of us have stereotypes of old age, but almost every generality about the older person is quickly countered by personal experience with an older adult. Many processes that take place in a person as they advance in years are similar in broad strokes of what happens but also differ from one individual to another. This chapter provides an overview of physiological and psychosocial changes, with a special emphasis on the psychosocial aspects of aging as they are relevant to respectful interaction. We urge you to study the burgeoning literature of aging further, because the questions and clinical issues surrounding the care of older patients are complex.

REFLECTIONS

In Chapter 1, you completed a values clarification exercise. One way to establish our values and goals is to envision our older selves and think about what we hope to accomplish during our lifetime.
   Close your eyes and imagine yourself at the age of 85.
- What do you imagine you will be like? Look like?
- What roles will you have? How will they differ from your roles today?
- When you tell your life story, what will the highlights be?

Rapid societal changes taking place around older adults give them greater opportunity for divergent roles than ever before. While some older adults may be home bound, many are actively involved outside of the home as employers, employees, volunteers, or members of community organizations. Today's older adults write books, start new businesses, run marathons, travel, attend college, raise grandchildren, and have active social media accounts. Consider that Joseph R. Biden, the 46th President of the United States, is the oldest President sworn in at 78 years and 61 days!

Despite many opportunities for older adults, the downside is that if they are unable to take advantage of these opportunities, as many are, they may be burdened by a greater feeling of being left out of the action than were their predecessors. One of the authors was saddened by a patient's remark that he had stopped subscribing to a magazine for older adults because it made him too depressed; everyone his age looked younger and did more than he could do. Our experience is that health professionals can play an important role in helping each older person make the best of their opportunities so that their potential for a meaningful old age is optimized.

Views of Aging

Aging in its broadest sense refers to the "changes that occur during an organisms' life-span."[5] It is a multifactorial process and the rate at which various changes take place is highly individualized. Extensive gerontological research has documented the interaction among genetics, environmen- tal influences, lifestyles, and disease processes.[6] Aging also intersects with gender and culture, attaching different social meanings, expectations, attitudes, and evaluations.[7] Theories of aging span the fields of biology, psychology, and sociology. These theories, along with experience and the cultural and societal views of aging, influence how health professionals understand the aging process and how they engage in their work with older patients and their families. You will expand your knowledge of aging theories in various areas of coursework that prepare you to work with the older adult population. The text that follows highlights a few of these theories to support your learning in this area.

BIOLOGICAL THEORIES

Biological theories of aging share the concept, "aging results from a decline in the force of natural selection."[8] There is no known way to stop or reverse the aging process. As adults age, their bodies change and progressively lose function. This increases an individual's vulnerability to both disease and environmental threats. There are two main types of biological aging theories, genetic (programmed theories) and stochastic (damage theories). Genetic theories propose that "aging is genetically determined and organisms have an internal clock that programs longevity."[8] Stochastic or damage theories propose, "chance error and the accumulation of damage over time cause aging. Stochastic theories include wear and tear, error catastrophe, free radical theory, DNA damage hypothesis, loss of adaptive cellular mechanism, and the mitochondrial theory."[8] In other words, our cells, organs, and systems face progressive decline due to genetics, damage, and the environment we live in. However, this is just one of a host of diverse aging concepts and theories.

SOCIAL THEORIES OF AGING

We interact with older adults in the context of societies, cultures, and communities. What people see or read in the media or hear from adults plays a critical role in shaping their perceptions of older people.[6] Thus, it is important to promote representations of older adults in the full range of their activities and health states. Think for a moment about an older adult you know, perhaps a grandparent. Is this individual active and engaged or immobile and frail? Is the person perhaps pleasant and tech-savvy? Or irritable and old fashioned? Or pleasant and old fashioned? Our individual and societal experiences with older adults contribute to our views, which is why it is essential to learn as much as we can regarding healthy aging. Doing so prevents ageism in health care.

REFLECTIONS

Children and even older adults themselves can hold negative attitudes about the older adult population in large part due to mass media. Ageism leads to stereotypes of older adults as forgetful, incompetent, or cranky and can have far-reaching consequences such as discrimination, disrespect, and even elder abuse, which we will discuss later in this chapter.[7]

As we discussed in Chapter 4, there are specific strategies that we can employ to limit the effects of bias (such as ageism) on our interactions with our patients. The first step is to become aware of our biases (often "implicit" and hidden). One of the resources provided in Chapter 4 is Project Implicit by Harvard Medical School[9] which has various association tests that users can complete. There is a specific implicit association test on distinguishing young and old faces that you may find informative. Chapter 4 also highlights the steps that we can take after we become aware of our biases. Once more aware of our biases, we can instead consider multiple different theories about and experiences of the aging process.

The *life-course approach* is a common societal perspective on aging.[6,10] This theory "recognizes the social, cultural, and structural contexts of a person's lifelong development."[10] Key principles guiding the life-course perspective include historical time and place, timing of events in a person's life, and human agency to make decisions. Appreciating how life events have affected the patient, such as an adverse childhood experience or service in the military during war, will help you understand how to best support and promote health in this older adult patient. According to societal theory, it is also essential to recognize the contribution of agency to health. *Agency* refers to an individual's "capacity to influence their own life and exert control over their actions and outcomes."[10] Agency is linked to physical, cognitive, and mental health. Adults who hold positive views of aging recover from disability at higher rates and are more likely to engage in behaviors that promote successful aging.[11] How an individual adapts to age-related change is important. The life-course approach is just one of several social theories focused on aging. Common elements include social engagement later in life and adaptation to age-related changes.

PSYCHOLOGICAL THEORIES OF AGING

Psychological theories of aging refer to both psychological changes as a result of aging and adaptive psychological mechanisms (or lack thereof) to counteract the losses associated with functional decline that results from aging.[12] Social sciences research is moving away from the focus on decline and dependency to adopting a more optimistic view of aging which focuses on the potential of human development. The World Health Organization (WHO) uses the term "active ageing" and has a policy framework to optimize "opportunities for health, participation and security in order to enhance quality of life as people age."[13] We will focus on two main models of successful aging.

The first model focuses on achievement/maintenance into the final decades of life (i.e. a focus on outcomes). Successful aging is thought to be defined by three criteria: (1) low risk of disease and disability, (2) high physical and cognitive functioning, and, lastly, (3) active engagement with close personal relationships and involvement in activities. This model however faces criticism for its focus on disability and the elitist approach to defining successful aging that only a privileged minority could attain.[14]

The second model focuses on the processes which allow us to adapt to the challenges conditions we face as we age. Rather than considering a final ideal state, there is increased attention paid to human beings' ability to adapt. While there are many theories that accompany this model of aging, the SOC model (which stands for selection, optimization, and compensation) is the most influential.[14] When there are new tasks or challenges which exceed available resources, the older adult relies on a process of selection and selects which challenge they will tackle. The individual also focuses on acquiring resources to improve function (optimization) or compensates when previously available resources are lost. The SOC theory challenges the passive approach to aging but rather highlights the capability of the older adult who has active influence over meeting their goals.[14]

Essential to these theories are the cognitive, emotional, and behavioral skills that support development, and in turn aging, over time. Cognitive plasticity, intelligence, emotional self-regulation, and behavioral regulation are vital skills that allow the older adult to cope and learn to adopt new health behaviors, roles, and routines to support healthy aging. One of the most positive views of aging is to see people who have lived a long time as a source of wisdom and experience. Recent interest in obtaining oral histories from older adults who have witnessed great and mundane historical events is evidence of this insight. The experience of older adults is of value to younger generations and fits well with Erikson's theory of development,[15] introduced in earlier chapters.

REFLECTIONS

Historic events in our society and culture greatly influence our lives. You often hear older adults reminisce about these events. For example, they may say, "I remember exactly where I was the day JFK was shot" or "It was a historic day when man landed on the moon." More recently, you hear people talk about the tragic events of September 11, 2001 and where they were as events unfolded. Perhaps you remember the events of 9/11 but have friends who were not born yet.

Name a historic event that influenced you and/or your family.
- How did it affect you and how you participated in your life roles?
- How did your family talk about this event?
- How has its meaning for your life and society changed over time, if at all?
- When you recount this event to the next generation, what will you say?

Needs: Respect and Integrity

Several basic psychological and social processes are evident in the widely divergent lifestyles of today's older adults. Erikson proposes that the success with which an older person can make psychological and social adjustments will depend on their ability to meet the most basic psychosocial developmental challenge of old age—that of integrity. In this last stage of human development, the person "understands, accepts, and loves the life he [or she] has led."[15] The person "possesses wisdom" and is willing to share this wisdom with the younger generation.[15] The little girl and older man in Fig. 13.1 perfectly illustrate this sharing of expertise across generations.

Health professionals are delighted, and sometimes awed, by an older person who expresses the breadth and depth of acceptance described by Erikson. These older adults readily accept the psychological and social adjustments that confront them. However, some older persons despair of being old, the psychological and social adjustments of old age overwhelm them, and they find little from their past to support them in their present situation. Key psychological and social processes assist or deter older persons from achieving a sense of wholeness and integrity in old age.

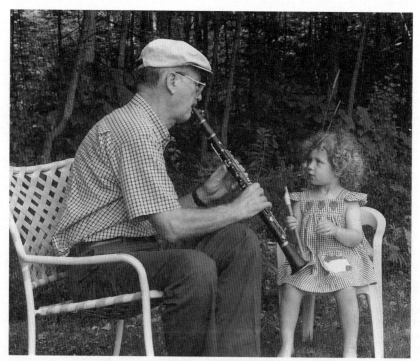

Fig. 13.1   Shared expertise across generations. © 1995 Joan Beard, from Family: a Celebration, edited by Margaret Campbell, Peterson's.

Studies of aging have given rise to the notion and understanding of healthy aging as a life-long process of optimizing opportunities to preserve and improve health and physical, social, and mental wellness; maintain independence; enjoy a high quality of life; and experience enhancing successful life-course transitions.[14] This includes optimizing physical, cognitive, and mental health and facilitating social engagement.[16] The definition of healthy aging provides avenues to overcome natural losses that occur with age. It is a model of health promotion, injury prevention, and effective disease self-management. Community health programming such as exercise programs, fall prevention, and yoga for the older adult all support the healthy aging model. Regardless of what clinical research or health care may define as "successful aging," many older adults have simply defined it as having the physical, mental, and financial means to engage in worthwhile endeavors.[16]

REFLECTIONS

- What theory best describes the attitudes of older adult patients you have treated or observed regarding relationships, gains or losses, health, etc.?
- How is the process of aging and the treatment of older adults described in your culture?
- How might your idea of healthy aging differ from that of an older patient and what might be a barrier to expressing genuine respect to this person?

Social Capital in Older Adulthood: Friendship and Family

As discussed in Chapter 4, the social determinants of health have a great deal of impact on population health.[17] One of the determinants which is particularly relevant to the older adult is social capital. Social capital is described as a resource that is accessed via social networks. Like the word "capital" implies, it is an investment in social relations which then in turn results in the sense of community, emotional support, good health, and perhaps even job or volunteer opportunities. Along with networks, there is also a degree of reciprocity and trust associated with social capital.[18] Social capital was revealed to be an especially valuable resource during the COVID-19 pandemic. Bonding ties (between families and friends) were particularly useful during the early stage of the pandemic and associated with fewer pandemic-related deaths.[19] (Consider friends and family members completing grocery shopping or picking up medication/prescriptions for the older adult in their lives to save them from unnecessary trips to the grocery store and pharmacy.) It is easy to see that, regardless of the form that it takes, even when there is no public health crisis, having social capital is associated with both improved mental and physical health.[18]

While relationships and contacts may change as we age, social capital continues to be an important part of our lives and our health as we age. However, the amount of contact older people maintain with their families and friends varies greatly. Many persons lose a valuable source of natural physical contact and companionship with the diminution of friendship and family ties, whereas others remain actively integrated into family and community circles.

The sequelae of the loss of contact and diminution of social capital for older adults were also evident during the pandemic. As of September 2021, there were over 650,000 deaths in the United States attributed to COVID-19 with more than 75% of the deaths in the 65 years and older age groups.[20] Older adults were especially susceptible to the disease due to a weaker immune system and greater potential of having a comorbidity/chronic condition such as heart disease, diabetes, and lung cancer, which were risk factors for complications from COVID-19. Due to these risks, older adults were advised to self-quarantine. Families were advised not to visit residents in skilled nursing facilities (SNFs) due to the risk of transmitting the disease and rapid spread to other residents. While legitimate, the consequences of these public health measures were isolation, loneliness, and decreased social participation for older adults.[21] Many health care providers described how patients, especially older adult patients, valued contact with them during the pandemic. Telehealth visits quickly became a treasured part of the day for many older adults.

Even after social distancing measures are a thing of the past, when you treat older adult patients, you should take time to assess how many needs for social contact are being met by friends and family. You will understand a lot about their conduct during their time with you. It is not unusual for people to transfer their needs to health professionals once they have lost other relationships.

FRIENDSHIPS

Until the present ultra-mobile way of life in the United States, the acquisition of a single set of friends continued throughout early life and tapered off when one settled down in a community. One's job seldom changed during the entire period of employment, and as a result, the community (and the friends therein) remained the same up through old age. This is of course vastly different. Today, the average worker will hold 12.4 jobs in their lifetime.[22] In one sense, the older model of one lifetime job (and associated friends) was a secure mode of existence, but reliance on lifelong friendship carries with it the risk that, if these friends all die, the person will be left alone. Many people who have depended on lifelong friendships find it difficult to make new acquaintances at 70 or 80 years of age. An older person whose friendships are centered on their occupational relationships may find that, after retirement, the friend is very much alive, but their friendship is dead. Conversely, a distant friendship may thrive after retirement because energy once directed elsewhere can now be devoted to the friend. In this sense, the basis of a friendship is an important determinant of its longevity. For older adults, events such as illness, new living arrangements, and mobility problems may make maintaining friendships difficult.[23]

Even though the number of close friends decreases with age, older adults who are active in their communities report more friends than those who are unable to be socially involved or opt not to be.[24] Friendships have been demonstrated to influence a person's psychological well-being and health outcomes.[25] In working with patients, you can understand some important things by exploring who the person's friends are and how friendships are generated and sustained. It is also helpful to keep in mind that low income, poor health, lack of transportation, and infrequent information access are linked to social isolation in the aging adult population.[26] Supporting older adults in social engagement who face some of these barriers improves health and quality of life.

FAMILY

Participation in families is one of the most lasting and significant roles a person assumes. As we discussed in Chapters 7 and 12, the family structure is changing. However, for the most part, in long-term couple relationships, couples usually have an opportunity to spend time alone together. When children become a part of the relationship, attention is transferred to them, and, in many families, much of the communication for years to come takes place in the presence of at least one child. Frequently in these older adults, only after the children have left home or the working years end is the couple alone again. Some couples find this to be an opportunity to engage in activities together that they put off in their younger years. Of course, these plans may be disrupted when grown children return to live at home sometimes with their own children. As discussed in Chapter 12, there are great gains to be made from living in multigenerational homes—for all involved, including the older adult.[27]

In the present oldest old population (those 85 years and older), there are many who are in committed relationships or were formerly in a long-term relationship. Being in a relationship that is now changed due to the aging process can pose challenges for the older adult. You may work with an older adult who is unable to cope with financial and other home management business affairs because that was their partner's role in the relationship. You may also work with an older adult who never grocery shopped or prepared a meal from scratch because their partner took on those responsibilities. Generally, there is a balance of tasks that most longtime intimate partners develop. When one partner can no longer perform an essential role because of illness or injury, the other partner may become overwhelmed by the need to complete additional tasks. Loss of a spouse or partner can be extremely difficult, not only emotionally, but also because of the disruption to the surviving older adult's patterns, roles, and routines. Some turn to children, nieces, or nephews for help. Older adults often turn to friends and siblings when they find themselves alone. A sibling has the added benefit of a shared history as evident in the following poem:

Homecoming
I

> *after 45 years*
> *of writing letters*
> *& calling, Estelle sent word*
> *to find a contractor—*
> *she wants a home*
> *built next to her sister*
> *the house, brick & modern*
> *is an oddity—*
> *sits prominently among shotgun houses,*
> *cows, chickens, fish ponds, bait shops*
> *& trailer homes*
> *Celeste walks the clay red road*
> *to her Oakland-California-sister—*
> *they have forty-five years to catch up on*

II

> *Estelle & Celeste talk of the other two sisters*
> *who died in their early 70s—*
> *bring out boxes of black & white worn photos*
> *Estelle rakes arthritic fingers*
> *through Celeste's hair*
> *conjuring memory*
> *she parts the white/yellow-stained strands—*
> *braids her sister's hair.*

ANDREA M. WREN[28]

A discussion of aging and family relationships must include an assessment of who is most likely to provide support for older people in times of illness. Social support systems for people who are partially or totally dependent include both family caregivers and informal ones (friends, neighbors, or members of a religious or other types of community). As we discussed in Chapter 7, families provide most of the care for older relatives. Many families struggle to provide this care, as is evident in the following example:

> *Dad may be desperately ill, demanding constant attention and unable to join the family and guests at dinner. Mom may be afflicted with Alzheimer's and can't follow a conversation. Grandma may be bedfast. And in as many cases as not, the woman of the house does the*

caretaking even though she is poor, busy with a job to stay above subsistence level, preoccupied with her own children, and untrained. In such circumstances—God forbid—there is no extra room for the ill or aged, and little patience or reason for hope. Caring in the home is still the great overlooked medical-social problem among all classes in the United States.[29]

High levels of caregiver stress can sometimes lead to elder abuse. The WHO defines elder abuse as, "a single, or repeated act, or lack of appropriate action, occurring within any relationship where there is an expectation of trust which causes harm or distress to an older person." *Elder abuse* can be physical, sexual, emotional, or financial and is prevalent all over the world.[30] Ten percent of those over the age of 65 will experience some form of abuse and these numbers continue to rise.[31] It can occur in any setting an older person engages in and can be engaged in a relationship in which the older adult is trusting of another person or identity. Alternatively, the older adult can be targeted based on their age or disability. Elder abuse can take several forms[32]:

1. *Physical abuse*: Encompasses the use of force that can result in injury, pain, or impairment.
2. *Sexual abuse*: "Sexual abuse is defined as non-consensual sexual contact of any kind with an elderly person. Sexual contact with any person incapable of giving consent is also considered sexual abuse."[32]
3. *Psychological/emotional abuse*: The person is debased and intimidated verbally, threatened, isolated, or belittled. Anguish and distress can also be inflicted via nonverbal acts.
4. *Neglect/abandonment*: Failure or refusal to provide adequately for a vulnerable elder's safety, physical needs, or emotional needs; the desertion of a vulnerable elder by anyone with a duty of care.
5. *Financial/material exploitation*: Monetary or material theft, fraud, or undue influence to gain control over an older person's money or property.
6. *Self-neglect*: "Self-neglect generally manifests itself in an older person as a refusal or failure to provide himself/herself with adequate food, water, clothing, shelter, personal hygiene, medication (when indicated), and safety precautions."[32]

Elder abuse often is not reported or is underreported because the older person (or others) fear retaliation or believe that nothing will be done to change the situation. Just as with a child whom you suspect is being abused or neglected, you are legally responsible to report suspected elder abuse. It is important to note that you do not need to prove that abuse is occurring. If you suspect abuse or neglect, follow your institutional guidelines or call Adult Protective Services and the abuse will be investigated.[33] Unfortunately, elder abuse is not isolated to the home setting. It occurs in institutional settings as well, such as group homes, nursing homes, adult day care, or even hospitals.

Where "Home" Is

A major challenge for older people is to decide where to make their homes. Aging brings an increased risk for disability, isolation, and financial stress that affect housing decisions.[25] Key components of independent living for older adults include physical health, cognitive health, functional ability, and social ability (including driving and access to the larger community).[26] Security, accessibility to services, transportation, and physical considerations are key variables in older adult housing decisions. As we discussed, family and friend ties are vital to healthy aging. The desire to be near friends or relatives also often weighs heavily for people who have a choice of location and aging in place can also prolong positive social relationships.[34] The preference of many older adults is to age in place. Aging in place is defined by the Centers for Disease Control and Prevention as "the ability to live in one's own home and community safely, independently, and comfortably, regardless of age, income, or ability level."[35] Unlike decades ago, when moving to a nursing facility was the final housing change for older adults,[36] today many older adults achieve their goal of aging in place. Through the support of formal and informal caregivers, environmental adaptations, and supportive technology, the proportion of older adults living alone continues to increase.[34]

Senior apartment communities, intentional retirement communities, and other age-friendly communities are housing alternatives for persons who do not remain in their own homes (or move in with or near relatives) but that allow them to age in place.[37,38] With the dramatic rise in the number of baby boomers who are reaching old age, a burgeoning new industry of "continuing care centers" is expanding. They may be for-profit or not-for-profit sponsored and provide the opportunity for older people to move into an independent living apartment or townhome, graduate to partial assistance, and eventually have full medical and other supports of nursing home arrangements.

For older persons with functional disabilities or those who need more assistance with daily living activities than can be provided at home by family or professional caregivers, an assisted living or SNF may become their last place of residence. The most common reason for admission to an SNF is the inability to perform activities of daily living. The primary medical conditions associated with SNF admission are dementia and stroke.[39] According to the 2020 Census, 1.6 million individuals were living in SNFs.[40] Of this population, many are women although this percentage is declining.[41] Not all admissions to SNFs are for the rest of a patient's life and lengths of admission are also declining.[41] Some older adults are admitted to SNFs for short-term rehabilitation so that they can regain strength and function to return to independent or partial assisted living.

REFLECTIONS

Imagine you are seriously injured and told that you must live in an SNF for 2 months.
- What would you miss most about your current living situation? Why?
- What about the move would be hardest for you to cope with?
- What supports would make such a move easier for you?

You will benefit from bearing in mind that these challenges may have already occurred for the older adult simply because they are old rather than because of illness or injury. In many Western societies, the loss of a long-established place of residence, of consequence to anyone, is felt deeply by the older person because self-respect and the power to command the respect of others depend in part on remaining independent. Although many patients experience the loss of independence as temporary, older adults usually realize that each loss can be a step toward more dependence. Moving out of one's home permanently symbolizes dependence with a capital D.

Each move of residence may have greater significance for older adults than for those of any other age group. For example, a woman who has been forced to move into her daughter's home and who then requires admission to the hospital for elective surgery that results in placement in an SNF for rehabilitation certainly has grounds for feeling completely "undone" by the number of moves she has had to make in a short period. Thoughtful health professionals take these factors into consideration and are patient in helping the older person adapt accordingly.

REFLECTIONS

A key to respectful interaction with an older person is to promote as much stability in the place of residence as possible.
- How could you gather information from the patient about what might increase their comfort and stability while admitted to an inpatient setting (whether it be a long-term acute care or SNF)?
- Which members of the interprofessional team could you collaborate with to help meet the older adult patient's needs for stability?
- Are these needs specific to an older adult patient?

Challenges and Opportunities of Changes With Aging

Not all adults have the privilege of living into older adulthood and enjoying the fruits of their labor which may include retirement after years of hard work and perhaps watching children and grandchildren grow. As we discussed in Chapters 4 and 12, life expectancy in the United States differs by both race[42] and education.[43] However, for those who do grow into older adulthood, aging brings with it both opportunities and challenges.

A CHANGING SELF-IMAGE

The discussion so far in this chapter offers ample evidence that humans have the potential to continue to develop throughout the life span, and self-esteem can remain high or even grow stronger in the older years. Some recognize talents they never knew they had or refocus their energies on other hobbies or projects.

Some persons do not even notice changes in how they look, seeing only what they want to see in the mirror (Fig. 13.2). Others may cling to a former visual image and begin to reject the

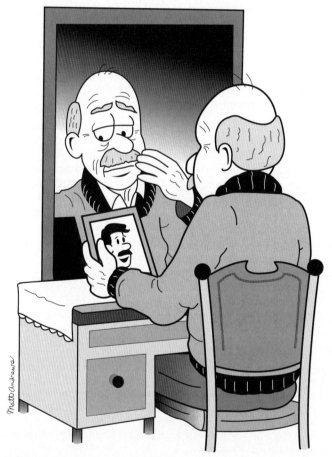

Fig. 13.2 "I haven't changed a bit."

changes brought about by aging. They might even see themselves as has-beens questioning their value in society, or get angry or depressed because they cannot perform as they did in the past. Much of this is perpetuated by mass media including the film and print industry which values youthful images, particularly of women. Tina Fey and Amy Poehler hosting the 2014 Golden Globes awards famously joked about George Clooney in the movie Gravity stating *"It's the story of how George Clooney would rather float away into space and die than spend one more minute with a woman his own age."*[44] While this joke was about the ageism and sexism of Hollywood, retirement from any long-held job or career focus often poses a threat to self-image (and, subsequently, to self-esteem) in many older adults.

With almost all adults employed in the workforce at some time in their lives, more people than ever before will face the challenge of retirement. While the average American reports that they planned to retire by the age of 62, this number differs by generation. While Generation Y has plans to retire by the age of 59, baby boomers plan to work longer with an expected retirement age of 68.[45] Many predict that this forecast is accurate, and the baby boomer generation may indeed not retire at the traditional age of 65. This stems from concerns about funding shortfalls in Social Security and Medicare, possible cuts in government programs for older people, and cuts in traditional benefit pension plans that previously provided a fixed income in old age. For most, retirement not only involves a substantial reduction in income but also signals a change in daily activity.

As the person looks forward in time to retirement, a central issue becomes replacing time spent in work with other productive activities. One of our colleagues calls retirement a "preferment" because you can finally spend your time doing things you prefer to do. However, the disappearance of work potentially leaves much of the older adult's landscape unfilled. At a minimum, retirement precipitates change in the person's regular activity pattern.[46] Four basic tasks are purported to comprise essential postjob satisfaction: social activity, play, creativity, and lifelong learning.[47]

To maintain their self-imposed status as productive members of society, almost all older adults need to be engaged in ongoing activity. This may be a job, a hobby, a volunteer service, or a club. In fact, most volunteer hours are contributed by Americans beginning in midlife and continuing into old age in many areas that US social policy fails to address adequately, such as the provision of basic human services.[48] Regardless of the activity chosen, older adults need to have something to look forward to and to know they are needed in a certain place at a certain time. Research suggests that involvement in volunteer activities may significantly improve the health and well-being of older individuals through lower rates of depression, increased life satisfaction, retention of functional abilities, improved physical activity, and cognitive activity.[49–51] However, not all older adults are able to be involved in such activities, and there are some good reasons why:

- They may be shy about meeting new people, particularly if they have maintained one set of friends and acquaintances for many years.
- They may possess too many physical, cognitive, or mental health impairments to participate in ongoing activities.
- They may have no way to get to them.
- They may not be able to afford to go.
- They may be afraid to go out alone or at night.
- They may be marginalized or discriminated again by select groups

One or more of these reasons may also prevent them from seeking ongoing health care. Fortunately, the narrative of the aging adult is changing, and older adults are achieving major milestones later and later in life. As the average age of our society grows, older people will become involved in continuous activities. For example, politics is one area in which the population older than 65 years has gained a powerful voice. Political involvement facilitates progress in legislation regarding personal interests and provides a broader perspective for legislation regarding society.

PHYSICAL CHANGES OF AGING

A higher percentage of older adults are remaining in good health longer than ever before; however, as addressed earlier in this chapter, all adults experience physical changes over the life span. The most common functional limitations in older adults are brought about by reduced strength and endurance, joint problems, and increased risk for falls and household accidents.[52,53] These functional problems are often associated with both physiologic and cognitive changes. Examples of physiologic age-related changes include bone loss, cartilage thinning, decreased cardiac reserve capacity, muscle weakness, sensory changes, and changes in touch, temperature, and pain perception.

Examples of cognitive changes include neuroanatomic changes in the brain that lead to decreased memory, attention, and a general decline in fluid intelligence (the ability to process novel information). With aging, the pattern of intelligence changes. The older adult demonstrates improvements in their crystallized intelligence (the ability to apply knowledge gained over time), and thus balance the loss in fluid intelligence, which aids older adults in deciding how to respond to certain situations.[12]

Visual changes include declines in acuity, speed of focusing, and accommodation in vision. With aging, adaptation to darkness usually declines, too. Hearing losses are greatest in the high-frequency range and are more prevalent in men than women. There is a steady loss in perception of body movement or kinesthesia. The older person may "adjust" to the losses gracefully. An example is an exchange that one of the authors had with her 92-year-old neighbor. As she walked into his living room, where the television announcer was blaring the Boston Red Sox's latest home run, she was surprised to see Tom planted in front of a blank screen. "Tom!" she shouted above the clamor, "There's no picture!" "Picture went about a month ago!" he shouted back. "Can't see the screen anyway!" Tom, despite his good humor, would probably concede that the savings on the television repair were not worth the price of his failing eyesight. Your sensitivity to a patient's feelings about these losses can have profound effects on the extent to which the patient feels respected by you. Understandably, your attention to and authentic care regarding a patient's sensitivity about such matters are critical components of showing respect.

We will not discuss musculoskeletal or neurological changes in the aging process in further detail because many health professionals learn this elsewhere. Posture, balance, strength, endurance, and other physical expressions of aging will vary, but overall wear and tear on the body will affect all adults in their later years. Your role as a health professional is to recognize normal aging and be able to contrast it with signs of pathology. An older adult or family member may mistake a clinical condition for normal aging and think "Oh, I am just getting older," when there may be a treatable condition that can be managed clinically to help the patient avoid disease and disability. For example, depression is often under identified in the older adult. It is commonly mistaken for apathy related to age.

Multiple studies demonstrate that exercise has a positive impact on human beings of almost any age. Regular activity can reverse the decreased mobility that contributes to disease and disability in old age.[54] Furthermore, exercise has been shown to promote modest positive changes in cognitive functioning in this phase of the life span.[54] Given demonstrated improvements in so many areas, a prescription for activity seems indicated for most older adults. *Self-efficacy* (conviction to organize and implement effective strategies to deal with potential stressors) is also a positive predictor for aging well. Self-efficacy when linked with activity helps maintain cognitive function, resilience, and social engagement.[55,56]

One way of dealing with all the physical changes that are a normal part of aging, as well as those that accompany chronic and acute illness and injury, is to share experiences with others who understand what the person is going through. Your sensitivity to changes, offering the person opportunities to talk about illness and loss and especially what changes mean for their feeling of well-being, is an avenue to respectful interaction, too.

MENTAL CHANGES OF AGING

A few minor differences in mental capacity and functioning among all who are older are noteworthy. If attended to, they can enhance the health professional's success in working with older people.

All patients benefit from the security of a set schedule, and this may be especially true for many older persons. The security arises from the knowledge that, at least in this one small area, they are in control of the environment. Some older people continue to exercise complete control over the details of their existence, whereas others gradually lose this opportunity. Even if this control extends no further than the patient telling the taxi or ride-share service driver to hurry because they are scheduled to be in speech therapy in 15 minutes, that person's self-respect will have been bolstered by exercising this type of agency.

Being able to count on an established schedule is also a way for an older adult to maintain a proper orientation to the environment. Some hospitalized older adult patients become confused about the time of day and the date because they have few clues to orient them compared with the person who works 5 days a week or a peer who has more ongoing routine activity.

An older person's sense of security, control, and orientation can be further enhanced if, in addition to being treated at the same time each day, the routine of a treatment or test is kept reasonably stable from one day to the next. If the treatment or testing situation varies significantly every day, the patient may feel that nothing about it is familiar; it may be an anxiety-producing experience every time the person reports to the health professional. Anxiety can greatly decrease the person's performance and have a detrimental effect on both the relationship with you and the patient's progress. The ideal situation is to create a balance between the patient's need for stability and their continuing interest in life and need for stimulation.

CARING FOR OLDER ADULTS WITH COGNITIVE IMPAIRMENTS

Cognitive impairment in the older adult can take many forms, and it is important that you study them in more depth than is appropriate to address in this book. However, impairment in one particular aspect of an older adult's life, instrumental activities of daily living (IADLs), has been shown to be correlated with the presence of dementia and may be one of the early signs of cognitive changes.[57,58] If there is impairment in one of the following four IADLs, a thorough mental status evaluation should be performed: (1) medication/health management, (2) money/financial management, (3) telephone management/communication device use, and (4) transportation management. We engage you in a general discussion about cognitive impairment and provide some general guidelines for respectful interaction with people with neuropathology that directly affects thought and speech processes.

Acute confusion or disorientation can be caused by a variety of factors, such as an infection, a fluid or electrolyte imbalance, or a cerebral vascular accident. It is important to determine the cause of confusion in an older adult patient and not just ascribe it to "being old." Often, a useful approach is to not support the older person's constantly confused ideas, unless correcting them causes them to become violent, further disoriented, or deeply agitated.

If an old man thinks he is in a hotel, you should try to correct him using a gentle reassuring voice and manner. If he confuses you with someone else, his mistake can be corrected by showing him your name badge and repeating your name. Chances are that he will be less frightened if the people around him are willing to help him clear up his mind, if only for a few minutes. It is a good general rule of respectful interaction to correct the person. However, you should also remember to listen with interest and politeness to the patient. Listening will help you determine the depth of the confusion, ascertain the wisdom of trying to correct it, and, in some cases, discern that the patient is making sense within a context not immediately evident.

Respect requires that the confused person should always be treated kindly. Spoken correction or redirection should never be condescending but rather should reflect the gentle authority that gives the patient a sense of security.

If the confusion is the result of a disease such as Alzheimer's disease or another form of dementia, many of the same principles apply. Some additional strategies for communicating with patients with dementia are as follows: use broad opening statements or questions, try to establish commonalities, speak to them as equals, speak at a normal rate and without exaggerated intonation, eliminate distractions, repeat when necessary and according to whether the listener misunderstood versus forgot what was said, and try to recognize themes in what the patient is trying to share with you.[59]

Sometimes medication can help an agitated patient relax or in other ways be more comfortable, although with older adults it is best to be cautious with the use of medications. Goals must be adapted according to what patients can comprehend. Some patients may be unable to remember the simplest tasks from one testing or treatment period to the next and may never grasp the most elementary verbal instructions. Others, however, will be able to follow astonishingly complex procedures. It is your responsibility and opportunity in such situations to approach each person as an individual and to not take for granted that all confused utterances are signs of organic brain changes. In some cases, the confusion will increase no matter what is done. However, none of these complications should deter you from first attempting, in a kind way, to correct inaccuracies. With a great number of patients, this humane act is the key to respectful interaction.

OPPORTUNITIES IN AGING

While we have spent most of this chapter on the challenges associated with aging, there are of course many benefits to getting older. One author offers this list of the "10 good things about getting older"[60]:

1. I've become less emotional and more thoughtful with my decisions.
2. I no longer sweat the small stuff.
3. I can go shopping for what I need in my favorite store: my basement.
4. I've become kinder to myself.
5. Liking myself.
6. I no longer drool over—or covet—fashion must-haves.
7. I have so many good stories to tell.
8. All my years of living make me sound smart.
9. I no longer need to keep up with the Joneses.
10. It's safe (and fun) to flirt.

In many ways, the list of 10 good things about aging highlights the process oriented or selection, optimization, and compensation view of aging[14] and leverages the resources that come with aging to face challenges. Even the physical signs of aging come with increasing perspective and confidence. As Helen Mirren says: *"The weird thing is, you get more comfortable in yourself, even as time is giving you less reason for it. When you're young and beautiful, you're paranoid and miserable. I think one of the great advantages of getting older is that you let go of certain things."*[61]

Assessing a Patient's Value System

Self-respect is a consciously prized value for older people because they often perceive, correctly, that they are subject to loss of self-respect in an ageist society. The mechanics of adjusting a hearing aid, setting a schedule, or correcting a confused-sounding statement must all be done in a way that supports the older person's value system. Otherwise, the person is reduced to nothing more than an object to be efficiently manipulated. Chapter 1 listed some of the primary societal, cultural, and personal values cherished by people in the United States. Older people as a group can be expected to hold the same range and variety of values; no value can be ruled out automatically based on age. However, the topics treated in this chapter can help you understand why so many older adults adhere to some values more than others.

Security, both financial and physical, may also be highly prized by older adults because, again, for many of them the hold on it is more tenuous. Further, continued independent functioning is valued dearly when transition to an SNF is a threat or when activities that can be performed alone become increasingly limited. Listening for which values the older patient expresses as their most precious and then trying to set treatment goals accordingly will greatly enhance your success. This will also help you understand the patient's (and family member's) experience and expectations and build partnerships for shared decision-making. In working with older people, the most important challenge confronting you is resisting the tendency to stereotype them. Society's expectations of its elders, many of which are inaccurate and outdated, are propagated through literature, television, and other popular media.

REFLECTIONS

Some states have instituted mandatory age-based testing for older drivers. This testing varies from state to state but ranges from vision examinations to on-road assessments.

Your patient is seeing you today for his well visit and states, "I am 75 in a few weeks, so I will have to pass the registry test to keep my license. It's not fair. Not only is that policy ridiculous, it is completely ageist! No one asks those tweeting, cell-phone wielding 20-year-olds to retake their test."

- How might you reply to this patient?
- How do you feel about the issue of age-related mandates?
  In thinking about this topic, consider the link between driving and independence in American society.
- How do limitations in this instrumental activity of daily living support or restrict participation for the older adult?

You can learn to appreciate individual differences among aged persons by increasing your contact with people who are older. Programs sponsored by both private and religious organizations, and the government offer volunteer opportunities ranging from transportation to recreational activities to providing hot meals for homebound persons. In some cities, senior activity centers, assisted living facilities, and other institutions where older persons live or spend considerable time welcome those who are interested in volunteering their services or visiting older people. Whether through volunteer services, organizations, or contact as a health professional, your challenge is to develop an acutely discriminating eye and appreciation for individual differences.

Summary

Care of older adults must be based on a sound understanding of the physiologic and psychosocial aspects of aging. The major developmental tasks of older adulthood are to find integrated meaning and satisfaction with life as it becomes increasingly difficult to keep up with everything that goes on in a quickly changing world. The chief goal of professional care is to maintain and support the patient's self-esteem by affirming their strengths and discovering hidden resources. By keeping in mind older patients' emotional and social needs, you can help them retain dignity and self-respect while being mindful not to overlook physical causes for changes in behaviors or attitudes. Overall, the secret to respectful interaction with older adults is to keep their age-related challenges, characteristics, and changes in mind while also supporting and encouraging their abilities, wisdom, and individuality.

References

1. John Adams as quoted in Wallis CL, ed. *The Treasure Chest: A Heritage Album Containing 1064 Familiar and Inspirational Quotations, Poems, Sentiments, and Prayers From Great Minds of 2500 Years*. New York: Harper and Row Publishers; 1965:12.
2. United States Census Bureau. *Quick Facts United States*. https://www.census.gov/quickfacts/fact/table/US/RHI125219; 2021
3. *US Census*. Demographic turning points for the United States: population projections for 2020 to 2060. https://www.census.gov/content/dam/Census/library/publications/2020/demo/p25-1144.pdf; 2020.
4. Colby SL, Ortman JM. *The Baby Boom Cohort in the United States: 2012 to 2060 Population Estimates and Projections, Current Population Reports*. US Census; 2014. Available at: https://www.census.gov/content/dam/Census/library/publications/2014/demo/p25-1141.pdf.
5. Pinto da Costaa J, Vitorinob R, Silvad GM, et al. A synopsis on aging—theories, mechanisms and future prospects. *Ageing Res Rev*. 2016;29:90–112.
6. Michel P. *Prevention of Chronic Diseases and Age-Related Disability*. Cham: Springer; 2019.
7. Levy SR. Toward reducing ageism: PEACE (positive education about aging and contact experiences) model. *Gerontologist*. 2018;58(2):226–232.
8. Lipsky M, King M. Biological theories of aging. *Dis Mon*. 2015;61:460–466.
9. *Project Implicit*. Retrieved from: https://implicit.harvard.edu/implicit/.
10. Hasworth S, Cannon M. Social theories of aging: a review. *Dis Mon [Serial Online]*. 2015;61:475–479.
11. Brothers A, Diehl M. Feasibility and efficacy of the aging plus program: changing views on aging to increase physical activity. *J Aging Phys Act [Serial Online]*. 2017;25(3):402–411. Available from MEDLINE Complete, Ipswich, MA.
12. Wernher I, Lipsky M. Psychological theories of aging. *Dis Mon [Serial Online]*. 2015;61:480–488.
13. *World Health Organization*. Ageing: healthy ageing and functional ability. https://www.who.int/western-pacific/news/q-a-detail/ageing-healthy-ageing-and-functional-ability; 2020.
14. Villar F. Successful ageing and development: the contribution of generativity in older age. *Ageing Soc*. 2012;32(7):1087.
15. Erikson EH. *Childhood and Society*. 2nd ed. New York: WW Norton; 1963.
16. National Prevention Council. *Healthy Aging in Action*. Washington, DC: U.S. Department of Health and Human Services, Office of the Surgeon General; 2016.
17. Braveman P, Gottlieb L. The social determinants of health: it's time to consider the causes of the causes. *Public Health Rep*. 2014;129(1_suppl2):19–31.
18. Ferlander S. The importance of different forms of social capital for health. *Acta Sociol*. 2007;50(2):115–128. https://doi.org/10.1177/0001699307077654.
19. Fraser T, Aldrich DP, Page-Tan C. Bowling alone or distancing together? The role of social capital in excess death rates from COVID19. *Soc Sci Med*. 2021;284:114241. https://doi.org/10.1016/j.socscimed.2021.114241.
20. *Centers for Disease Control and Prevention*. COVID-19 mortality overview. https://www.cdc.gov/nchs/covid19/mortality-overview.htm; 2021.
21. Wu B. Social isolation and loneliness among older adults in the context of COVID-19: a global challenge. *Global Health Res Policy*. 2020;5(1):1–3.
22. *US Bureau of Labor Statistics*. National longitudinal surveys frequently asked questions. https://www.bls.gov/nls/questions-and-answers.htm; 2021.
23. Brossie N, Chop W. Social gerontology. In: Robnett RH, Chop WC, eds. *Gerontology for the Health Care Professional*. 3rd ed. Burlington, MA: Jones & Bartlett Learning; 2015:17–50.
24. Blieszner R, Ogletree AM. We get by with a little help from our friends. *J Am Soc Aging*. 2017;41(2):55–62.
25. Chen Y, Feeley TH. Social support, social strain, loneliness, and well-being among older adults: an analysis of the health and retirement study. *J Soc Pers Relatsh*. 2014;31(2):141–161.
26. Hand C, Retrum J, Ware G, et al. Understanding social isolation among urban aging adults: informing occupation-based approaches. *Occup Ther J Res*. 2017;37(4):188–198.
27. Muennig P, Jiao B, Singer E. Living with parents or grandparents increases social capital and survival: 2014 General Social Survey-National Death Index. *SSM Popul Health*. 2017;4:71–75. https://doi.org/10.1016/j.ssmph.2017.11.001.
28. Wren AM. Homecoming. *Afr Am Rev*. 1993;27(1):157.

29. Marty ME. The "God-forbid" wing: in a world without easy remedies, who takes care of Dad? *Park Ridge Center Bull.* 1999;11(15).

30. *World Health Organization.* World Health Organization elder abuse key facts. https://www.who.int/news-room/fact-sheets/detail/elder-abuse; 2021.

31. Patel K, Bunachita S, Chiu H, Suresh P, Patel UK. Elder abuse: a comprehensive overview and physician-associated challenges. *Cureus.* 2021;13(4).

32. *National Center on Elder Abuse.* Types of abuse. https://ncea.acl.gov/Suspect-Abuse/Abuse-Types.aspx; n.d.

33. *National Center on Elder Abuse.* Reporting abuse. https://ncea.acl.gov/Suspect-Abuse/Reporting-Abuse.aspx.; n.d.

34. Evans IE, Llewellyn DJ, Matthews FE, et al. Living alone and cognitive function in later life. *Arch Gerontol Geriatr.* 2019;81:222–233.

35. *Centers for Disease Control and Prevention.* Healthy places. https://www.cdc.gov/healthyplaces/terminology.htm; 2009.

36. Tobin S, Lieberman M. *Last home for the aged.* San Francisco, CA: Jossey-Bass; 1976.

37. Jolanki OH. Senior housing as a living environment that support well-being in old age. *Front Public Health.* 2021;8:914.

38. Jeste DV, Blazer I, Feather J, et al. Age-friendly communities initiative: public health approach to promoting successful aging. *Am J Geriatr Psychiatry [serial online].* 2016;24:1158–1170.

39. Van Rensbergen G, Nawrot T. Medical conditions of nursing home admissions. *BMC Geriatr.* 2010;10(46).

40. *US Census Bureau.* New 2020 census results show group quarters population increased since 2010. https://www.census.gov/library/stories/2021/08/united-states-group-quarters-in-2020-census.html; 2021.

41. Applebaum R, Mehdizadeh S, Berish D. It is not your parents' long-term services system: nursing homes in a changing world. *J Appl Gerontol.* 2020;39(8):898–901. https://doi.org/10.1177/0733464818818050.

42. *U.S. Department of Health and Human Services. Centers for Disease Control and Prevention. National Center for Health Statistics. National Vital Statistics System.* https://www.cdc.gov/nchs/data/vsrr/VSRR10-508.pdf; 2021.

43. *Robert Wood Johnson Foundation.* Overcoming obstacles to health. https://www.rwjf.org/en/library/research/2008/02/overcoming-obstacles-to-health.html; 2008.

44. Reid J. *Three Jokes That Made Tina Fey and Amy Poehler Golden Globe Legends;* 2021. Retrieved from: https://www.primetimer.com/features/three-jokes-that-made-tina-fey-and-amy-poehler-golden-globe-legends.

45. Konish L. *This is the Age When Americans Say They Plan to Retire;* 2021. Retrieved from: https://www.cnbc.com/2021/09/15/this-is-age-when-americans-say-they-plan-to-retire.html.

46. Jonsson H, Kielhofner G, Borell L. Anticipating retirement: the formation of narrative concerning an occupational transition. *Am J Occup Ther.* 1997;51(1):49–56.

47. Vaillant GE. *Aging Well: Surprising Guideposts to a Happier Life From the Landmark Harvard Study of Adult Development.* Boston, MA: Little, Brown; 2002.

48. Turner JA, Klein BW, Sorrentino C. Making volunteer work visible: supplementary measures of work in labor force statistics. *Mon Labor Rev.* 2020:1–20. Retrieved from https://www.bls.gov/opub/mlr/2020/article/making-volunteer-work-visible-supplementary-measures-of-work-in-labor-force-statistics.htm.

49. Moen P. Reconstructing retirement: careers, couples, and social capital. *Contemp Gerontol J Rev Crit Discuss.* 1998;4(4):123–125.

50. Fried LP, Carlson MC, Freedman M, et al. A social model for health promotion for an aging population: initial evidence on the experience corps model. *J Urban Health.* 2004;81(1):64–78.

51. Yuen HK, Huang P, Burik JK, et al. Impact of participating in volunteer activities for residents living in long-term-care facilities. *Am J Occup Ther.* 2008;62:71–76.

52. Gill TH, Guralnik JM, Pahor M, et al. Effect of structured physical activity on overall burden and transitions between states of major mobility disability in older persons. *Ann Internal Med.* 2016;165:833–840.

53. McGrath RP, Ottenbacher KJ, Vincent BM, Kraemer WJ, Peterson MD. Muscle weakness and functional limitations in an ethnically diverse sample of older adults. *Ethn Health.* 2020;25(3):342–353.

54. Chu D, Fox KR, Chen L, et al. Components of late-life exercise and cognitive function: an 8-year longitudinal study. *Prevent Sci.* 2015;16(4):568–577.

55. Robnett RH, Chop WC. *Gerontology for the Health Care Professional.* 4th ed. Burlington, MA: Jones & Barlett Learning; 2018.

56. Son JS, Nimrod G, West ST, Janke MC, Liechty T, Naar JJ, Julie S. Promoting older adults' physical activity and social well-being during COVID-19. *Leis Sci.* 2021;43(1-2):287–294.

57. Cornelis E, Gorus E, Beyer I, et al. Early diagnosis of mild cognitive impairment and mild dementia through basic and instrumental activities of daily living: development of a new evaluation tool. *PLoS Med.* 2017;14(3):1–22.

58. Marshall GA, Rentz DM, Frey MT, et al. Executive function and instrumental activities of daily living in MCI and AD. *Alzheimers Dement.* 2011;7(3):300–308.

59. Small J, Perry JA. Training family care partners to communicate effectively with persons with Alzheimer's disease: the TRACED program. *Can J Speech-Language Pathol Audiol.* 2012;36(4):332–350.

60. Rosas A. *10 Good Things About Getting Older,* 2015. Retrieved from: https://www.aarp.org/health/healthy-living/info-2017/10-good-things-about-getting-older.html.

61. Patterson C. *Helen Mirren Guardian Shows Women Can Age Beautifully But We Shouldn't Have To,* 2014. Retrieved from: https://www.theguardian.com/commentisfree/2014/oct/29/helen-mirren-women-age-beautifully-tv-bosses#:~:text=When%20you're%20young%20and,re%20older%20and%20it's%20ironic.%E2%80%9D.

Some Special Challenges: Creating a Context of Respect

Introduction

In this section of the book, we explore two types of special challenges we think warrant your attention. Chapter 14 addresses relevant considerations you will want to bear in mind while working with patients who are dying and with their loved ones. Patients and their families almost always show evidence of the disruption life-limiting illness has on their present lives and future dreams. The news also may bring challenges, unleash new hopes, and expose unexercised strengths during this time. You have an opportunity to examine these issues and how they affect patients and their families. You will learn about priorities that you as a health professional can set for such patients, their families, and yourself to show them respect at end of life.

In Chapter 15, we examine select situations that health professionals sometimes identify as difficult. In this chapter, our goal is for you to think expansively about your potential for respectful interaction when you encounter complex patients and situations. Example situations include caring for patients with a history of violent behavior and supporting members of the interprofessional care team who make errors in care delivery. Regardless of the situation, effective communication is essential to health care delivery; therefore we summarize key evidence-based guidelines that will help you show respect in difficult conversations. Our hope is that these will serve as guideposts throughout your career, providing an opportunity to both optimize patient care outcomes and cope with the emotions that result from difficult conversations.

CHAPTER 14

Respectful Interaction: When the Patient Is Dying

Prelude

My holocaust survivor of a patient who lost everyone he loved in the death camps must die alone. I am unable to get a priest to offer anointing and sacrament of the sick—instead it is completed over Face Time. The wife of a patient sobbed to me that she hasn't seen her husband in 6 weeks while he was hospitalized with COVID-19—and that's the longest they've been apart in 65 years of marriage. And now he's unresponsive.

KRIS M.[1]

Of all the challenges you will face, your work with people with life-limiting illness will provide some of the most challenging moments in your career and the greatest opportunities to use your skills of communication and collaboration in health care delivery. The speaker in the prelude to this chapter is a nurse working with COVID-19 patients in an intensive care unit, but she could be any kind of health professional in almost any hospital in the United States working with these critically ill patients over the past several years. The underlying distress that she is expressing is that patients died, and perhaps still are dying, in ways that were clearly not the sort of death most people would choose—isolated and separated from family and the rituals that accompany dying. Beyond the unique barriers that COVID-19 created in the care of the dying, another challenge is the confusing terminology surrounding death and dying.

Even with the simplest of terms, such as the word "dying," there can be different understandings. Thus it is helpful to start with clarification of some commonly used terms when referring to patients with a life-limiting illness or injury. *Terminally ill* is a term that is commonly seen in the literature to describe people who are dying. Persons who suffer from a degenerative illness may live for many months or years. Another person with a different condition may die within days or weeks. Still, both fall under the heading of terminally ill.

Like all labels, it allows people in this group to be identified according to their needs. At the same time, we refrain from using it in this chapter. One difficulty with the term is its generality. Thus we use the term *life-limiting illness* to indicate that the patient, and those who care for them, have good reason to believe that the present illness or injury will limit the patient's life, leaving the time frame open to the various trajectories of dying. Lynn and Adamson originally developed a model of the dying trajectory of elderly patients to allow time to plan and deliver the appropriate type of care and for advance planning or adjustment for imminent death if that is the case.[2] For example, the course of illness for three prototypical trajectories near the end of life are as follows:

- a sudden death from an unexpected cause (such as motor vehicle accident, myocardial infarction, or stroke);
- a steady decline from a progressive disease with a terminal phase (such as cancer); and
- an advanced illness marked by slow decline with periodic crises and eventual sudden death (such as chronic lung disease or congestive heart failure).[3]

During the COVID-19 pandemic, health professionals initially had little experience with the illness trajectory of this novel virus. As more and more people died from COVID-19, patterns emerged not only regarding the signs and symptoms of imminent death but also how supportive care was delivered to dying patients such as the practice of using speaker functions on phones to allow families to say good-bye to critically ill loved ones or chaplains using video chat functions on iPads to deliver their last rites from a distance as mentioned in the prelude to this chapter.[4]

The reverse problem—that is, not recognizing the trajectory of an illness—is also true. Some diagnoses resist the label of a life-limiting illness such as Alzheimer's disease in its later stages. Many health professionals, patients, and family members view Alzheimer's disease as a chronic, degenerative illness that progresses over many years, which in fact is generally the case. However, by not recognizing the life-limiting aspects of later stages of Alzheimer's disease, patients and families are far less likely to reap the benefits of care afforded to the dying. As with all types of patients, the key is to look for the distinguishing factors that make this person's situation unique and respond respectfully to the needs that arise out of that individual person's experience. Overall, patients with advanced illness who are approaching the end of life "… are entitled to access to high-quality, compassionate, evidence-based care, consistent with their wishes, that can reasonably be expected to protect or improve the quality and length of their life. Ensuring that access and delivering that care humanely and respectfully is a central clinical and ethical obligation of health care professionals and systems."[3] Toward achieving these goals, a first step in any health professional's understanding of a patient's situation is to gain some general idea of how the dying process and death are viewed within the larger society.

Dying and Death in Contemporary Society

Dying is first and foremost a personal experience. However, there are some general ideas about what a "good death" means such as adequate pain management, being with loved ones and having time to say one's good-byes, not leaving financial burdens or the burden of difficult decisions regarding life-sustaining treatments and exercising choice over where to die.[3,4]

All persons share some awareness that the end of the dying process is the death event. What does this mean to a person? In the minds of some patients or their families, a known diagnosis and somewhat predictable range of symptoms make them feel robbed of the "natural" flow of life. The dying process may feel unnatural, an imposition.

A life-limiting condition generates new fears and concerns. Fortunately, for others, it is also an opportunity to conduct long-neglected business, put one's affairs in order, or pursue a postponed adventure. Anticipation of the death event, too, creates its own concerns, fears, and hopes. For most people, death remains perhaps the ultimate mystery. An understanding of the connection between the dying process and the end point of death are essential for health professionals as they care for patients with life-limiting illnesses. The next section explores various understandings of the dying process.

Dying as a Process

In most cultures, stories are passed down from one generation to the next that inform our understanding of death. Today, mythic or other types of origin stories coexist with scientific understanding of the dying process. Of course, not all cultures or even those who exist within a particular culture have the same understanding of life and death. Consider how your relationship with a patient could be affected by differing beliefs about the existence of an after-life.

In today's rich diversity of patients an essential step in creating a therapeutic relationship based on care is to try to gain some understanding of dying as a process to be viewed apart from death itself. This provides a starting place for further deliberation about how to respect what a patient or family says, how they behave, and what their attitudes are toward various aspects of their interaction with you and others during the dying process. In addition to paying attention to cultural and social understandings of the dying process and death, it is important to realize that there is also confusion about what it means for a patient to be dead because of different clinical measures to determine death. In 1981 the President's Commission for the Study of Ethical Problems in Medicine and Biomedical and Behavioral Research reinforced the concept of brain death originally proposed more than 50 years ago in 1968 by an ad hoc committee at Harvard Medical School, that is, a person who is dead is: "An individual who has sustained either (1) irreversible cessation of circulatory and respiratory functions or (2) irreversible cessation of all functions of the entire brain, including the brain stem, is dead. A determination of death must be made in accordance with accepted medical standards."[5] The National Conference of Commissioners on Uniform State Laws adopted this two-pronged definition of death (Uniform Determination of Death Act) and health officials at the state level across the country worked to get this definition passed into statute. This definition was approved by the American Medical Association in 1980 and by the American Bar Association in 1981.

Although this definition of death is widely adopted in the United States, there is still no uniform legal definition of death. There are practical reasons for standardizing scientific criteria for determining death in the law, "so that one is dead regardless of the jurisdiction in which one has resided, or to which one has traveled."[6] Furthermore, "knowing when an individual is dead is, of course, important for many social functions: when a spouse becomes a widower, when life insurance has to pay claims, when health insurance does not have to pay claims, and so on. It is also critical to know when someone has died in order to procure organs for transplantation..."[6]

Recently, there has been considerable debate regarding the distinctions between these two sets of physiological criteria for determining death with most of the controversy surrounding death of the brain. The "brain-death" criteria remain confusing to medical personnel, families, and philosophers.[7] New controversies surrounding brain-death have appeared such as:

> ... whether there is a right to refuse apnea testing (a test to determine if a patient can breathe without the support of a ventilator), which set of criteria should be used to measure the death of the brain, how the problem of erroneous testing should be handled, whether any of the current criteria sets accurately measures the death of the brain, whether standard criteria include measurements of all brain function, and how minorities who reject whole-brain-based definitions should be accommodated.[8]

It appears that the issue of establishing a uniform definition of death is far from settled and continues to raise vexing questions for health professionals, patients, and families.[9]

Denial of Mortality

It is often said that Western societies are death denying. What can that possibly mean when all around us people are dying every day from illness, accidents, violence, old age, war, and other causes? Probably the best explanation is that although there is evidence everywhere of our mortality, we do our best to hold the inevitable at arm's length.

In many parts of Western culture, the treatment of the dead body is one expression of a need to deny death its power. The dead body is painted and dressed to make it appear alive, although a sign of life, such as a sigh or fluttering eyelash, would cause most people to rush screaming from the room. For the most part, however, denial has simply become subtler. For example, a subtle denial that death is the end of the dying process is manifested in the incredible scenes of violence and killing viewed in films and on television in dramas, cartoons, and the news. The highly popular novels, television shows, and films about the "undead"—that is, vampires and zombies—are another indication of the fascination mainstream American culture holds with death and its denial. Distancing that keeps death at arm's length for as long as possible even during one's dying process is another method of denying the finality of death. This attempt to stave off the inevitable is also experienced by loved ones and poignantly is conveyed in the following quote from a 51-year-old woman who learned that her best friend was dying of cancer:

> *Before one enters this spectrum of sorrow, which changes even the color of trees, there is a blind and daringly wrong assumption that probably allows us to blunder through the days. There is a way one thinks that the show will never end—or the loss, when it comes, will be toward the end of the road, not in its middle . . ..*[9]

At the same time, the health care team can be helpful in assisting both patients and loved ones not to become stuck in prolonged denial, such as happened in the following:

> *My husband, John, age 55, was handed his diagnosis of liver cancer by a newly graduated doctor—John's own had just retired. "As I'm sure you know," the young man had blushingly begun, and John said simply, "Yes." We walked out of the office holding hands and cold to the marrow.*
>
> *Near the end, I started looking for signs that the inevitable would not be inevitable. I watched a few leaves that refused to give up their green to the season. I took comfort in the way the sun shone brightly on a day they predicted rain—not a cloud in the sky! I even tried to formulate messages of hope in arrangements of coins on the dresser top—look how they had landed all heads up... what were the odds? I prayed, too, in a way that agnostics do at such times. Sorry I doubted you "dear God, help us now."*[10]

REFLECTIONS

- What, if anything, do you think the doctor or other members of the health care team could have done at the outset to help set this bereaving wife on a different course or later as her spouse's life-limiting illness grew increasingly evident?
- Think back to Chapter 7 and review the content on enduring uncertainties and re-valuing significant relationships that accompany life-limiting illness. How would better appreciation of these aspects of the couple's situation helped the health care professionals involved care for them?
- Reflect on your own experiences with death and dying. How might those inform your work as a health professional, positively or negatively?

Denial mechanisms are so widespread in almost all Western societies that we gave special attention to it here, but, obviously, there are other considerations and responses to dying and death that we turn your attention to now.

Responses to Dying and Death

Individual responses to a life-limiting diagnosis are influenced by a variety of factors, including age, life experiences, religion, and culture. Death may be a commonplace occurrence to one person who lives in a neighborhood with high levels of violent crime and sudden deaths. For other people, death might be such a rare occurrence that they do not experience a death until their young adulthood. Even with a wide range of experience with death, most people generally dread the thought of gradual and certain loss. The news of a life-limiting diagnosis, for oneself or a loved one, is almost always disquieting. In this chapter, you have an opportunity to think about what your own and your patients' possible responses to dying and loss are and the challenges to which this inevitable part of life gives rise.

Common Stresses and Challenges Demanding Response

What would be your biggest challenges if you learned that you were dying? Most people can vaguely imagine and project what they would dread most; once the diagnosis is made, however, the reality of their specific situation intrudes. Then a patient's previous notions about a disease or injury and the known experiences of others who have had it combine to create a vivid picture of what the patient believes to be ahead. The following are some of the most commonly expressed concerns about death and dying.

ANTICIPATION OR FEAR OF FUTURE ISOLATION

Separation from the routine and regularity of life and familiar faces can have a disorienting effect on many people as noted by the wife of the patient in the prelude to this chapter. Often a prolonged dying process involves a gradual loss of function, habits, acceptance by others, and familial, social, and societal roles. Some patients may experience overwhelming grief regarding these losses sometimes defined as *anticipatory grief* that includes "... the mourning, coping, planning and psychological reorganization that are stimulated... in response to the awareness of impending loss."[11]

The fear of separation from the familiarity of home and routine as a way of ordering one's life becomes a reality for many. At the heart for most is a deeper fear of abandonment by loved ones and caregivers. Anxiety about this may be expressed in comments such as "They are starting to ignore me"; "My family is busy with other things"; and "They spend more time with the woman in the next room, but of course they know I'm dying." Many persons are aware of the practice of being admitted to the hospital to die or of having to spend the final period of their lives in a care facility, and some contribute to their isolation by rejecting visitors. During the COVID-19 pandemic, families were generally not allowed to visit dying relatives in the hospital. Although family members were not voluntarily withdrawing from loved ones, the absence of loved ones at such a critical time was deeply felt by patients, families, and health professionals alike. Rethinking the necessity of visiting restrictions aimed to protect the public were re-evaluated as vaccinations became available.[12]

You can "treat" (allay) the patient's fears of isolation by your own presence. You cannot always ensure patients that their loved ones will not voluntarily leave them when the going gets rough, because sometimes families or friends do withdraw from the person. Observing this tapering from supportive relationships is often trying for you, let alone the patient. Relationships are bound to be altered during this time; some friends and relatives disappear because of indifference, despair, pain, or exhaustion, and those who do not become more cherished.

PROSPECT OF PAIN AND OTHER SYMPTOMS

Those who have known others who experienced a painful end to life cannot be sure that their own dying will not be equally distressful or worse. Recall that one of the core elements of a "good death" includes control of pain and other symptoms.[13] Fortunately, assessment of physical, emotional, and spiritual pain has advanced in modern health care delivery. In the late 90s, pain was declared the fifth vital sign along with temperature, pulse, respirations, and blood pressure measurements.[14] Thus there is a great deal more attention paid to the quality of assessing and managing pain whether chronic or acute. Modern modes of health care intervention for pain today take a holistic approach to the physical pain of dying, though it is still a challenge in some settings to get positive pain relief.

Other symptoms can be equally distressing such as *dyspnea*, the subjective experience of breathing discomfort, which is one of the most common symptoms experienced by critically ill patients.[15] Other symptoms or health issues such as constipation, oral ulcers, or discomfort from wounds or skin breakdown should be addressed with appropriate therapy and preventive measures whenever possible so that they do not add to the patient's suffering at end of life.[16]

Anxiety and depression can have a heightened effect on pain and other symptoms whereas distraction and feelings of security tend to diminish the suffering associated with pain. Therefore the patient's suffering may be decreased by your reassurance, presence, compassion, and caring, as discussed in Chapter 2 and elsewhere. However, remember to take individual patient's preferences into account as personal notions of a good death and symptom management are individualized.

RESISTANCE TO DEPENDENCE

Real or feared loss of independence during illness or injury is often a challenge. The extensive literature in end-of-life care supports that patients fear loss of autonomy and loss of dignity. They are concerned about pain management, inability to control bodily functions, and worry about placing undue burden on family or caregivers. Continued independence within whatever sphere of decision-making a person can exercise when in the dying process usually remains a high priority. Proof that they have thought about this is shown in their expressions of astonishment at having reached a point in their symptoms they had previously believed would be totally unbearable. Indeed, everyone has ideas beforehand of what he or she believes to be the "outer limits" of what one could bear: loss of bowel and bladder control; sexual impotence; inability to feed oneself, to communicate verbally, or to think straight; unconsciousness; or other loss. Often (though not always), patients' acceptance changes after a period of fighting and grieving the specific loss. In other words, patients can adapt to the "new normal" in the dying process.

Patients' experiences of real or imagined isolation, pain, and increasing dependence are basic, but there are other concerns as well, such as the dread of suffocation and the fear that one's loved ones will not be adequately provided for. A person who dies suddenly in a car accident or plane crash or from a myocardial infarction may have long harbored these fears but did not have a period of prolonged illness during which these concerns surfaced. Those who have time to anticipate their death must find a way of dealing with these fears and concerns. One common way to encourage patient's think about the type of care they would like to receive is to engage in *advance care planning*. Such planning includes:

The whole process of discussion of end-of-life care, clarification of related values and goals, and embodiment preferences through written documents and medical orders. This process can start anytime and be revisited periodically, but it becomes more focused as health status changes.

Ideally, these conversations (1) occur with a person's health care agent and primary clinician, along with other members of the health care team; (2) are recorded and updated as needed; and (3) allow for flexible decision making in the context of the patient's current medical situation.[3]

The "recorded conversations" mentioned in #2 above refer to advance directive documents such as a living will and the appointment of a health care agent that indicate the patient's wishes about end-of-life care. You can access free advance directive forms through various websites. Some websites even provide a link to information for a specific state as laws regarding advance directives vary state-to-state (aarp.org/caregiving/financial-legal/freeprintableadvancedirectives). There are also tools that encourage discussion about a wider range of goals for end-of-life care. For example, Five Wishes is a guide developed by an association of physicians, nurses, and lawyers and is recognized as a legal document in 40 states and the District of Columbia.[17] Five Wishes allows patients to explore and determine (1) who they wish to make decisions for them (i.e., a health care proxy or surrogate), (2) what medical treatment(s) they wish to receive or deny, (3) what will make them comfortable at the end of life, (4) how they wish to be treated by loved ones and care providers, and (5) what they want to share with others as they near the end of life.[17]

You can be instrumental in making suggestions to help patients carry out their wishes if you get a hint that they desire to do so by offering advice about accessing planning tools and templates that are freely available on the Internet from health care organizations and professional associations. In so doing, you are also assisting the patient's family so that they do not have to bear the unexpected burden of responsibility for making decisions about medical, financial, and funeral choices that occur when end-of-life planning is not completed.[18]

In summary, during their dying process, people must rely on their own best inner resources and the support of family, friends, and health professionals to sustain them as they face their challenges. Any hesitance, embarrassment, or disdain you show when a person expresses a concern, even one that seems unfounded to you, will exacerbate the suffering associated with it.

Reckoning With What Death Might Mean

Different cultures and individuals treat the moment of transition from alive to dead differently, but for many, it is not something to relish. What is the range of expressions about what will happen when death comes? Often as death nears, people turn to religion and ritual to facilitate their final passing. "Death and dying often draw out profound questions of spirituality, even among those who would not normally consider these questions."[19] Reflect on the content in Chapter 4 as all forms of religious experience are influenced by a person's cultural, familial, and ethnic backgrounds meaning beliefs about death and rituals such as prayer may be shaped and interpreted by the patient.

Many people believe that after this life, there is something else. The varieties of religious or philosophical beliefs are many, regarding the relationship of this life to the next. Predominant beliefs in many religions, especially but by no means only those associated with Eastern religions such as Hinduism, propose that "death" is a process of birth and rebirth (e.g., reincarnation). The last step is not extinction but perfection, at which time one is absorbed into a "place" or into a "being" in which complete unity of all beings is realized. Depending on the religion, the type of being one will become after physical death, and the opportunity for the final step into ultimate unity may or may not depend on the type of life one lived on earth during an embodied human lifetime. In Islam, one may be transported through several levels of paradise depending on the type of life one has lived.

Some people believe in the resurrection of souls only, whereas others believe that the actual human body will be restored, usually in an improved form. There is one version of a literal, sudden bodily resurrection (sometimes referred to as the "rapture") in which those—both dead and still

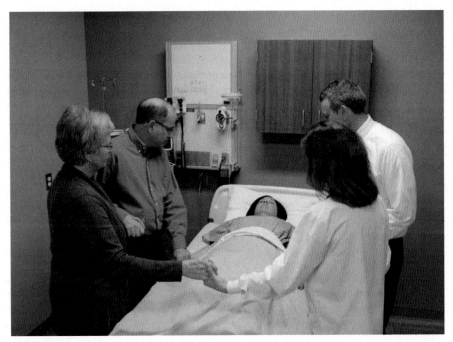

Fig. 14.1   Patients and families often engage in rituals during the dying process. Courtesy Maren Haddad.

living—who have lived holy lives will be immediately transported to heaven, whereas others will be left behind forever to suffer the consequences of their sins. Other Christians have different versions of what it means to be "resurrected," although all share this basic belief.

You will meet individuals who talk with anticipation about "going to meet the Lord," whereas others are sure their lives will not meet the standards of acceptability and they will be consigned to suffering of some kind. Knowing that any of these beliefs about immortality may influence the way an individual interprets the impact and meaning of their own impending death, you can be better prepared for comments from patients or for rituals a patient and family engage in during the dying process (Fig. 14.1). However, a significant number of people today do not view death as a precursor of immortality in any form. You must be prepared to interact in a respectful way with patients and family members (who may not hold the same beliefs as the patient) who have very different ideas about what happens, if anything, after death.

REFLECTIONS

Before proceeding, think about conversations you may have had with patients or others who hold different positions than yours about what happens after death.
- Which beliefs do you hold, if any?
- How might your beliefs influence your approach to patients who are dying?
- How would you respond to a patient who holds different beliefs than yours about what happens after death? How could you be affirming or comforting?

These concepts about death can help you understand patients and their families when they share their feelings and ideas about death and how to prepare for it. However, many health professionals feel ill-equipped and shy about discussing spiritual or religious beliefs with patients and their families. Providing spiritual care requires self-reflection on one's spiritual beliefs, self-awareness, introspection, and recognition of one's own vulnerability.[20] It is likely that ongoing personal development is necessary to become comfortable in addressing spiritual care needs with patients. When you can enter such sensitive conversations with equanimity and express genuine interest in what the person wants or needs to say about death and their spiritual beliefs, you will be showing respect for that person. When meeting a patient's spiritual needs go beyond routine care and support, it is essential to refer patients and families to trained spiritual care providers.

Coping Responses by Patients

Although denial is initially a common coping response, the concerns associated with dying and the death event usually become more sharply focused over time, and you can anticipate other emotional–psychological responses as well. For many, the first response is acute shock or disbelief. Coping also may take many other forms, such as periods of depression, anger, and hostility, bargaining behavior, or acceptance.[21] Patients who undergo a long process of dying are likely to feel all of them from time to time and many times over. On one day, a woman denies her impending death; on another, she makes secret bargains with God about how long she will live; on the following days, she feels the relief of acceptance followed by a deep depression, and so on. Although the danger with any such framework is that you or your colleagues may tend to pigeonhole a patient according to the categories provided, we have found them to be a useful general set of benchmarks for thinking about what a patient is experiencing.

The patient's basic personality structure is an important factor in determining which kinds of responses will predominate, too. How each person deals with stress and copes is different. "Most people rely more heavily on one or two things. No style is right or wrong, however some coping styles may be more or less effective in particular life situations."[22]

To further prepare yourself for working with patients with different cultural and religious beliefs from your own, we suggest you pause here to engage in a reflection on your own life.

REFLECTIONS

Try to think about how you respond to stressful situations in your life.
- Can you imagine what you might be like as a patient or family member faced with the challenge of a dying loved one?
- If you have, in fact, had to face it, try to recall your major types of responses.
- Which of your responses were most productive? Least productive?

Narrative reflection is a resource many use to process the dying experience and cope with end of life. As mentioned in Chapter 6, the writings of novelists, poets, memoirists, and others can be a useful tool for patients and families. Many have recorded their experiences in this powerful period of life, and it is to your advantage to avail yourself of these narrative accounts in preparation for your professional encounters with people who are dying.

Coping Responses by the Patient's Family

The best and worst aspects of family relationships are exposed when a family member is gravely ill or dying. You will witness a range of behaviors from the most intimate, loving characteristics of family relationships to complicated, lifelong destructive patterns. Regardless of the familial response, the interprofessional care team must recognize the family as essential participants in the death and dying process. Although each families' situation is unique, the great majority of families are brought closer together by an end-of-life experience, and their mutual support during this time is touching to observe. If the patient has not yet been told of the life-limiting nature of the condition, family members may whisper to you in doorways, trying to involve you in elaborate schemes to ensure continued deception. At times, you may feel torn as to who needs your expertise and support more, the patient or the family member. At the busiest time of day, they may stop you to tell you something, only to burst into tears. You may wonder, why is it important for them to be there? One reason could be that it allows them to cope more effectively with their own stresses and make sense of what is happening in their lives.

Families cope with uncertainty, stress, and anxiety when caring for a person with a life-limiting illness in various ways. Some family members pull back and try to get some distance. Others want to get closer to the patient and more involved. Some family members try to maintain control by planning. Still, others become overly optimistic.[22] We include these examples of different coping styles here to help you to understand your own coping mechanisms and those of the people under your care.

Symptoms of acute grief may take the forms of a tendency to sigh, complaints of chronic weakness or exhaustion, and loss of appetite or nausea. In addition, a family member may be preoccupied with what a person looks like, express guilt or hostility, and change their usual patterns of conduct. Except in extreme situations, family members are so integral to the ongoing life and preferences of the patient that the patient feels lost without this support. They can be an essential element of communication for and about the loved one. Recall also, as noted in Chapter 7, that the definition of family has been broadened to include others beyond kin or legal spouses/partners who are significant in the life of a patient.

In many instances, patients and families will need the expertise of key members of the interprofessional care team such as social workers, counselors, and chaplains to help them make important decisions in this unique moment of their lives. Your willingness to access and collaborate effectively with these colleagues can extend your own effectiveness considerably.

Coping Responses by Health Professionals

Health professionals cope with death on a more frequent basis than those outside of health care. Experiences in caring for dying patients are not always negative but may contain positive experiences that involve creating close bonds with a patient, feeling satisfied that good care was provided, working with members of the hospice team, being prepared and good communication.[23] Negative experiences include family discord, challenging care, and feeling helpless in the face of patient suffering.[23] Clinical inexperience can have a profound influence on a health professional's ability to provide quality care to dying patients. For example, it is hard for novice health professionals to watch the physical deterioration that accompanies a life-limiting illness. Also, symptom control for dying patients differs from standard treatment in delivery, dosing, etc. Therefore opportunities to learn about effective symptom control and comfort measures for patients who are dying should be sought out from experienced health professionals especially those with expertise in palliative care and hospice.

Health professionals react to a patient's death in a variety of ways, some healthy, some unhealthy. Positive coping mechanisms of health professionals as they faced dying patients were sorely tested during the COVID-19 pandemic. Some coping strategies that were helpful to health professionals were to strive for effective communication especially with the interprofessional team, learn from experience in dealing with dying patients including collaborating with patients and families to reduce the moral burden of decision-making regarding care, share experiences and emotions with colleagues, and take breaks from intensive care delivery when possible.[24]

Information Sharing: What, When, and How

In addition to your role as one who respects the patient and family through listening and responding caringly to them, two additional priorities are appropriate when a patient is dying. They include information sharing and helping patients balance hope with reality. What types of information do patients and families need to know? Start with the patient's diagnosis and prognosis. The key is for the entire interprofessional care team to be attentive and ready to communicate those things they each have a right to, and are ready to, know. For the most part, modern medical policies and practices support the position that patients have a right to information about their health status. There is also a conviction that the duty not to harm is best realized by disclosure—the truth "sets free." Thus the emphasis on involving the patient and those they deem appropriate into the shared planning of goals is especially important in the dying process.

The value of openness and shared decision-making is by no means shared universally. At the very least, you can be attentive to clues you are receiving from the patient and family as to whether directly sharing this information with the patient is a culturally informed way for members of the health care team to proceed.

Whatever combination of considerations make up the interprofessional care team's decisions, most are now telling patients with life-limiting conditions their diagnoses, usually in direct terms with emphasis on keeping communication channels open after the initial discussion.[25] In the end, there is no substitute for personalized, sensitive communication by all members of the interprofessional care team, initially and throughout the patient's course of interaction with them.

REFLECTIONS

- Do you think you would want to be told the news that you have a life-limiting condition that the physicians have just discovered? If yes, try to imagine the physical setting, people you would hope were (or were not) present, and key points you would want to know in this initial exchange.
- What would you like to have happen to you over the course of your dying that would most help you feel that you were being treated with respect from the start?
- What (if any) role would health professionals play in this process?

Seldom will it be within the boundaries of your role to personally shoulder the sole responsibility of a life-limiting diagnosis. Typically, the interprofessional care team will discuss and plan for the time to speak to a patient about the diagnosis, prognosis, and goals of care. As part of that team, you should listen to the patient's story with focused attentiveness. Your attention to patient and family questions will provide some relief to their anxieties because it will show that you care and respect even their most unusual concerns. It also conveys your willingness to keep communication channels open. Using language and words the patient understands is imperative. Without this translation from medical/clinical terminology to everyday language, nothing will make sense in the conversation.

Talking with a patient and family about a life-limiting prognosis has its own challenges because almost always the prognosis is not known with absolute certainty. Today physicians often talk about probability: "You have a 50% chance of a 5-year survival." This approach allows certain information to be transmitted to the patient and may permit the patient to learn what typically happens to people in similar situations. At the same time, probabilistic information does not answer the key question of "What, exactly, does this mean for me?"

Although an exact time of death is hard to predict, recall the various trajectories of dying presented at the outset of this chapter and how the dying process depends on the type of illness or condition(s) the patient has. Regardless of the illness trajectory, helping the person and family adjust to losses in function, or "little deaths" as they are experienced, is a continuing challenge. Your respectful caring requires being attuned to the losses while affirming the patient's remaining strengths.

Helping Patients Maintain Hope

In the first part of the chapter, we emphasized the importance of recognizing and understanding patients' challenges during this unique period of their life.

When a patient is dying, the focus of hope will change over time, from a hope for cure to a hope for meaningful activities in the remaining life left to this person. Hope may be directed toward events such as seeing a loved one or pet another time, visiting a favorite place, or hearing a familiar piece of music played.

Some hopes are less tangible: that one will be able to keep a positive spirit or sense of irony to the end, that one will hold to their faith and beliefs, or that a tradition will be carried on in one's absence. Previously sought long-term goals are put into perspective, and the patient focuses their hopes on the most important ones, knowing that some will no longer be attainable.[26]

Families also adjust their hopes for what is possible given the new circumstances. As one husband wrote when he learned that his wife was not going to recover from her early bouts of ovarian cancer:

> There is a transition between the certainty of living and the acceptance of dying. When there is such acceptance, there is a kind of emotional purgatory. The cartoon character stands still in space beyond the edge of a cliff and awaits the fatal fall. That is where things were for us in early October. There were choices, however, even in this purgatory. They remained a moment to live in… if only a moment. After that we will go on with our lives. Before it was over and before I began my desperate search for a new life, there would be a time for us as a family that was like none other. Most important was that we manage the pain. The first priority was comfort. The second priority was to get Lezlie back home not so much so that she could die there as that she could live there before she left.[27]

How can you show respect in terms of supporting hope? Hope itself depends significantly on the attitudes of health professionals, as well as on those of family and friends when the patient dares to disclose a hope. We have witnessed tender scenes between family or friends and the patient when one dares to say, "I was hoping…" Your listening for clues can help maintain the person's feeling of worth and provide a human context into which hopes may be more freely expressed. Health professionals also often can play a significant role in helping the patient realize some specific hopes by making a few important telephone calls to the right people, by mentioning the patient's wishes to the family and others, or by other similar means.

Most people faced with dying hope that they will be treated kindly, that everything reasonable will be done to make them comfortable, and that meaningful human interaction will not disappear. You can do your best in your role to support those general hopes.

The Right Care, in the Right Place, at the Right Time

The site, timing, and focus of caring interventions have been the source of much discussion and policy in health care. An important factor is considerations arising from an improved understanding of physiological and other responses to pain or other disturbing symptoms associated with many life-limiting conditions, and where the interventions can best be delivered. When asked about 80% of Americans reported that they would prefer to die at home (Fig. 14.2). In the year before the COVID-19 pandemic, more people died at home for the first time since the 1970s

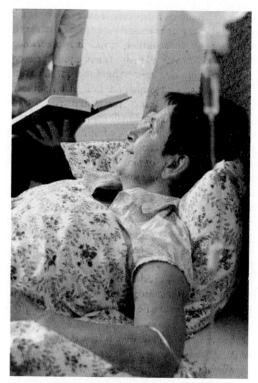

Fig. 14.2   Most Americans would prefer to die at home in familiar surroundings although circumstances may require a different care setting. © KatarzynaBialasiewicz/iStock/Thinkstock.com.

where we have reliable data.[28] Then, the pandemic changed where people died to the hospital because the intensive care available there was required for many patients. As the pandemic continues, some patients affected by COVID-19 will die in intensive care units, many in ordinary medical/surgical units in hospitals and even more in skilled nursing facilities.[12]

There are many barriers to dying at home beyond the need for intensive care including the emphasis on cure regardless of prognosis, lack of understanding about what palliative care or hospice can offer to patients with a life-limiting illness, and fear and anxiety on the part of family as to their roles and responsibilities for a dying loved one. Regardless of the actual setting of care delivery, palliative care and hospice are of importance to all patients with a serious or life-limiting illness or injury.

PALLIATIVE CARE

Palliative care traditionally was thought of as what health professionals can offer when cure no longer is possible. In other words, it becomes appropriate when all else has failed. From Hippocrates' time onward the suggestion was that if cure was no longer possible, the disease had gone beyond the "art of medicine" and should not be interfered with by the doctor. So, all too often palliation meant that dying patients received little medical intervention. At the same time, you can understand that the idea of palliative care is important because, applied appropriately, it allows you to have better insight into how to maximize the quality of life, attending to patient's own fear, distress, timing, and life situation.

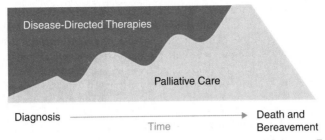

Fig. 14.3 Conceptual shift for palliative care. From National Academies of Sciences, Engineering, and Medicine. *Models and Strategies to Integrate Palliative Care Principles into Care for People With Serious Illness: Proceedings of a Workshop.* Washington, DC: The National Academies Press; 2018:3. https://doi. org/10.17226/24908.

Today the growing focus on appropriate end-of-life care has shed new light on what palliative care entails. Palliative care goes well beyond the traditional "hand-holding at the bedside" so often portrayed in the pictures before modern medicine could offer so much. Comfort can be achieved for patients through many varieties of intervention, such as medications, respiratory therapies, surgical procedures, acupuncture and other alternative therapies, and psychological and spiritual counseling, to name a few. Contemporary palliative care is defined as follows:

> *Palliative care is specialized medical care for people living with a serious illness. This type of care is focused on providing relief from the symptoms and stress of the illness. The goal is to improve quality of life for both the patient and the family.*[29]

Palliative care is growing and expanding in the United States and other countries. "As of 2019, 72% of hospitals with 50 or more beds report a palliative care team, up from 67% in 2015 and 7% in 2001. These hospitals serve 87% of all hospitalized patients in the US, an increase from 82% in 2015."[29] Along with this heightened consciousness and technology focus, there also has been a rethinking about the traditional assumption of a progression from "treatment" to "palliation" as the patient's dying ensues as is suggested by the inclusion of "at any stage" of a serious illness in the Center to Advance Palliative Care definition given previously. Using cancer as a model, the National Academy of Medicine (formerly the Institute of Medicine) in the United States proposes that treatment geared to cure versus treatment geared to palliation does not progress in a tidy, linear way (Fig. 14.3). Different combinations of education about how to prevent deterioration or the appearance of new symptoms, responsiveness to rehabilitative needs, acute care interventions, and comfort measures all may remain appropriate from the beginning to the end of a serious illness or eventually when the patient begins the dying process.[30]

HOSPICE

The modern hospice, which began in England and spread to Canada, the United States, and many other countries, provides treatment and care expressly designed to meet the needs of patients who are expected to die within 6 months. Hospice is holistic in its approach to caring for patients, family members, and their friends. Hospice services are available for all types of patients with life-limiting conditions such as end-stage cardiac or renal disease, Alzheimer's disease, progressively deteriorating neurological conditions, cancer, and chronic obstructive pulmonary disease.

Hospice focuses on comfort measures when cure or remission is no longer possible. The hospice setting is characterized by interprofessional care team approaches. When there is a family, it (and not the patient alone) is the unit of care. Family perspectives on end-of-life care for elders with advanced-stage cancer in different settings showed significantly more favorable experiences of their loved ones dying outside of the hospital setting with hospice services than those whose loved ones died in hospitals. Hospice is far better equipped to provide symptom relief, communication with health professionals, emotional support, and less aggressive treatment.[31]

Hospice services are "without walls"; that is, they are designed to provide care within the home with devices such as hotlines, care networks, and respite programs for caregivers or a designated hospice care facility or a skilled nursing facility. There are also inpatient hospice programs some of which took on a particularly onerous and important role during the COVID-19 pandemic when the number of dying patients in a hospital became overwhelming to the intensive care staff members.

> *Our nurses [in-patient palliative care] went to the bedside of every patient that died. They cared for the patient in a dignified way. This alleviated the stress from the frontline doctors and nurses. It allowed them the valuable time to spend with patients in need. We also collaborated with transport and the morgue team to track all the patients. The hospice counselors provided emotional support and telephone counseling to the families of the deceased. Our staff (hospice) assisted families with funeral plans and coordinated with funeral homes. After each pronouncement, patients were treated with the utmost reverence and respect. It was the last act of kindness that we could do for so many suffering with the virus. Hospice provided education and support to the nursing staff.[1]*

You are entering the health professions at a time when the attention devoted to the core concepts of quality end-of-life care will assist you in doing a better job than your forbears did in providing care for dying patients.

When Death Is Imminent

At some point during a life-limiting illness, it becomes apparent that the person will die soon. Persons who do not suffer from a prolonged illness as such also face the moment of imminent death: the accident victim or the young person seriously injured in battle or other violence.

INDIVIDUALIZED PATIENT- AND FAMILY-CENTERED CARE

The patient whose death is imminent should not be barraged with routine requests and procedures that no longer matter. As one woman sitting by her dying father's bedside asked dismayingly, "Does it matter, really, if his bowels haven't moved on the last day he will probably be alive?"

Attempts to relieve pain by medication, massage, and other therapeutic means may have been started long before, and these should be continued unless the patient asks that they be withdrawn. Some people, knowing that they are experiencing the final days of their lives, find the stupor induced by heavy medication more troublesome than uncomfortable symptoms.

However, maximizing comfort goes beyond alleviating pain. It involves the relief of real or potential suffering. Suffering is a far more inclusive, personalized concept than pain, and your assistance in helping patients and their families have a final time together as free of pain and suffering as possible is a laudable goal. Families do many things to try to provide a meaningful and peaceful transition. We have seen families who read to their loved ones, bathe them, sing songs they loved, or fill the room with flowers. A friend of one of the authors sneaked her 2-month-old daughter up to the hospital room so that her husband could witness his wife nursing their child for one last time. A religious leader may be called in for instruction or rituals. Specific activities will vary from person to person influenced by personal preference and cultural, ethnic, religious, or other beliefs. When they exist, respect requires you to alter your treatment procedures to honor them.

Caregivers in the health care environment can be facilitators by allowing the family and friends their final day or days together, remaining "on standby" if needed. This might mean breaking typical hospital rules and readjusting one's schedule. It also means knowing whom should be called if the patient's condition worsens and death appears near.

SAYING GOOD-BYE

Many people find it difficult to say good-bye to a friend or other loved one who is going away. It is often more difficult still when the person is dying—so much so that good-byes are seldom said, especially by the health professional to the patient and the patient's family. This is, however, something that you can do to show respect for the people and their situation when many other forms of interaction have been suspended.

This encounter also allows the patient and their family to express similar feelings. There is often a real sense of closeness and gratitude felt toward the health professional, and to be able to show it is a great relief. In addition to what the exchange does for the patient and family, it is important to realize how much it can help in your own grieving. Giving patients and families an opportunity to express gratitude to you may sound odd, but it is one way in which some patients and families can be assisted in their own grieving. When they observe that the health professional receives their thanks humbly, they will appreciate this show of human caring.

However, you should also prepare for the patient and family to reject your attempts to show respectful caring during this intense period of their lives. Sometimes when a person is close to dying, he or she shuts out many people. Such a patient may not want to have anything more to do with you. There are many possible reasons for this:

1. Many have great difficulty saying good-bye under any circumstance.
2. The person has accepted their death and no longer needs any people around, except the closest few of whom you are not one.
3. The patient and their family may direct their anger about the death toward you and other members of the team.
4. You are inextricably linked to the whole setting in which suffering and the dying process have taken place. So much anguish may be associated with you and your professional environment that it is painful for the patient or family to be in your presence.

In short, when your final efforts and good intentions are neither wanted nor welcomed, you may feel hurt by these sudden or unexpected rebuffs and can do little more than forgive the person responsible for them. At times when hurt is present, support from your interprofessional colleagues becomes vital. Sharing feelings of failure, rejection, or bewilderment with an understanding colleague can lend insights into the reasons listed earlier, supporting reflective practice and clinician well-being.

Summary

This chapter considers some basic, key factors that can be helpful to you in your attempts to show respect in the extreme life situation in which death is approaching for a patient in your care. The patient needs your professional skills, compassion, and wisdom in this situation. At the same time, you are confronted with your own uncertainties and fears about dying and death along with the irony that, no matter what you do, the result for this patient will be death. Your part in making the remainder of life for a dying patient as rich and worthwhile as possible may be the motivation you will need to sustain that person and their loved ones.

References

1. Kris M. Wiki Wisdom Forum. Frontline Nurses: Wisdom from Nurses So We Never Again Mishandle a National Healthcare Crisis. Wiki Wisdom; 2020:6. wikiwisdom.net/frontline-nurses.
2. Lynn J, Adamson DM. *Living Well at the End of Life. Adapting Health Care to Serious Chronic Illness in Old Age.* Washington, DC: Rand Health; 2003.
3. Institute of Medicine. *Dying in America: Improving Quality and Honoring Individual Preferences Near the End-of-Life.* Washington, DC: National Academies Press; 2015.
4. Moore B. Dying during COVID-19. *Hastings Cent Rep.* 2020:14. https://doi.org/10.1002/hast.1122.
5. President's Commission for the Study of Ethical Problems in Medicine and Biomedical, and Behavioral Research. Defining death: A report on the medical, legal and ethical issues in determination of death. July 1981, Library of Congress card number–81-600150, Washington, DC, p. 2.
6. Ross LF. Respecting choice in definitions of death. *Hastings Cent Rep.* 2018;48(6):S53–S55, p. S53. https://doi.org/10.1002/hast.956.
7. Belkin G. A path not taken: Beecher, brain death and the aims of medicine. *Hastings Cent Rep.* 2018;48(6):S10–S13, p. S10. https://doi.org/10.1002/hast.944.
8. Veatch R. Controversies in defining death: a case for choice. *Theor Med Bioethics.* 2019;40:381–401, p. 381. https://doi.org/10.1007/s11017-019-09505-9.
9. Caldwell G. *Let's Take the Long Way Home.* New York: Random House; 2010.
10. Berg E. *The Year of Pleasures.* New York: Random House; 2005.
11. Garand L, Lingler JH, Deardorf KE, DeKosky ST, Schulz R, Reynolds III CF, Dew MA. Anticipatory grief in new family caregivers of persons with mild cognitive impairment and dementia. *Alzheimer Dis Assoc Disord.* 2012;26:159–165, p. 160. http://dx.org/10.1097/WAD.0b013e31822f9051.
12. Anneser J. Dying patients with COVID-19: what should hospital palliative care teams (HPCTs) be prepared for? *Palliative Supportive Care.* 2020;18:382–384, p.382. https://doi.org/10.1017/S147895152 0000450.
13. Krikorian A, Maldonado C, Pastrana T. Patient's perspectives on the notion of a good death: a systematic review of the literature. *J Pain Symptom Manage.* 2019;7(33). https://www.jpsmjournal.com/article/S0885-3924(19)30451-8/fulltext.
14. Pasero C, McCaffrey M. Pain ratings: the fifth vital sign. *Am J Nursing.* 1997;97(2):15.
15. Campbell ML. 2018. Ensuring breathing comfort at the end of life: the integral role of the critical care nurse. *Am J Crit Care.* 2018;27(4):264–269.
16. Wang Y. Nursing students' experiences of caring for dying patients and their families: a systematic review and meta-synthesis. *Front Nursing.* 2019;6(4):261–272, p. 269. https://doi.org/10.2478/FON-2019-0042.
17. *Five Wishes.* https://www.fivewishes.org.
18. Banner D, Freeman S, Damanpreet K, Meikle M, Russell BKM, Sommerfeld EA, Flood D, Schiller CJ. Community perspectives of end-of-life preparedness. *Death Stud.* 2019;43(4):211–223. https://doi.org/1 0.1080/07481187.2018.1446060.
19. Bayliss J. Rethinking loss and grief. In: Nyatanga D, ed. *Why Is It So Difficult to Die?* 2nd ed. London: Quay Books; 2008:241–254.
20. Chahrour WH, Hvidt NC, Hvidt EA, Viftrup DT. Learning to care for the spirit of dying patients: the impact of spiritual care training in a hospice setting. *BMC Palliative Care.* 2021;20(115):2021. https://doi.org/10.1186/s12904-021-00804-4.
21. Balber PG. Stories of the living dying: the Hermes listener. In: Corless I, Germino BB, Pittman MA, eds. *Dying, Death, and Bereavement: A Challenge for Living.* 2nd ed. New York: Springer Publishing; 2003.
22. Purtilo R, Robinson E. *Maintaining Compassionate Care: A Companion for Families Experiencing the Uncertainty of a Serious and Prolonged Illness.* Boston, MA: MGH Institute of Health Professions, Inc; 2007:34 Available at: https://www.mghihp.edu/sites/default/files/publications/compassionate-care-booklet.pdf.
23. Cagle JG, Unroe KT, Bunting M, Bernard BL, Miller SC. Caring for dying patients in the nursing home: voices from frontline nursing home staff. *J Pain Symptom Manage.* 2017;53(2):198–207.
24. Kuek JTYK, Ngiam LXL, Kamal NHA, Chia JL, Chan NPX, Abdurrahman ABHM, et al. The impact of caring for dying patients in intensive care units on a physician's personhood: a systematic scoping review. *Philos Ethics Humanit Med.* 2020;15(12):1–16. https://doi.org/10.1186/s130300-020-00096-1.

25. Brighton IJ, Bristowe K. Communication in palliative care: talking about end of life, before end of life. *Postgrad Med J.* 2016;92:466–470.
26. Purtilo RB. Attention to caregivers and hope: overlooked aspects of ethics consultation. *J Clin Ethic.* 2006;17(4):358–363.
27. Surman O. *After Eden: A Love Story.* New York: iUniverse; 2005.
28. Emery G. *Home Is Now the Most Common Place of Death in the US;* 2019. https://www.reuters.com/article/us-health-dying-choices-idUSKBN1YF2Q6.
29. Center to Advance Palliative Care. www.capc.org/about/palliative-care.
30. National Academies of Sciences, Engineering, and Medicine. *Models and Strategies to Integrate Palliative Care Principles into Care for People With Serious Illness: Proceedings of a Workshop.* Washington, DC: The National Academies Press; 2018:3. https://doi.org/10.17226/24908.
31. Wright AA, Keating NL, Ayanian JZ, et al. Family perspectives on aggressive cancer care near the end of life. *JAMA.* 2016;315(3):284–292.

Respectful Interaction in Complex Situations

The reader will be able to

- Identify three potential sources of difficulties that create barriers to a respectful health professional and patient interaction;
- Discuss how disparities in power within the health care context can lead to anger and frustration for all involved;
- Identify attributes and behaviors of patients, such as manipulative, sexually provocative, or aggressive behaviors, that may challenge the health professional's ideal of respectful care in all its forms;
- Recognize patients with "high need," and understand how the interprofessional care team can collaborate to effectively meet the care demands of this population;
- Describe strategies to cope with the emotions that result from difficult conversations;
- Reflect on personal expectations of what it means to be a "good" health professional and how this affects interactions with patients;
- Describe environmental factors that may contribute to difficulties in health professional and patient interaction;
- Understand the connection between difficult conversations, moral distress, and moral resilience;
- Recognize strategies and tools for supporting moral resilience and clinician well-being;
- List and evaluate guidelines for managing and, when possible, preventing difficult interactions to optimize health professional and patient relationships and health care outcomes; and
- Identify 10 strategies for effectively managing difficult conversations in health care.

Prelude

We had a fair amount of COVID patients, and right outside these patients' windows were demonstrators, protesting against the vaccine. It was hard to not be angry. To have gone from being a healthcare hero, to having people not believe us, or believe in science, or think this is all fake, has been infuriating. Now that we are in the thick of it, that anger is still there, but it is different. The anger is shaded by devastation and sadness.

C. KRETSCHMAR[1]

Difficult situations are part of everyday life in health care. Patients and families present for care when they are most vulnerable, and the interprofessional care team is often responsible for communications that bring both joy and sorrow. There are patient care situations in which you will come away with a great sense of satisfaction and others that may elicit profound frustration. As a health professional, you must be prepared for all types. This chapter focuses on difficulties inherent in the health professional and patient interaction that have not specifically been addressed elsewhere in this book or that bear reemphasizing. We suggest that you refer to Chapters 2 and 4 to review the content on establishing relatedness, recognizing boundaries, building trust, and respecting differences in a diverse society. You will need to use these insights and skills in your work with patients who challenge your conceptions of what it means to be a "good" health professional. Moreover, you will have an opportunity to think about other factors that can create great tension in the health professional and patient interaction, such as disparities in power, bias, role expectations, or an unsafe working environment that can cause harm to the health professional or patient. We devote this chapter to some summary statements about how to work more effectively with complex patients, families, and organizations and offer ways to effect change in "difficult" situations.

Sources of Difficulties

Generally, when you enter a relationship with a patient, you have good reason to expect that things will go well, or if there are problems, you expect that they can be resolved. However, there are situations in which even your best efforts cannot make things right. When this happens, a common response is to look for a place to lay the blame. For example, you might wonder what else you could have done for the patient, or you might reason that the patient was not ready for treatment, or you might become defensive and decide that the patient was disruptive, maladjusted, or any number of other negative labels. Refer to the quote that opened the chapter regarding the complexity of caring for patients throughout the COVID pandemic. Especially note the last sentence, indicating the emotions that health professionals go through when faced with difficult situations. A frequent assumption in health care is that it is the patient or family who is difficult, when in reality complex circumstances are often the source of the difficulty. Difficulty relating to a patient or group of patients may originate in the health professional, in the interaction itself, or within the setting where the interaction takes place.

SOURCES WITHIN THE HEALTH PROFESSIONAL

As emphasized throughout this book, you bring a wealth of experiences, education, biases, and values to your interaction with patients and their families. These factors can affect how you react to a particular patient. For example, recall the discussion on transference and countertransference in Chapter 2. A patient may remind you of your former stepfather, whom you particularly feared and disliked. This experience can arouse intense emotional reactions in the present relationship. In addition, your personality and how you deal with stress will play a large part in how you manage patient care situations that are interpersonally difficult.[2] In fact, your personality, more than your professional or demographic background, may explain why you react negatively to some patients and certain situations and have little difficulty with others.

For the health professional, the most reliable indicator of a negative emotional response is an unfavorable gut response or sense of discomfort in encounters with a patient.[3] If you are attuned to monitoring your feelings, you can try to assess how much anger, fear, or guilt you bring to the interaction and try to manage those feelings before trying to manage the patient. After you identify the emotions you are experiencing, two questions often follow: "Why is this happening?" and "Where is this emotion coming from?"

Although it is a widely held belief, which has certainly been emphasized in this book, that health professionals should be nonjudgmental in their relationships with patients, it is a fact that health professionals often find some patients more difficult to work with than others. In general, patients who do not respect or affirm the health professional's recommendation can be considered "bad patients." The patient's rejection of the health professional's help can be easily misread as a rejection of the health professional. This rejection can take many forms, ranging from complaints to incessant demands, manipulative behavior, ingratitude, or basic unwillingness to follow advice or treatment. The literature categorizes "difficult patients" as patients who are needy, demanding, manipulative, help-rejecting, self-destructive, and racist.[4] Patients with these characteristics may evoke strong negative feelings (including guilt, hostility, and aversion). They may attempt to intimidate, devaluate, and ignore recommendations. They also may become aggressive and frighten or sometimes even threaten or physically harm health professionals. Still, others may make unacceptable sexually explicit or bigoted remarks that undermine the relationship or challenge the safety or comfort of health professionals or others in the health care environment.

During your program of study to become a health professional, the ideal that is reinforced is that you should be able to function effectively in a wide variety of patient situations. Many professional programs now integrate clinical simulations and other trainings to assist interprofessional teams with developing competencies in difficult encounters.[5] Long before you have a full complement of skills and a breadth of experience with which to deal with difficult situations, you may blame yourself for failing to meet the needs of a challenging patient encounter. For this reason, it is important to remember that new situations can raise old doubts or uncertainties at any period in one's career.

SOURCES WITHIN INTERACTIONS WITH PATIENTS

Patients who are overly demanding, oppositional, manipulative, hostile, aggressive, violent, self-destructive, or who neglect self-management (do not adhere to treatment generally) can be labeled as problematic. The label of "difficult patient" is one that warrants considered reflection by the provider and the interprofessional care team. Separating pathology from personality can be challenging, particularly in care of the patient with persistent mental illness. Regarding patients as "good" and "bad" uses an interactionist approach, since patients are not passive recipients of care but active agents in the interaction process with the health care team. As Aronson notes, "When we call patients and families 'good', or at least spare them the 'difficult' label, we are noting and rewarding acquiescence. Too often, this 'good' means you agree with me and you don't bother me and you let me be in charge of what happens and when. Such a definition runs counter to what we know about truly good care as a collaborative process."[6]

It is also important to note that by the time a patient interacts with you for their care or appointment, they have already interacted with a myriad of individuals on their way to, or in, the health care system. Some patients might drive over 100 miles to an appointment, while others will take three trains, two buses and then walk a mile all before arriving at check-in. Others who are in the inpatient setting will have interacted with the food service delivery crew, their roommate's family, and the patient transport associate. They may arrive to your interaction tired, frustrated, in pain, hungry, stressed, angry, or embarrassed. Research supports that health professionals who attend to the patient's and family's emotions, seek to understand the patient's context, show authentic empathy, and engage in shared decision-making have an enhanced ability to handle difficult conversations.[7–9]

The focus of the health professional's dislike can easily move from dislike for the consequences of inappropriate or unacceptable attitudes or behavior to dislike for the person who is a patient. For example, patients with illnesses that are socially unacceptable are often labeled as difficult even if their behavior is a model of adherence. Similarly, patients who are judged to be responsible in some way for their illness or injury, such as people who are obese or addicted to tobacco or other substances, are often also labeled as less worthy of respect than patients who are "blameless" for their present health condition. These patients have one thing in common: either because of the nature of their health problems or the way they respond to the health professionals involved in their care and treatment, they withhold the legitimacy that makes health professionals feel good about who they are and what they do.

Thus a large part of the label a patient receives depends on our role expectations of patients in general and of patients with specific characteristics. One of the most basic expectations of patients is adherence with agreed-on treatment. *Adherence* is defined as the extent to which a person's behavior—taking medication, following a diet, and/or executing lifestyle changes—corresponds with agreed recommendations from a health care provider.[10] Adherence is multidimensional and affected by multiple factors, including patient factors, socioeconomic factors, clinical condition-related factors, therapy-related factors, and health care system-related factors. *Nonadherence* is largely viewed in health care literature as a problem to be resolved: we assume patients are not following professional advice because they do not understand or have some misconception that prevents them from understanding. Major efforts, then, are directed toward getting patients to understand so they will adhere to treatment. This often includes attending to the social circumstances in which patients live their lives.[11] If health professionals approach the problem of nonadherence by trying to understand the factors in patients' lives that mediate their cooperation, efforts can be made to change factors that are amenable to change or adjust treatment to meet the reality of a patient's life.

HIGH-NEED PATIENTS

According to the CDC, about 68 million adult patients in the United States are living with two or more chronic conditions.[12] These patients, as well as others with complex needs, have recently been the focus of attention in the study of health care delivery and expenditure. The literature suggests that the top 1% of patients who use health care resources account for more than 20% of health care expenditures, and the top 5% account for nearly half of US spending on health care.[13] *High-need patients* have been defined as those with "complex conditions and circumstances requiring multiple services that, for the most part, are not currently delivered easily or effectively by the health care system."[14] Subgroups of high-need patients include adults over the age of 65 with multiple chronic conditions, functional disability, or advanced illness; the frail elderly; and young adults with a disability or behavioral health conditions. Care for high-need patients is often categorized as fragmented, with acute-on-chronic health conditions and preventable health utilization service.[15] Social risk factors include low socioeconomic status, low health literacy, social isolation, community deprivation, and housing insecurity.[16]

Because of the functional difficulties many of these patients experience with activities of daily living and navigating the health care system, they warrant collaborative and integrated interprofessional care. Multidimensional care models that attend to the medical, functional, behavioral, and social needs of patients with high needs can help improve the cost and quality of care delivery.[17]

SOURCES IN THE ENVIRONMENT

The health professional and patient interaction takes place in a particular context. Increasingly, today's health care delivery settings place increased stressors on providers, patients, and families, and this context can be the source of difficulty in an interaction. For example, if the environment is strange and frightening, the patient or health professional may react in a fearful or angry manner. An apt example is how the COVID-19 pandemic and fear of exposure to the virus significantly reduced access and utilization of health care, particularly in minoritized groups.[18] Fig. 15.1 illustrates that for many patients, a health care facility can be an extremely threatening place. Taken in this context, even a simple activity such as bathing can be viewed as menacing. Rader[19] noted that for a person with apraxia (inability to execute purposeful, learned motor acts despite the physical

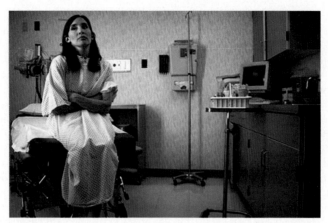

Fig. 15.1   Patients often feel overwhelmed and out of place in health care settings. © Photodisc/Photodisc/Thinkstock.com.

ability and willingness to do so), agnosia (inability to recognize a tactile or visible stimulus despite being able to recognize the elemental sensation), and aphasia (loss of language function either in comprehension or expression of words)—symptoms often found in patients who have had a cerebral vascular accident—the standard nursing home bathing experience may be perceived as horrific. Consider the following limitations and place yourself in the patient's position.

> *A person the nursing home resident does not recognize comes into her room, wakens her, says something she does not understand, drags her out of bed, and takes off her clothes. Then the resident is moved down a public corridor on something that resembles a toilet seat, covered only with a thin sheet so that her private parts are exposed to the breeze. Calls for help are ignored or greeted with, "Good morning." Then she is taken to a strange, cold room that looks like a car wash, the sheet is ripped off, and she is sprayed in the face with cold and then scalding water. Continued calls for help go unheeded. Her most private parts are touched by a stranger. In another context this would be assault.*[19]

An environment can be equally strange and intolerable to the health professional. For example, we have noted in earlier chapters that, in community health practice, health professionals may go into the unknown realm of the patient's living environment. One of us recalls a home visit to a small, run-down house literally butted up against the back fence of the holding pens for cattle at the stock market. The smell of manure was overwhelming both outside and inside the house. The elderly woman who lived there (and the subject of the home visit for management of diabetes) seemed oblivious to the odor. In fact, she had just finished hanging a load of clean sheets on the line to dry in her tiny backyard!

Other environmental factors that make care difficult include the esthetics of a space, crowding, noise, and climate. Similar stresses can arise in a hectic and crisis-ridden environment. Patients who are kept waiting in an overcrowded emergency department or office are more likely to be frustrated and hostile to health professionals when they are finally seen. Understaffing often leaves health professionals feeling frustrated and dissatisfied as they attempt to meet the needs of too many patients with too little time and too few resources. Overworked staff worry about the effect of stretching themselves too thin and the impact of this can have on patient care.

As discussed in Chapter 3, building resilience for professional practice in today's ever-changing health care delivery settings is an individual, team, and organizational commitment. Professional

TABLE 15.1 ■ **Strategies Used by Health Professionals to Manage Emotions Related to Difficult Conversations**

Category	Strategies
Self-care	Identify personal emotions before conversation Breathe deeply Take breaks or use self-calming techniques Find an outlet to decompress (exercise, writing) Talk about experience with others Acknowledge individual and system-level limitations
Preparatory and relational skills	Anticipate family's needs Consider how patient/family would most prefer to hear the news Rehearse conversations ahead of time Speak slowly; allow silence Adapt approach based on patient/family responses/emotional cues
Empathic presence	Put yourself in patient's/family's shoes Imagine the context of the patient/family health care journey Remember primary role to support patient/family
Team approach	Include other team members in conversation to broaden expertise offered to patient/family Consult with more experienced peers and mentors before conversation Debrief with other team members after conversation
Professional identity	Lead with compassion Separate emotion from responsibility Leave professional problems at the workplace

From Luff D, Martin EB, Mills K, Mazzola NM, Bell SK, Meyer EC. Clinicians' strategies for managing their emotions during difficult healthcare conversations. *Patient Educ Couns*. 2016;99:1461–1466.

demands can result in physical and psychological exhaustion that can drain health professions and result in compassion fatigue. *Compassion fatigue* is "emotional, physical and psychological exhaustion due to exposure to chronic work-related stress."[20] For health professionals exposure to suffering, trauma, and constant use of empathy can leave the care provider feeling depleted with a reduced sense of professional accomplishment. The issue of compassion fatigue has received considerable attention because of the increasing rates in practice (particularly as a result of the COVID pandemic), the growing evidence that it impacts both quality patient care and long-term clinician well-being, and the construct of the role of health care in society.[21] Creating a repertoire of strategies for attending to the emotions that may arise from difficult patient encounters is one way to prevent compassion fatigue and realize more success in these interactions. Luff and colleagues[22] identified several common strategies that experienced health professionals use to assist them in problem-solving through difficult conversations. They include self-care, development of preparatory and relational skills, empathic presence, use of a team approach, and reliance on one's professional identity. These strategies are summarized in Table 15.1.

Disparities of Power

We have noted several times in this book that patients are placed in a position of diminished power upon entering the health care environment. The numerous losses that patients face because of illness or trauma include independence, social status, ability to fulfill responsibilities, and other expressions of identity. Often these losses, combined with health disparities when people enter a health care institution, contribute to feelings of powerlessness. A common reaction to powerlessness is anger, and a common target of anger is the most accessible and least-threatening health professional involved with the patient.[23] Thus students are often the target for a torrent of rage from a patient that has little to do with the student or his or her abilities. Few studies have explored patients' perceptions of this inequity in power, but in one study of mental health workers and patients, both groups reported an awareness of the struggle to gain or retain power and control. Patients noted that when health professionals demonstrated respect, took time with them, and were willing to give them some control and choice in their own care, feelings of anger were reduced.[24] Not surprisingly, the human presence is what is most valued.

Role Expectations

Because we are socialized not to use negative terms such as "bad," we substitute euphemisms to describe patients with the attributes listed earlier. They are described as disruptive, unmotivated, maladaptive, and manipulative. Patients who are perceived to be difficult to treat evoke intense negative affective responses in the health professional that can work against establishing a positive, constructive relationship.[25] Furthermore, there is also a strong possibility that the professional's language exerts a powerful impact on thought and, consequently, action. Negative words lead to negative thoughts and actions regarding difficult patients. An example from rehabilitation medicine highlights the impact of language.

Most rehabilitation staff members have encountered patients who resist their best efforts to engage them in therapeutic activities. These patients seem to not want to be in rehabilitation. They may view therapies as trivial, irrelevant, uninteresting, or too demanding, and they must be constantly coaxed to attend therapy sessions; if they do attend, they do not participate. Staff members become quickly frustrated with patients who do not share the "rehabilitation perspective" that places a high premium on attaining optimal independent functioning within constraints imposed by the patient's condition.

Any patient behavior that is inconsistent with expected patient role behavior (read "good patient behavior") could negatively influence the care of the patient. Not only might you be tempted to diminish your efforts in the care of a nonadhering patient, but you might also resort to distancing yourself from the patient. Unfortunately, avoidance and distancing may result in the reinforcement of deviant behavior as a patient response to nonsupportive care. In extreme cases, health professionals have been known to respond to patient challenges with their own version of negative behavior. In a national study of transplant coordinators, a full 62% revealed a belief that a hostile or antagonistic patient should not receive an organ transplantation.[26] The irony and tragedy in such findings are that expressions of anger and frustration (behavior that can be labeled as *hostile*) may be a natural response by patients to chronic illness.

Most health professionals can control these kinds of strong emotional reactions and continue, at least marginally, to meet their obligations to the patient. The result is a sort of "grudging attention" (i.e., the patient gets the minimal care that he or she needs and nothing more). Grudging attention occurs because of a combination of factors. Once a negative label is attached to a patient, it is difficult for health professionals to look past it and process other data about the patient. Negative labels often get "passed on" until a patient develops a bad reputation.[27] It is as if we see only one aspect of the patient. Couple these stereotypes about the difficult patient with idealistic role expectations of health professionals as caring, nonjudgmental, and capable of reaching every patient, and the result is an interaction devoid of everything but going through the motions.

Although it is important to work toward the goals of acceptance and constructive problem-solving, sometimes the only solution is to do what you must for the patient and then leave. This is exactly what happened in the case of a sexually aggressive patient who made lewd propositions and repeatedly exposed himself to his caregivers. The health professionals in the below case responded with grudging attention.

Mr. Leland was getting only the absolute necessities—no extras. After all, who wants to sit down and chat with someone who talks about nothing but his sex life—or keeps asking about yours? Once our professional responsibilities were met, we avoided Mr. Leland. He could not fail to notice this, and as a result, his demands for attention become angrier and more disruptive.[28]

REFLECTIONS

- If you were assigned to care for Mr. Leland and he continued to talk explicitly about sex after you asked him not to, what would be your next step?
- What are some possible negative outcomes of "grudging attention" for the patient or the health professional staff?

Going through the minimal motions of care is a temporary and ineffective solution to a much larger problem. Often it results in guilt on the part of the health professional and can result, as in the case of Mr. Leland, in an escalation of the behavior that led to avoidance in the first place. Although the following quote refers to nurses, the same can be applied to all health professions: "If patients interpret a nurse's manner as uninterested, or if they overhear pejorative comments, they fear that they will not be cared for adequately. It is as valuable to examine staff's behaviors as it is to understand a patient's motivations."[29]

Difficult Health Professional and Patient Relationships

In this section, we introduce you to patients who share some of the attributes that have been identified as difficult by most health professionals. As you examine some of the character traits, behaviors, and nature of the health professional–patient interactions we hope you will gain insight into your own values and attitudes and reflect on how you will respond.

WORKING WITH PATIENTS WHO ARE SELF-DESTRUCTIVE

Sometimes, the most difficult patient is not the one who commits actions that are outrageous or inappropriate but who shrinks from constructive action and resorts to self-harm behavior. These behaviors can range from persistent substance use, to self-injury, to inadequate or total lack of self-management. In the case of self-destructive patients, the perception of difficulty rests to some extent on the invalidating effects of the patient's behavior on the other health professionals caring for them. In the eyes of the professionals, intervention should include accountability on behalf of the patient. When they fail to accept the help that is offered to them, the primary treatment goal is thwarted and the health professional's role as a therapeutic agent can feel invalidated. A recent consideration that has added to the complexity of the role of the health professional in society is the frustration and invalidation that health professionals felt during the COVID-19 pandemic. Increasing amounts of misinformation, politicization of information, and the way that misinformation impacted the spread of COVID-19 were an added burden for providers. As one health professional notes

When I get in my car it takes me at least 10 minutes to start my car. Because I have to process everything that I've gone through and then realize that once I start my car I'm entering into this world where people are coming up with these hoaxes. Like, this is not the first pandemic. This is not going to be the last. Right? Viruses and bacteria are real, there's not a conspiracy and these conspiracy theories are making our fight on the front lines harder.[30]

Challenges to scientific knowledge, expertise, and trust will likely continue to demand the attention of health professionals in their roles as care providers and citizens.

WORKING WITH PATIENTS WITH A HISTORY OF VIOLENT BEHAVIOR

Many health professionals feel inadequately prepared to deal with patients who have a complex medical condition that is complicated further by a history that involves violent behavior. The case of Darrin Block and Austin Greder involves a seriously ill patient and behavior that is generally unacceptable in an acute care institution.

CASE STUDY

Darrin Block was a nurse on the step-down unit at an urban medical center. Because of the medical center's location in a large city, the intensive care unit got more than its fair share of victims of gunshot wounds. Most of these patients were male, young, unemployed, and knew their assailants. Many were members of gangs and had to be admitted under aliases for their own protection. Austin Greder fit this description exactly. He was a 21-year-old high school dropout who had been shot by a rival gang member. Austin's major sources of support were his mother and girlfriend. He was admitted to the surgical intensive care unit in serious condition but had begun to recover, so he was moved to a medical/surgical step-down unit. His wound was not healing as well as the treatment team expected. Since his admission to the step-down unit, the staff had referred to Austin and his numerous visitors as "nothing but trouble." Austin's girlfriend, Alicia, had practically taken up residence in Austin's room. One time, Darrin walked into Austin's room and found him and Alicia involved in what appeared to be sexual activity. Darrin left in confused embarrassment but was somewhat angry, too. He did not expect to walk in on a sexual encounter and did not think he should have to apologize. After this incident, Darrin asked Alicia to leave whenever he entered the room to provide care. In response, Austin became angry and dismissive to Darrin, refusing to let him perform wound care and asking for one of the other nurses to care for him. To make matters worse, Austin posted a photo on Snapchat of Darrin with the caption "my nurse hating on my girlfriend." Darrin thought the right thing to do was set limits on Austin's behavior because things were clearly getting out of control. However, he was fearful of retaliation by Austin's friends outside of the safety of the hospital. He had heard more than one other member of the interprofessional care team talk about being confronted in the parking garage by a "gang member."

REFLECTIONS

- Put yourself in Darrin Block's position. What would you do the next time the patient refused wound care?
- What resources might there be in the hospital to assist Darrin and the interprofessional care team in working with Mr. Greder to "set limits"?

Patients can challenge the notion of what it means to be a "good" health professional. They make us realize that, although we are generally able to effectively help patients, sometimes we fall far short even with our best efforts. In the following section, we offer various techniques that may help you in working with difficult patients of all types. We also share some ideas about changing a difficult working environment.

Showing Respect in Difficult Situations

When patients are uncooperative, manipulative, angry, or reject help, health professionals may become frustrated or defensive which can negatively impact clinical outcomes.[31] You will have to be responsive to your own feelings of disgust, fear, anger, and doubt to manage patients' unacceptable behavior and utilize strategies to reengage the patient–provider relationship. (Fig. 15.2).

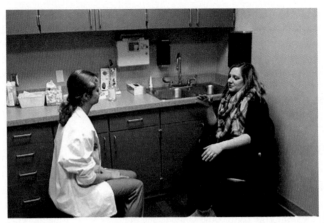

Fig. 15.2   Patients and health professionals sometimes must engage in difficult discussions. Courtesy Maren Haddad.

REFRAMING

An appropriate place to start is to show respect by initially refusing to believe that you are dealing with a person whose character is flawed. Reframing the interaction is important to recognize that the patient has complex health and social needs. The behaviors and attitudes may be the result of a treatable or modifiable factor. For example, one of your first determinations is to make certain that the patient has received a thorough, understandable explanation of the treatment or therapy in question. The patient may also be unmotivated or uncooperative if he or she has not been shown the respect of participation in establishing personally meaningful goals. Framing language to be empowering is also essential. Language focused on the patient's strengths, which are hope oriented, and free from derogatory slang (e.g., frequent flyer) convey respect and set the stage for a productive conversation built on trust.[32]

STRUCTURE AND CONSISTENCY

As a rule, for all types of difficult situations, structure and consistency in communication in every aspect of patient care are important.[33] A key component of a deliberate, consistent approach is setting limits. Setting firm limits is a part of setting boundaries with all patients but with additional safeguards given the extremity of the situation. By setting forth clear, consistent expectations in a nondefensive manner, you can help strengthen the patient's inner control. Be open to negotiation. Listen for opportunities to find out what is important to the patient.

When you are involved in setting limits, respect for the patient must govern the interaction. You should ask yourself whether the limits you set are arbitrary—that is, do they stem from your need to be in control or punish the patient—or whether the patient' welfare would indeed be best served by establishing external limits. Any plan to set limits should be agreed on by all members of the interprofessional care team to avoid the potential for a patient to "split" the staff (i.e., divide staff into all good or all bad). Good communication lines among all members of the team are essential.

FOCUS ON BEHAVIORS

It is also helpful to focus on a patient's unacceptable behaviors rather than on the person. This allows for open communication and avoids negative labeling that tends to stick to patients and obscure the real problem. One way to avoid negative labeling of patients is to be honest with them and tell them exactly how you feel. A good rule is to be candid, compassionate, and humble. Again, your honest comments should be directed at the patient's behavior and not at the patient. This way you can share your reactions and still not humiliate the patient. Look for opportunities to give plenty of positive feedback for desired behaviors. Also, focus on the here and now rather than long-term aspects of behavior. If all else fails, a behavioral contract can be developed to focus on specific actions. A contract, sometimes called a *patient care agreement*, "outlines the expectations, plans, and responsibilities of the patient and the consequences for noncompliance."[33]

CONTRIBUTE TO A RESPECTFUL ENVIRONMENT

On a broader basis, you can encourage the development of an environment that is respectful of everyone. Such a setting encourages patients to ask questions and challenge the system's rules and practices. If just a single member of the health care team prompts the patient legitimately to question their care, the rest of the team could come to see the patient as "difficult." Having patients ask about the care they receive and make decisions about their care must be considered the normal, desired state. The safety of health professionals also should be encouraged in a respectful environment. There must be practices and policies in place to give staff members basic protection from harassment, abuse, discrimination, and other threats. You may find yourself in an environment that is amenable to change through education and support for staff. In fact, the support of supervisory staff in the form of validation and insight is an essential component of an environment that fosters positive health professional and patient interactions.

From the Difficult to the Ethical: Moral Distress and Moral Resilience

Ethical tensions in clinical practice present a particular type of difficult conversation that health professionals must have with patients, families, and interprofessional colleagues. Ethics has been defined as "a moral compass that aids navigation of the often difficult terrain of everyday practice in contemporary health care environments."[34] Health professionals use their ethical decision-making to navigate difficult conversations when diverging health care choices and values turn from clinical to ethical. The compounding effect of managing ethical tensions and difficult conversations on a day-to-day basis can lead to moral distress. Moral distress was first theorized in health care and nursing by Jameton in 1984. Moral distress occurs when the health professional knows what the morally appropriate course of action is but meets external barriers, internal resistance, or a high level of uncertainty.[35] Recent studies of moral distress in health care have demonstrated its correlation with job dissatisfaction, turnover, burnout, depression, poor patient outcomes, and increased institutional costs.[36,37]

The COVID-19 pandemic led to heightened states of moral distress due to high levels of uncertainty, high-demand work environments, positive and negative emotions, staffing limitations, rapid care redesign, and emotional exhaustion amongst health care providers. Regardless of the health care delivery setting, it is essential to recognize moral distress early so that action can be taken to prevent the buildup of distressing situations (moral residue) and to problem solve effective solutions. Developing moral resilience is one way to mitigate the detrimental effects of moral distress and foster adversity in everyday practice.[38] Moral resilience is defined as "the capacity of an individual to sustain or restore their integrity in response to moral complexity, confusion, distress, or setbacks."[39] Research demonstrates the importance of processing traumatic experiences with challenging cases and resolving distress related to the moral injury that arises from making or witnessing difficult treatment decisions.[40] As discussed in Chapter 3, effective self-care, mindful practice, communities of practice, and organizational support systems can all bolster resilience and clinician well-being. Ethics education, ethical decision-making models, and taking the time to reflect on and explore moral aspects of difficult situations are key strategies to build moral resilience.

Difficult Conversations

Communication is the most common procedure in health care. It is so central to a respectful relationship that Chapters 8 and 9 are devoted directly to aspects of it. Unlike other procedures, there are no easy checklists or algorithms for executing communication because each conversation involves different individuals, topics, and contexts. However, studies show that health professionals who practice difficult conversations improve the quality and outcomes of their communications and national organizations endorse skilled communication as a key component of advancing a culture of well-being and ethical practice.[41]

The text that follows summarizes 10 evidence-based guidelines for showing respect toward patients and families in difficult conversations[23,28,41–50]:

1. *Timeliness matters.* Many people avoid difficult conversations because the topic may be hard to discuss, or those involved may have difficult behaviors. Do not avoid or wait too long. Most individuals appreciate information that is timely, clear, and direct.

2. *The setting matters.* One would think this might go without saying; however, in busy health care environments, health professionals are more likely to have hallway conversations and forget that patients and families need the proper space and place to hear important messages. Aim to always talk at the bedside or in a private space.

3. *Establish goals for the conversation and practice in advance.* If you are on an interprofessional care team, make sure all members of the team understand the goals before the meeting. Ask yourselves "what is the one message we want the patient or family member to take away from this conversation." As part of planning, expect, rather than avoid uncertainty and complexity. Encourage your interprofessional colleagues to remove the "difficult" label or not use it in the first place.

4. *Start the conversation by communicating the big picture and why all involved should care.* Respectfully acknowledge the emotions in the room with candor. Commit to seek shared decision-making and mutual purpose. Often, patients and families are seeking to be heard by those caring for them. Reassure them that you do by using phrases like "I heard you say ___, can you share with me more what you mean by that?"

5. *Remember that the caring function is as important as other interventions.* Make an empathetic statement such as, "I know you must be frustrated or disappointed." This kind of response tells the patient that you understand. In the words of Brene Brown "empathy is a strange and powerful thing. There is no script. There is no right or wrong way to do it. It is simply listening, holding space, withholding judgment, emotionally connecting, and communicating that incredibly healing message of you are not alone."[49]

6. *Talk less and listen more.* Generally, if you are talking more than half of the time, you are talking too much. Ask open-ended questions such as "What is your understanding of the situation?" or "What are your fears?" and "What are your hopes?" This helps you understand the patient or family perspective. Next share your point of view. Avoid trying to persuade; rather, work together to solve problems and achieve shared decision-making.

7. *State facts and observations to remain as objective as possible.* Avoid the use of derogatory labels as a means of reducing your frustration or anger. Label the encounter, not the patient. It is also helpful to use "I" statements versus "you" statements. For example, instead of saying "Your mental health is not good, you cannot think clearly" say "Given the care team's observations of your disorganized thinking, I am concerned about your mental health."

8. *Set realistic expectations.* To achieve shared decision-making and advance patient health, treatment adherence must be based on realistic expectations. Do not expect to change aspects of the patient's situation beyond your control. Instead, work to understand the patient's context, priorities, and goals and try to help change the underlying social and institutional conditions or attitudes that lead to nonadherence in high-need populations.

9. *Ensure safety.* When interacting with an aggressive patient or family, always ensure personal safety for yourself, members of the interprofessional care team, and the patient. Monitor body language and tone of voice that can quickly escalate to a threatening stance. If a patient or family member is hostile, diffuse the situation by allowing him or her to vent uninterrupted. Then strive to understand the problem, affirm what can be done, and follow through. Bring in additional resources such as ethics consultants and security personnel as needed. Affirm policies and practices (e.g., the patient rights and responsibilities statement) that are in place in your institution to encourage mutual respect.

10. *Conclude by clarifying expectations and summarizing the conversation.* Document the plan so that all members of the interprofessional care team know the direction of care and any emotional support that the patient, family, or team may require.

Although all your efforts as a health professional should be directed at acknowledging negative biases and keeping them in check, you may find that you cannot operate in the best interest of a given patient, no matter how much you try. If it comes to letting a patient go, be certain that you are referring him or her to a capable professional and not abandoning the person. Respect includes everybody, but as humans, we come in all shapes and forms, so the wise health professional recognizes that unresolvable difficulties with patients and situations will arise.

Professionals' Mistakes and Making Apology

An additional difficult situation that is unfortunately all too common in health care is dealing with errors in patient care, whether they are the result of individual mistakes or generated by system-level problems. Errors include challenges between the individual health professional and patient involved, as well as within the broader system in which the error occurred.

In recent years, significant literature in the health professions has emerged on the topic of the response of health professionals to a patient when a mistake related to the patient's care is made by individual professionals or because of a systems error in the health care institution. Communication breakdowns, diagnostic errors, poor judgment, and inadequate skill have all been found to result in patient harm and death.[51] The number of deaths and serious injuries that occur in the United States each year alone is staggering. Recent literature estimates an incidence of approximately 250,000 deaths per year associated with medical errors and preventable adverse events in hospitalized patients.[52] Some authors have suggested that if medical error was categorized as a disease, it would be the third most common cause of death in the United States.[51] Errors that have serious negative consequences for the patient must be disclosed to the patient or his or her family, and appropriate restitution must be made. However, disclosure of an error is generally difficult for health professionals.

There are numerous reasons why disclosure of errors to a patient and his or her family is so difficult for health professionals. One is that health professionals often think they are immune to error, so they find it hard to admit that an error has occurred. The second reason is that it is experienced as a sign of failure. Third, until recently, there have been few mechanisms in place for health professionals to talk freely with peers about the circumstances surrounding an error because of shame and irrational legal fears. Finally, disclosing an error to a patient and following the disclosure by apologizing requires a great deal of humility and skill on the part of the health professional. The case of Melanie Lieberman and Laura Keenan deals with the various facets of disclosure of an error that resulted in harm to the patient.

It was an exceptionally busy night on the medical/surgical floor where Melanie Lieberman worked. To make matters worse, one of the nurses called in sick at the last moment and the supervisor was unable to get a replacement for the first 4 hours of the 7 p.m. to 7 a.m. shift. Melanie had responsibility for twice the number of patients that she usually would during the beginning of the shift, the busiest time during the 12 hours she would be on duty. One of the patients under Melanie's care was Laura Keenan, who returned to the unit in the early evening from surgery for a mastectomy and breast reconstruction. Melanie was able to manage a full assessment of Laura at the beginning of the shift, but after that, she was occupied with medications, dressing changes, pages, and phone calls from physicians for new orders on a transfer from the emergency department. When Melanie sped past Laura's room, she did look in once or twice to affirm that the patient was resting quietly but she did not have time to complete a more thorough assessment. When the replacement nurse finally arrived at 11 p.m., Melanie offered up a quick report to her colleague on the patients he would assume responsibility for the rest of the shift and then went straight to Laura's room. Melanie realized after taking Laura's blood pressure and pulse that something was wrong. A quick look at the dressings covering the reconstruction indicated that Laura was bleeding and likely suffering from hypovolemic shock. Melanie knew that the most common postoperative problem for breast reconstruction patients was bleeding and she had not checked for the most obvious signs of this complication. After summoning additional assistance to monitor Laura, Melanie rushed to contact the surgeon and supervisor and upon returning learned that in her brief absence Laura's vital signs indicated worsening shock. Melanie increased the rate of the intravenous fluid and reinforced the dressing, all the while mentally berating herself for missing such an obvious problem. She knew she was overstretched but thought she could handle the workload. Now her lack of monitoring for a predictable problem was going to require another trip to the operating room for Laura and perhaps life-threatening consequences if the surgical team did not get the bleeding stopped fast enough. As if things were not bad enough, Melanie knew that she would have to talk to Laura's family and explain what happened. She dreaded this more than anything. Nothing like this had ever happened to Melanie before.

- Review the case and indicate where you think the error of lack of monitoring could have been prevented. In other words, would you have handled the situation differently from the way Melanie did give the same set of circumstances?
- What are the system-level problems that contributed to the error?
- What are the individual-level issues that contributed to the error?

The type of error in the case of Melanie Lieberman and Laura Keenan is a combination of the failure of the individual, in this case the nurse, to meet basic standards of postoperative care and system-level problems, including staffing issues. To prevent errors from occurring in the future, health professionals must view errors as a learning opportunity that is different from the "shame-and-blame culture that focuses only on individual responsibility or culpability."[53]

Melanie's error is not uncommon. Neither is her reaction to the expectations of negotiating the rough terrain of owning up to her share of the responsibility and disclosing what happened in a manner that is meaningful to the patient and her family. She knows that this will mean taking accountability and communicating a genuine apology. The right apology, at the right time, in the right context can do wonders for reestablishing trust, allowing patient, family, and health professional to move forward. The science of safety, including root cause analysis and the development of safety culture tools and systems, helps support the health professional when an error occurs. They serve to break the silence surrounding such events in clinical practice. Institutional supports are in place for health professionals to report, resolve, and reflect on errors. These supports begin with members of the interprofessional care team and extend to supervisors and employee assistance programs. Many organizations have offices of quality and safety that will provide on-call support, including incident debriefing. These supports are key to ensuring efficient, effective, and high-quality patient outcomes, while at the same time ensuring that both individual health professionals and systems learn from mistakes.

Summary

This chapter makes suggestions about respectful interaction with types of patients whom many health professionals find difficult to treat without negative feelings or behaviors intruding on the relationship. The context in which the relationship takes place also can cause difficulties and add to frustration, anger, and other negative responses by both parties. The environment often plays a significant role in one of the most difficult health professional and patient situations, the occurrence of an error and its aftermath. Despite such challenges, your responsibility to show respect for the patient as a person remains and can be expressed through attempts to use strategies that provide an opportunity to minimize the negative aspects of the relationship and optimize care outcomes. Attention to clinician well-being and tools for effective communication help support health professionals in navigating difficult conversations and situations.

See Section 6 Questions for Thought and Discussion to apply what you've learned in this section to a variety of case scenarios.

References

1. Kretschmar C. Commentary: *From the Front Lines: A Nurse's Story of Caregiving in the Time of COVID.* Seacoastonline, January 2, 2022. https://www.seacoastonline.com/story/opinion/columns/2022/01/02/commentary-covid-19-wentworth-douglass-nurse-caregiving-pandemic-vaccine-intubate-patients/9071224002/. Accessed January 22, 2022.
2. Santamaria N. The relationship between nurses' personality and stress levels reported when caring for interpersonally difficult patients. *Aust J Adv Nurs.* 2000;18(2):20–26.
3. Herbert CP, Seifert MH. When the patient is the problem. *Patient Care.* 1990;24(1):59.
4. Sokol D. Dealing fairly with racist patients. *BMJ.* 2019;367:l6575; Theofanidis D, Fountouki A. The difficult patient: a qualitative investigation exploring the "labels" set by hospital nurses. *Nosileftiki.* 2021;60(1):81–88.
5. Eukel HN, Morrell B, Holmes SM, Kelsch MP. Simulation design, findings, and call to action for managing difficult patient encounters. *Am J Pharm Educ.* 2021;85(7):552–563. https://doi.org/10.5688/ajpe8327.
6. Aronson L. "Good" patients and "difficult" patients—rethinking our definitions. *N Engl J Med.* 2013;369:796–797, p. 797. https://doi.org/10.1056/NEJMp1303057.
7. Rock LK. Communication as a high-stakes clinical skill: "just-in-time" simulation and vicarious observational learning to promote patient- and family-centered care and to improve trainee skill. *Acad Med.* 2021;96(11):1534–1539.
8. Jackson JL, et al. Capturing the complexities of "difficult" patient encounters using a structural equation model. *J Gen Intern Med.* 2021;36(2):549–551.
9. Tanoubi I, Cruz-Panesso L, Drolet P. The patient, the physician, or the relationship: who or what is "difficult", exactly? An approach for managing conflicts between patients and physicians. *Int J Environ Res Public Health.* 2021;18:12517.
10. World Health Organization. *Adherence to Long-Term Therapies: Evidence for Action.* Geneva: World Health Organization; 2003.
11. Fernandez-Lazaro CI, García-González JM, Adams DP, et al. Adherence to treatment and related factors among patients with chronic conditions in primary care: a cross-sectional study. *BMC Fam Pract.* 2019;20:132.
12. Boersma P, Black LI, Ward BW. Prevalence of multiple chronic conditions among US adults, 2018. *Prev Chronic Dis.* 2020;17:200130. https://doi.org/10.5888/pcd17.200130.
13. Cohen DJ, Davis MM, Hall JD, et al. *A Guidebook of Professional Practices for Behavioral Health and Primary Care Integration: Observations From Exemplary Sites.* Rockville, MD: Agency for Healthcare Research and Quality; 2015.

14. Salzberg CA, Hayes SL, McCarthy D, et al. *Health System Performance for the High-Need Patient: A Look at Access to Care and Patient Care Experiences.* New York: The Commonwealth Fund; 2016.
15. Bilazarian A. High-need high-cost patients: a concept analysis. *Nurs Forum.* 2021;56(1):127–133.
16. Berkman ND, Chang E, Seibert J, Ali R, Porterfield D, Jiang L, Wines R, Rains C, Viswanathan M. *Management of High-Need, High-Cost Patients: A "Best Fit" Framework Synthesis, Realist Review, and Systematic Review. Comparative Effectiveness Review No. 246. (Prepared by the RTI International–University of North Carolina at Chapel Hill Evidence-based Practice Center under Contract No. 290-2015-00011-I.) AHRQ Publication No. 21(22)-EHC028.* Rockville, MD: Agency for Healthcare Research and Quality; 2021.
17. Long PM, Abrams A, Milstein G, et al. *Effective Care for High-Need Patients: Opportunities for Improving Outcomes, Value, and Health.* Washington, DC: National Academy of Medicine; 2017.
18. Núñez A, Sreeganga SD, Ramaprasad A. Access to healthcare during COVID-19. *Int J Environ Res Public Health.* 2021;18(6):2980. https://doi.org/10.3390/ijerph18062980.
19. Rader J. To bathe or not to bathe: that is the question. *J Gerontol Nurs.* 1994;20(9):53.
20. Xie W, Chen L, Feng F, et al. The prevalence of compassion satisfaction and compassion fatigue among nurses: a systematic review and meta-analysis. *Int J Nurs Stud.* 2021;120. https://doi.org/10.1016/j.ijnurstu.2021.103973.
21. Haefner J. Self-care for health professionals during coronavirus disease 2019 crisis. *J Nurse Pract.* 2021;17(3):279–282.
22. Luff D, Martin EB, Mills K, et al. Clinicians' strategies for managing their emotions during difficult healthcare conversations. *Patient Educ Couns.* 2016;99:1461–1466.
23. Mittal D, Ounpraseuth ST, Reaves C, et al. Providers' personal and professional contact with persons with mental illness: relationship to clinical expectations. *Psychiatr Serv.* 2016;67(1):55–61.
24. Breeze JA, Repper J. Struggling for control: the care experiences of "difficult" patients in mental health services. *J Adv Nurs.* 1998;28(6):1301–1311.
25. Fowler J. From staff nurse to nurse consultant: survival guide part 10: surviving 'difficult' patients. *Br J Nurs.* 2020;29(6):380.
26. Neil JA, Corley MC. Hostility toward caregivers as a selection criterion for transplantation. *Prog Transplant.* 2000;10(3):177–181.
27. Juliana CA, Orehowsky S, Smith-Regojo P, et al. Interventions by staff nurses to manage "difficult" patients. *Holist Nurs Pract.* 1997;11(4):1–26.
28. Wasan AD, Wootton J, Jamison RN. Dealing with difficult patients in your pain practice. *Reg Anesth Pain Med.* 2005;30(2):184–192.
29. Nield-Anderson L, Minarik PA, Dilworth JM, et al. Responding to the "difficult" patient: manipulation, sexual provocation, aggression—how can you manage such behaviors? *Am J Nurs.* 1999;99(12):26–34.
30. Austin EJ, Blacker A, Kalia I. "Watching the tsunami come": a case study of female healthcare provider experiences during the COVID-19 pandemic. *Appl Psychol Health Well-Being.* 2021;13(4):781–797.
31. Drossman DA, Rudy J. Improving patient-provider relationships to improve health care. *Clin Gastroenterol Hepatol.* 2020;18(7):1417–1426.
32. Carroll SM. Respecting and empowering vulnerable populations: contemporary terminology. *J Nurse Pract.* 2019;15:228–231.
33. Morrison EF, Ramsey A, Synder B. Managing the care of complex, difficult patients in the medical-surgical setting. *Medsurg Nursing.* 2000;9(1):21–26.
34. Jones-Bonofiglio K. Navigating moral distress *Health Care Ethics Through the Lens of Moral Distress. The International Library of Bioethics.* Vol. 82. Cham: Springer; 2020:138. https://doi.org/10.1007/978-3-030-56156-7_10.
35. Doherty RF. *Ethical Dimensions in the Health Professions.* 7th ed. St. Louis, MO: Elsevier Saunders; 2021.
36. Giannetta N, Sergi R, Villa G, Pennestrì F, Sala R, Mordacci R, Manara DF. Levels of moral distress among health care professionals working in hospital and community settings: a cross sectional study. *Healthcare.* 2021;9:1673. https://doi.org/10.3390/healthcare9121673.
37. Antonsdottir I, Rushton CH, Nelson KE, Heinze KE, Swoboda SM, Hanson GC. Burnout and moral resilience in interdisciplinary healthcare professionals. *J Clin Nurs.* 2022;31(1–2):196–208.
38. Rushton CH, Swoboda SM, Reller N, Skarupski KA, Prizzi M, Young PD, Hanson GC. Mindful ethical practice and resilience academy: equipping nurses to address ethical challenges. *Am J Crit Care.* 2021;30(1).

39. Brigham T, Barden C, Dopp AL, Hengerer A, Kaplan J, Malone B, Martin C, McHugh M, Nora LM. A Journey to Construct an All-Encompassing Conceptual Model of Factors Affecting Clinician Well-Being and Resilience. *NAM Perspectives*. Discussion Paper. Washington, DC: National Academy of Medicine; 2018. https://doi.org/10.31478/201801b.

40. Litam SA, Balkin RS. Moral injury in health-care workers during COVID-19 pandemic. *Traumatology*. 2021;27(1):14–19.

41. Hughes MT, Rushton CH. Ethics and well-being: the health professions and the COVID-19 pandemic. *Acad Med*. 2021;97(35):S98–S103. https://doi.org/10.1097/ACM.0000000000004524.

42. Browning DM, Solomon MZ. The initiative for pediatric palliative care: an interdisciplinary educational approach for health care professionals. *J Pediatr Nurs*. 2005;20:326–334.

43. Farrell M. Difficulty conversations. *J Libr Adm*. 2015;55:302–311.

44. Hinkle LJ, Fettig LP, Carlos WG, et al. Twelve tips for just in time teaching of communication skills for difficult conversations in the clinical setting. *Med Teach*. 2017;39(9):920–925.

45. Cline C. Why some conflicts involving "difficult patients" should remain outside the province of the ethics consultation service. *Am J Bioeth*. 2012;12(5):16–18.

46. Hinkle LJ, Fettig LP, Carlos WG, et al. Twelve tips for just in time teaching of communication skills for difficult conversations in the clinical setting. *Med Teach*. 2017;39(9):920–925.

47. *American Association for the Advancement of Science*. Communication fundamentals. https://www.aaas.org/page/communication-fundamentals-0; 2017.

48. Gawande A. *Being Mortal: Medicine and What Matters in the End*. New York: Metropolitan Books; 2014.

49. Brown B. *Daring Greatly: How the Courage to be Vulnerable Transforms the Way We Live, Love, Parent, and Lead*. New York: Avery Publishers; 2015:125.

50. Stone D, Patton B, Heen S. *Difficult Conversations: How to Discuss What Matters Most*. New York: Penguin Books; 2010.

51. Makary MD, Daniel M. Medical error—third leading cause of death in the US. *BMJ*. 2016;353:1–5.

52. Rodziewicz TL, Houseman B, Hipskind JE. *Medical error reduction and prevention. 2022 Jan 4. StatPearls [Internet]*. Treasure Island, FL: StatPearls Publishing; 2022. PMID: 29763131.

53. Woods A, Doan-Johnson S. Executive summary: toward a taxonomy of nursing practice errors. *Nurs Manage*. 2002;32(10):45.

Questions for Thought and Discussion

Section 1 Creating a Context of Respect

Chapter 1—Respect in the Professional Role
Chapter 2—Professional Relationships Built on Respect
Chapter 3—Respect for Self in the Professional Role

1. What important ways is your education in the health professions like or different from other types of formal education?
2. We argue that respect is a particularly compelling value for persons practicing in the health professions. Do you agree with that argument? Discuss why or why not.
3. As you have learned, professional respect requires you to adapt to the challenges of everyday situations in health care practice. One such example is that everyone who provides patient care sometimes gets into a time bind for one reason or another. Cecilia has been caught short today because so many patients on her schedule needed a little extra time with her for them to feel she has given them their fair share of professional attention. As the afternoon progresses, she is becoming increasingly behind schedule and is aware that three patients are in the waiting area. Cecilia needs a solution to fit three patients into a time frame usually reserved for two before the unit closes. None of them knows the time when the others were scheduled to be seen.

   What should Cecilia do to show due respect for each person waiting to see her? Discuss why each of the following options offered here is or is not acceptable. You can combine some of the choices or add others of your own.

   a. Continue to take them in the order they were originally scheduled, cutting the time for each one, and explain the situation to each one privately.

   b. Tell all of them together what the situation is and let them decide among themselves the order in which they will be seen.

   c. Make an independent decision about who is most in need of care, and take them in that order, telling all three of them what you are doing and apologizing for what has happened.

4. You have become good friends with Callum, a professional colleague who works closely with you in your roles as supervisors on inpatient units in the hospital setting. He tells you that he is planning to invite everyone on the interprofessional team to an informal rounds session next Friday so that the team can process the recent change in visiting policies and talk about how to support each other's well-being at work. Callum says, "I am thinking it would be good for the team to get together and talk. I am going to order pizza and invite all the professional staff, but none of the support staff." Callum asks you, "What do you think?" As a co-worker and friend, how will you respond to your colleague Callum's question? What are the implications of excluding certain members of the team? How might this be of benefit or detriment to the teamwork on the hospital unit? Discuss the factors you will consider that support your decision to respond.

5. You have been asked by colleagues to run for office in the state organization of your profession. You are already busy with work and your personal commitments, yet you are tempted and honored to be recognized by your peers. List your most important priorities and decide what would be compromised the most by taking on this new position should you be elected. What values will determine whether you will choose to run for this office?

Section 2 Respectful Interactions in the Delivery of Care

Chapter 4—Respect in a Diverse Society
Chapter 5—Respect in Care Delivery Systems

1. You are the supervisor of an ambulatory clinic. You recognize an increase in the number of Mayan immigrants in your patient population. You are also surprised to learn that English is their third language. The Mayans speak Spanish as a second language and commonly do not read Spanish. Where should you start in preparing yourself and peers to care for these patients?
2. An 8-year-old girl presents at the emergency department with her mother. Both are recent immigrants from Afghanistan. The child has several unusual neurological symptoms, but when the physician recommends a lumbar puncture to rule out encephalitis, the child's mother refuses. When asked why, she explains that a "djinn" (a spirit in Islamic folk belief) is involved and the lumbar puncture will upset the djinn and her daughter will become more ill.[1] As a health professional involved in her care, how should you proceed?
3. Review an organizational chart from a clinical site preferably one where you worked or participated in experiential learning. Identify the various administrators such as the Chief Executive Officer and the lines of communication that link various departments and employees. Notice if the organizational chart includes such areas as quality assurance, risk management, compliance, and human resources and any information about reporting mechanisms. What does the organizational chart tell you about the organization? Are the lines of reporting and responsibilities clear and understandable?
4. You are asked to participate on the planning committee charged with designing the new waiting room for families in the emergency room at your institution. The architects report that they are eager for "front-line clinicians" to provide input. What suggestions will you provide to the architects, decorators, and administrators?

Section 3 Respect for the Patient's Situation

Chapter 6—Respecting the Patient's Story
Chapter 7—Respect for the Patient's Family and Significant Relationships

1. Find a standard "case study" in a professional journal. Rewrite it from the patient's perspective. Now, rewrite it from the family's perspective. How do these perspectives vary?
2. In groups of four, have one student act as a patient with an injury such as a fall from a ladder; have the second act as the interviewer trying to find out how the patient was injured and what sort of pain or other symptoms that patient is experiencing; have a third student act as the patient's family member who heard the fall and arrived to find the loved one on the ground; and have the fourth student observe and then critique the interview process. Change roles four times so that all get to play the patient, health professional, family member, and observer/critic. What do you discover about the patient's story with the different interview techniques? What works well, and what does not? What did you learn about how to best interact with the family member as a member of the team supporting the patient's care?

3. A patient asks you if she can bring her friend to treatment with her. You know that this patient has been asking a lot of questions and seems to be anxious. When the friend comes, she starts asking you some of the same questions that the patient asked you previously. Some are what you would take as private matters. You want to honor the patient's privacy and so are hesitant to respond. The friend states, "You know how anxious she gets. I just want to be able to reassure her, and I can't do that without knowing what is going on." You ask the patient what she would like you to share, and she just shrugs her shoulders. You really cannot tell whether the shrug is a passive resignation or something else. Not feeling completely comfortable with your answer, you say to them that you are not free to share information with anyone unless the patient is positive that it is OK. At that, she shrugs her shoulders again. What steps can you take to show this patient and her friend respect regardless of your concerns about the patient's privacy? What specific questions might you ask to better understand the role of this friend in supporting the patient's recovery?

4. A single woman in her 60s comes to you with symptoms you know are related to the stress of her position as the primary family caregiver for her elderly father who has Alzheimer's disease. You know the best thing for her is to have some respite from the situation. You first ask her about other family members who might share her responsibility, but she claims to have none who are willing or able to help share her burden. Her situation seems perilous to you, and you begin to think of a perfect society where she would not be stuck in this seemingly endless and intense situation. List all the things you can think of to design an environment for her and her father so that both can realize the respect they deserve.

Section 4 Respect Through Collaboration and Communication

Chapter 8—Respectful Interprofessional and Intraprofessional Communication and Collaboration

Chapter 9—Respectful Communication in a Technology-Driven Age

1. Form interprofessional teams or role-play different members of the interprofessional team in groups of five or six; assign roles such as timekeeper, recorder, and observer. Assume you all work within the same outpatient pediatric clinic. In 45 minutes, establish goals for a standard procedure for communicating with parents about vaccination that incorporates the unique perspectives of each member of the interprofessional team particularly regarding parents who are selective about vaccination or refuse to have their children vaccinated at the clinic where the team works. Who took the leadership position and why? Were all the appropriate members of the team present who would have helpful input and expertise for this planning session? Was everyone given an opportunity to be heard? What did the observer note that members of the team did not?

2. Think of a clinical situation that you participated in or witnessed where interprofessional communication (verbal or nonverbal) was essential to the outcome—for example, a situation that took a turn, for better or worse, because of the quality of the communication. In what ways was communication key to the outcome? If a negative outcome, what barriers were evident that prevented effective communication?

3. Write out instructions for a simple procedure such as using a cane or giving a subcutaneous injection that a patient might carry out at home. Share the instructions with a classmate and see if he or she is unclear about any of the written instructions. Work together to improve the clarity of the written instructions. What do other modes of communication such as email messages, texts, or telehealth patient interactions offer that basic, written instructions do not? Experiment with delivering the same instructions but in an electronic format. Which works better and why?

4. Effective communication requires a variety of skills on the part of the health professional. Which of the following communication skills do you find most challenging? What might you do to improve the skills you find challenging? Pick two in each category and reflect on your plan for addressing these as a health professional.
   - Use of clear, understandable language
   - Use of appropriate touch
   - Avoidance of jargon
   - Attention to tone and volume of voice
   - Respect for different conceptions of time
   - Gestures and body language
   - Facial expressions
   - Organization of ideas

Section 5 Respectful Interactions Across the Life Span

Chapter 10—Respectful Interaction: Working With Newborns, Infants, and Children in the Early Years
Chapter 11—Respectful Interaction: Working With School-Age Children and Adolescents
Chapter 12—Respectful Interaction: Working With Adults
Chapter 13—Respectful Interaction: Working With Older Adults

1. You are approached by a parent of a child in the pre-kindergarten setting where you work. The parent is concerned that her daughter is not identifying letters and numbers at the level she should and that she is not socializing with other children at the school. The parent says, "No one appears to be listening to me. This is exactly what happened with the boys." Her two older sons have learning disorders, and she is worried that her daughter may be at risk as well. How would you respond to this parent's concern?

2. You are the supervisor of an adolescent unit in a hospital. The patient, a 16-year-old named Sam, is mature for his age, and you have found him to be very thoughtful. Sam has cancer that you know has metastasized. His parents have decided with the surgeon that he should have an amputation, although all agree that the hope of saving him completely from the spread of the disease is negligible. One evening you notice that Sam is withdrawn. He says, "My parents and the doctor are going to cut off my leg, and they haven't even asked me what I think about it. I'd rather die than lose my leg."
   a. What should you do?
   b. To whom should you speak about this conversation? Why?
   c. How can the interprofessional care team best support Sam, and his family, guided by the principles of patient- and family-centered care?
   d. How does the principle of assent apply to Sam's case?

3. You are hurrying down the hospital corridor when you notice an acquaintance of your family, a firefighter in his middle 50s, who is apparently a patient. You express surprise at seeing him there because he has always been the picture of good health. He tells you that he has had a heart attack. Suddenly he begins to pour out a blow-by-blow description of the incident. As he talks, he becomes increasingly agitated and finally bursts into tears, sobbing, "It's all over. I'll never be able to go back to my job or anything. What am I going to do?"
   a. What can you say or do right then to calm this man's immediate anxious state?
   b. We learned about the responsibility of work roles in adult years. How is this patient's identity tied to his work role and contributing to his emotional state?
   c. Will you communicate this interaction to anyone? If so, to whom and why?
   d. How can the interprofessional care teamwork together to treat the middle-age person's anxiety about the long-term effects of illness on family, job, and self-esteem?

4. Young adulthood is often referred to as "the healthy years and the hidden hazards." What does this mean? What are the implications for the life span?

5. Given what you know about the theories of aging, which theory do you find aligns best with your chosen health profession?
   a. Why?
   b. How will it support healthy aging in the patients you will be treating?
   c. How do you think the baby boomer generation will change or inform theories of aging over the next decade?

6. An alert 92-year-old patient who has been in your care for several days arrives late for treatment one morning at your ambulatory care clinic. She explains that she missed her usual bus and had to wait in the rain and cold for the next bus to arrive. You begin to converse with her in your usual manner and quickly realize that something is wrong; she does not answer your questions appropriately. Once or twice, she mentions her son (whom you know was killed years ago while in the armed services). The patient's sentences are disconnected and incomplete.
   a. What possible reasons may there be for her apparent confusion?
   b. Where will you start in your attempt to diagnose her problem?
   c. Who on the interprofessional care team will serve as resources to you as you navigate this change in presentation?

Section 6 Some Special Challenges: Creating a Context of Respect

Chapter 14—Respectful Interaction: When the Patient Is Dying
Chapter 15—Respectful Interaction in Complex Situations

1. There can be disagreement among the interprofessional members of the health care about when it is appropriate to focus on palliative care for a patient with a life-limiting illness. The same could be said about the right time to begin hospice care. How might you encourage a reluctant member of the team to consider shifting a patient to hospice care? Let us assume that the patient and family have both expressed interest in shifting their focus to comfort and moving the setting of care to the patient's home.

2. Coping with death and dying is important for all those involved in the process—patients, family members, and health professionals. What are healthy coping measures that you as a health professional could employ in the face of the stress and loss that comes with caring for a dying patient and their family members?

3. You are working in an outpatient clinic in an economically depressed area of the city. A disheveled woman comes in with three young children behind her. One of the children begins to complain saying that she is hot. You are in the receiving area and see the woman hit the child so hard that the child stumbles to the floor and begins to scream. The woman looks at you in panic. You are already late for your next appointment. Your next patient is anxiously waiting to be seen and looks with scorn at the woman and you.
   a. What feelings does this scene trigger?
   b. What does this teach you about the possible difference between your emotional and "professional" reaction to this extreme situation?
   c. What principles of difficult conversations might serve as guideposts to you in this situation?
   d. What might you say to either the woman who hit the child or the observers of the incident to show respect to all involved? Instead of saying I would say "X," pair up with a partner and actually say the words out loud. Reflect on how you feel hearing yourself talk through difficult messages/conversations.
   e. How might you process this moral distress to ensure that you can be resilient in providing compassionate care?

4. You are a rehabilitation aide working in a skilled nursing facility. You arrived early to the unit this morning, helping a new patient ambulate to the bathroom when no one else was available to answer the call bell. The patient was so grateful for your assistance saying, "Thank God you came. I thought I would wet the bed!" You are in the nurses' station and see the charge nurse. You say, "That new patient in room 22 is so nice. I just walked them to the bathroom since everyone was in morning report." Your nursing colleague says, "Oh dear! Please don't tell me you let him weight bear on his right leg. He was put on bedrest last night." You are immediately stressed and concerned that you may have hurt the patient. You always read the electronic health record before working with a patient, but today that just did not happen. What are the factors that contributed to this error? What are the next steps for you and the team working with this client? What systems supports such as who manages patient needs during morning report or signage on the door of a patient's room indicating special precautions might be helpful to you, the team, and the patient?

Reference

1. Seelman C, Suuromond J, Stronks K. Cultural competence: a conceptual framework for teaching and learning. *Med Educ.* 2009;434:229–237.

Note: Page numbers followed by "*f*" indicate figures, "*t*" indicate tables, and "*b*" indicate boxes.